Cardiopulmonary Bypass

Third Edition

Cardiopulmonary Bypass

Edited by

Florian Falter
Royal Papworth Hospital, Cambridge

Albert C Perrino
Yale University Medical Center, New Haven, CT

Robert A. Baker
Flinders Medical Centre and Flinders University, Adelaide

The editors are very grateful to Dr Ghosh, who started this project and led the first two editions
from idea to printed book

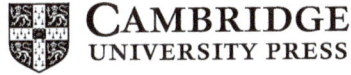

CAMBRIDGE
UNIVERSITY PRESS

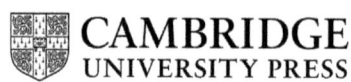

Shaftesbury Road, Cambridge CB2 8BS, United Kingdom

One Liberty Plaza, 20th Floor, New York, NY 10006, USA

477 Williamstown Road, Port Melbourne, VIC 3207, Australia

314–321, 3rd Floor, Plot 3, Splendor Forum, Jasola District Centre,
New Delhi – 110025, India

103 Penang Road, #05–06/07, Visioncrest Commercial, Singapore 238467

Cambridge University Press is part of Cambridge University Press & Assessment,
a department of the University of Cambridge.

We share the University's mission to contribute to society through the pursuit of
education, learning and research at the highest international levels of excellence.

www.cambridge.org
Information on this title: www.cambridge.org/9781009009621

DOI: 10.1017/9781009008143

First published 2009
Second edition 2015
Third edition 2022

A catalogue record for this publication is available from the British Library.

Library of Congress Cataloging-in-Publication Data
Names: Falter, Florian, editor. | Perrino, Albert C., Jr. editor. | Baker, Robert A,
    1960- editor.
Title: Cardiopulmonary bypass / edited by Florian Falter, Albert C. Perrino,
    Robert A. Baker.
Other titles: Cardiopulmonary bypass (Ghosh)
Description: Third edition. | Cambridge, United Kingdom ; New York, NY :
    Cambridge University Press, [2022] | Preceded by Cardiopulmonary
    bypass / edited by Sunit Ghosh, Florian Falter, Albert C. Perrino, Jr.
    Second edition. 2015 | Includes bibliographical references and index.
Identifiers: LCCN 2022010263 (print) | LCCN 2022010264 (ebook) |
    ISBN 9781009009621 (paperback) | ISBN 9781009008143 (epub)
Subjects: MESH: Cardiopulmonary Bypass–methods | Cardiac Surgical
    Procedures–methods
Classification: LCC RD598 (print) | LCC RD598 (ebook) | NLM WG 168.5 |
    DDC 617.4/120592–dc23/eng/20220511

LC record available at https://lccn.loc.gov/2022010263
LC ebook record available at https://lccn.loc.gov/2022010264

ISBN 978-1-009-00962-1 Paperback

Contents

Contributors

James H. Abernathy III
Associate Professor, Interim Executive Vice Chair, ACCM Chief, Division of Cardiac Anesthesiology Core Faculty, Armstrong Institute of Patient Safety, Department of Anesthesiology & Critical Care Medicine, Johns Hopkins University

Yasir Abu-Omar
Director, Cardiothoracic Transplantation and Mechanical Circulatory Support, University Hospitals Cleveland Medical Center

Robert C. Albright Jr
Consultant, Division of Nephrology and HTN Mayo Clinic Rochester; Professor of Medicine, Division of Nephrology and HTN, Mayo Clinic College of Medicine, Mayo Clinic, Rochester; Regional Vice President, Mayo Clinic Health System Southeast; Professor of Medicine; Consultant, Division of Nephrology and Hypertension

Ayyaz Ali
Vice Chairman of Cardiac Surgery and Surgical Director of Heart Transplantation and Mechanical Circulatory Support, Hartford Hospital

Jason M. Ali
Locum Consultant in Cardiothoracic and Transplant Surgery, Royal Papworth Hospital

Kyriakos Anastasiadis
Professor, Department of Cardiothoracic Surgery, Aristotle University of Thessaloniki

Simon Anderson
Clinical Perfusion Team Leader, Cambridge Perfusion Services, Royal Papworth Hospital

Polychronis Antonitsis
Associate Professor, Department of Cardiothoracic Surgery, Aristotle University of Thessaloniki

Helena Argiriadou
Cardiac Anesthesiologist, Assistant Professor, Aristotle University of Thessaloniki

Joseph E. Arrowsmith
Consultant Anaesthetist, Department of Anaesthesia & Intensive Care Medicine, Royal Papworth Hospital

Sherif Assaad
Associate Professor, Cleveland Clinic Lerner College of Medicine | Case Western Reserve University, and Staff Anesthesiologist, Department of Cardiothoracic Anesthesiology | Anesthesiology Institute, Cleveland Clinic

Martin Besser
Consultant Haematologist, Royal Papworth Hospital

Caitlin Blau
Perfusion Supervisor, Mayo Clinic

Jonathan Brand
Clinical Director and Consultant in Cardiothoracic Anaesthesia and Critical Care, James Cook University Hospital, Middlesbrough

Mark Buckland
Deputy Director, Head of Cardiothoracic Anaesthesia, Department of Anaesthesiology & Perioperative Medicine, Alfred Hospital and Monash University

Christiana Burt
Consultant Anaesthetist, Royal Papworth Hospital

Etienne J. Couture
Anesthesiologist & Intensivist, Institut universitaire de cardiologie et de pneumologie de Québec – Université Laval (IUCPQ-UL)

Amanda Crosby
Staff Perfusionist, University of Tennessee Medical Center

Edward M. Darling
Associate Professor, College of Health Professions, Department of Cardiovascular Perfusion, SUNY Upstate Medical University; Faculty/Clinical Coordinator

Filip De Somer
Professor in Perfusion Technology, University Ghent, Chief Perfusionist, University Hospital Ghent

Apostolos Deliopoulo
Perfusionist, Cardiothoracic Department, Aristotle University of Thessaloniki

André Y. Denault
Professor, and Anesthesiologist & Intensivist, Montreal Heart Institute, Université de Montréal

Timothy A. Dickinson
Assistant Professor of Surgery, CCP, Mayo Clinic; Director, Perfusion Services

Juan Pablo Domecq
Senior Associate Consultant, Division of Nephrology, Hypertension and Critical Care Medicine, Mayo Clinic, Rochester, and Mayo Clinic, Mankato; Assistant Professor of Medicine, Mayo Clinic College of Medicine

David Fitzgerald
Assistant Professor, Division Director, CVP Program, Medical University of South Carolina

Michael Franklin
Clinical Assistant Professor – Cardiothoracic Anesthesiology, University of Florida

Tom Gilbey
Anaesthetic Registrar and NIHR Academic Clinical Fellow, Department of Anaesthetics and Pain Medicine, King's College Hospital NHS Foundation Trust

Shahna Helmick
Program Director of Perfusion Education, University of Iowa Hospitals and Clinics

Joanne F. Irons
Senior Lecturer, University of Sydney; Staff Specialist Anaesthetist, Royal Prince Alfred Hospital

Gregory M. Janelle
Professor of Anesthesiology and Surgery and Associate Chair for Clinical Affairs, Department of Anesthesiology, University of Florida College of Medicine

Stéphanie Jarry
PhD candidate, Department of Anesthesiology, Montreal Heart Institute, Université de Montréal

Timothy J. Jones
Consultant Congenital Cardiac Surgeon, Birmingham Women's and Children's Hospital, University Hospitals Birmingham; Honorary Senior Lecturer, Institute of Cardiovascular Science, University of Birmingham

Gudrun Kunst
Professor of Cardiovascular Anaesthesia, Department of Anaesthetics and Pain Medicine, King's College Hospital NHS Foundation Trust & School of Cardiovascular Medicine and Sciences, King's College London; Consultant Anaesthetist and Professor of Cardiovascular Anaesthesia, British Heart Foundation Centre of Research Excellence

R. Clive Landis
Professor of Cardiovascular Research, and Pro Vice Chancellor and Principal, The University of the West Indies, Cave Hill Campus

Victoria Molyneux
Senior Clinical Perfusionist, Great Ormond Street Hospital for Children NHS Foundation Trust

Narain Moorjani
Consultant Cardiac Surgeon & Clinical Lead for Cardiac Surgery, Royal Papworth Hospital; Affiliated Assistant Professor, University of Cambridge; President, Society for Cardiothoracic Surgery in Great Britain & Ireland

Richard F. Newland
Senior Perfusionist & Clinical Lead for Perfusion, Flinders Medical Centre and Lecturer, Flinders University

Erik Ortmann
Chair, Department of Anaesthesiology, Schüchtermann-Heart-Centre

Jane Ottens
Chief Perfusionist, Ashford Hospital

Michael Poullis
Senior Fellow Cardiothoracic Surgery, Manchester Royal Infirmary

Luc Puis
Senior Perfusionist, University Hospital Brussels, Center for Heart and Vascular Diseases

Kenneth G. Shann
Director, Perfusion Services, Massachusetts General Hospital

Linda Shore-Lesserson
Professor of Anesthesiology, Zucker School of Medicine at Hofstra Northwell; Vice Chair Academic Affairs; Director, Cardiovascular Anesthesiology

Joseph J. Sistino
Professor Emeritus, Medical University of South Carolina College of Health Professions

Pingping Song
Assistant Professor, Department of Anesthesiology & Pain Medicine, University of Washington Medical Center; Medical Director, Cardiothoracic Intensive Care Unit

Bruce D. Spiess
Professor and Associate Chair (Research), University of Florida College of Medicine

Pascal Starinieri
Clinical Perfusionist, JESSA Hospital

Thoralf M. Sundt
Chief, Division of Cardiac Surgery, Director of Cardiac Surgery Clinical Service, and Edward D. Churchill Professor of Surgery, Harvard Medical School, Massachusetts General Hospital

Jessica Underwood
Perfusionist, Alfred Hospital; Director, Victorian Perfusion Specialists

Lindsay Wetzel
Cardiac Anesthesiologist, TriHealth Heart Institute - Seven Hills Anesthesia

Robert Young
Specialist Cardiothoracic Anaesthetist, Department of Anaesthesia, Flinders Medical Centre

Foreword

Six years after the publication of the second edition of *Cardiopulmonary Bypass*, Florian Falter, Robert Baker and Albert C Perrino have produced a substantial revision of this highly regarded text. Success in cardiac surgery requires each member of the team to be expert in the theory and capable in the practice of their individual discipline, but it also requires them to work together effectively as a team, often for long hours under considerable stress. It is thus very pleasing to see a strong new emphasis on teamwork, communication and human factors added to this already excellent book. This emphasis is reflected in the renewed authorship of each chapter, which (in most cases) now includes all three of the disciplines key to the management of cardiopulmonary bypass – anesthesia, perfusion and surgery. The list of editors and authors is a "Who's Who" of this field and reflects not only deep expertise in the relevant topics but also established ability to disseminate knowledge through lecturing and writing. The result, as one might expect, is a scientifically sound, clearly written and highly accessible text. It is a text that will (like the previous edition) be an excellent source of practical hands-on advice on how to apply the underpinning principles to the everyday practice of cardiopulmonary bypass within the dynamic context of cardiac surgery.

The number of chapters has increased from 16 to 20, but new material has been incorporated throughout. The themes of teamwork, communication, checklists and safety (both Safety-I and Safety-II) run through the entire book. As with the previous edition, the editors have achieved a consistency of style and message with a minimum of repetition. Thus, the book feels coherent and has a logical flow of ideas. As before, there is effective use of illustrations and tables and a good bibliography of selected references for each chapter. The book will continue to provide an outstanding introduction to this field of practice, both for surgeons and anesthetists, who primarily need to understand and contribute to the management of cardiopulmonary bypass or mechanical circulatory support, and for perfusionists who also have to set up and run the equipment. For those already expert in this field, it will provide a technically up-to-date source for revision of the relevant topics from a highly contemporary perspective.

The editors work in leading institutions in their respective countries (England, Australia and the United States). Each is known for leadership and innovation within their discipline. The same can be said for the chapter authors. It is unsurprising that the book carries a tone of authority that will leave readers confident in the reliability of the information and the soundness of the perspectives within it.

I offer the editors and the authors my hearty congratulations.

Alan Merry FANZCA, FFPMANZCA, FRSNZ
*Professor of Anaesthesiology, University of Auckland,
Specialist in Anaesthesia, Auckland City Hospital, New Zealand.*

Human Factors and Teamwork in Cardiac Surgery

Lindsay Wetzel, David Fitzgerald, Thoralf M Sundt and James H Abernathy III

Today we face many problems. Some are created essentially by ourselves based on divisions due to ideology, religion, race, economic status, or other factors. Therefore, the time has come for us to think on a deeper level, on the human level, and from that level we should appreciate and respect the sameness of others as human beings.

—*Dalai Lama*

In the current healthcare environment, there is an increasing focus on providing high quality patient care at ever lower costs while patients rightly expect excellent outcomes. Cardiac surgery in particular is dependent on several disciplines working together closely and having a good appreciation of the challenges facing each one. High quality outcomes are dependent upon a wide array of factors, ranging from patient specific issues, to provider acumen and technical skills, to ancillary support systems and increasingly to organizational factors.

Successful healthcare organizations understand the importance of using teams efficiently to accomplish difficult and complex tasks. Teams are assembled with a central, unifying objective in mind and specific roles are assigned to each member in order to achieve this goal. This allows members to play to their individual skill set and operate within their comfort zone. Advanced technology, streamlined techniques, and improved science, much of which is outlined in the chapters of this text, have no doubt improved practitioner skills and enhanced care. Importantly, a shared mental model gives what would otherwise be a group of skilled individuals working in isolation the ability to successfully tackle increasingly complex tasks together. Teams generally provide a purpose and a broader sense of meaning to each member, creating a sense of mutual support which can bind individuals together.

Teams are especially critical for avoiding errors and for responding to unexpected events that can result in catastrophic complications if not managed appropriately. The elite cardiac operating room represents a delicate symphony of quick decision-making, refined technical skill and sound judgment by each member of a large multidisciplinary team consisting of perfusionists, surgeons, anesthesiologists, fellows, residents, nurses, surgical technologists and other highly trained, capable healthcare providers.

A hallmark feature of successful teams is effective and open communication. The cardiac operating room is a high stakes environment where small breakdowns in communication and teamwork can have significant consequences on safe patient care and outcome. With that in mind, organizations that accredit healthcare providers, such as The Joint Commission in the United States, have pinpointed teamwork as being critical to thriving healthcare organizations that provide optimal patient care and minimize medical error.

Error

Before we understand teams, we must understand the root cause of error. It is increasingly recognized that most medical errors are avoidable. Rather than being related to a lapse of technical skill, poor medical decision-making, inadequate knowledge or suboptimal training, they are more commonly the result of a breakdown in effective communication, in teamwork or during transition of care. Addressing system-based issues, breakdowns in cognitive networks and advancing team-based approaches are essential to high quality care.

The famous human factors engineer, James Reason, described all systems as containing both active and latent failures. Active failures represent

Table 1.1. Overview of Safety 1 and 2

	Safety 1	Safety 2
Definition of Safety	That as few things as possible go wrong.	That as many things as possible go right.
Safety management principle	Reactive, respond when something happens or is categorized as an unacceptable risk.	Proactive, continuously trying to anticipate developments and events.
View of the human factor in safety management	Humans are predominantly seen as a liability or hazard. They are a problem to be fixed.	Humans are seen as a resource necessary for system flexibility and resilience. They provide flexible solutions to many potential problems.
Accident investigation	Accidents are caused by failures and malfunctions. The purpose of an investigation is to identify the causes.	Things basically happen in the same way, regardless of the outcome. The purpose of an investigation is to understand how things usually go right as a basis for explaining how things occasionally go wrong.
Risk assessment	Accidents are caused by failures and malfunctions. The purpose of an investigation is to identify causes and contributory factors.	To understand the conditions where performance variability can become difficult or impossible to monitor and control.

Reprinted from, From Safety-I to Safety-II: A White Paper, Hollnagel E et al. Retrieved from www.england.nhs.uk/signuptosafety/wp-content/uploads/sites/16/2015/10/safety-1-safety-2-whte-papr.pdf. Copyright 2015 by Erik Hollnagel, Robert L Wears, Jeffrey Braithwaite.

errors made by individuals at the service delivery end (the operating room team); latent failures are organizational deficiencies (hospital wide, governmental, manufacturers, etc.) that are lurking in the background contributing to active failures. Latent failures can be thought of as the holes in the Swiss cheese.

When errors occur, the majority of healthcare organizations focus on the active failures, the most obvious of failures, through investigations like root cause analyses or Morbidity & Mortality conferences. Questions typically asked are: "who made mistakes?" or "who didn't follow the rules?." This type of thinking with an emphasis on the negative has been coined "Safety 1." Safety 1 seeks to find the errors, the flaws, the vulnerabilities. An alternative perspective, however, has emerged called "Safety 2." In delivering complex, complicated healthcare we do a lot of good and most times, we do it correctly. We manage to do this despite operating in increasingly complex systems, with ever changing providers and more and more demanding patients. The reason things go right is not that people behave as they are supposed to but because people adapt to the conditions they work in to make outcomes better. Understanding how people and the systems they work in adjust in order to provide great care is how "Safety 2" is framed. Safety 2 embraces the variability in the healthcare delivery system and seeks to understand it. For example: Sally, a perfusionist, is sought-after for complicated cases. She is talented clinically, communicates well, shares what she is thinking, makes good decisions and is steady under pressure. Sally's resilience serves the team well and, when Sally is there, it performs better. Rather than punishing people for making poor decisions (Safety 1), Safety 2 seeks to understand what Sally does well and how this can be transferred to other situations.

The two different perspectives are best summarized in Table 1.1.

The Human Factors Perspective

Catchpole and McCulloch define human factors as: "Enhancing clinical performance through an understanding of the effects of teamwork, tasks, equipment, workspace, culture and organization on human behavior and abilities and application of the knowledge in clinical settings." Or, stated more simply, "The science of improving human performance and well-being by examining all the effectors of human performance."

Insights into the human factors perspective show us that stress and fatigue, shortcomings in human

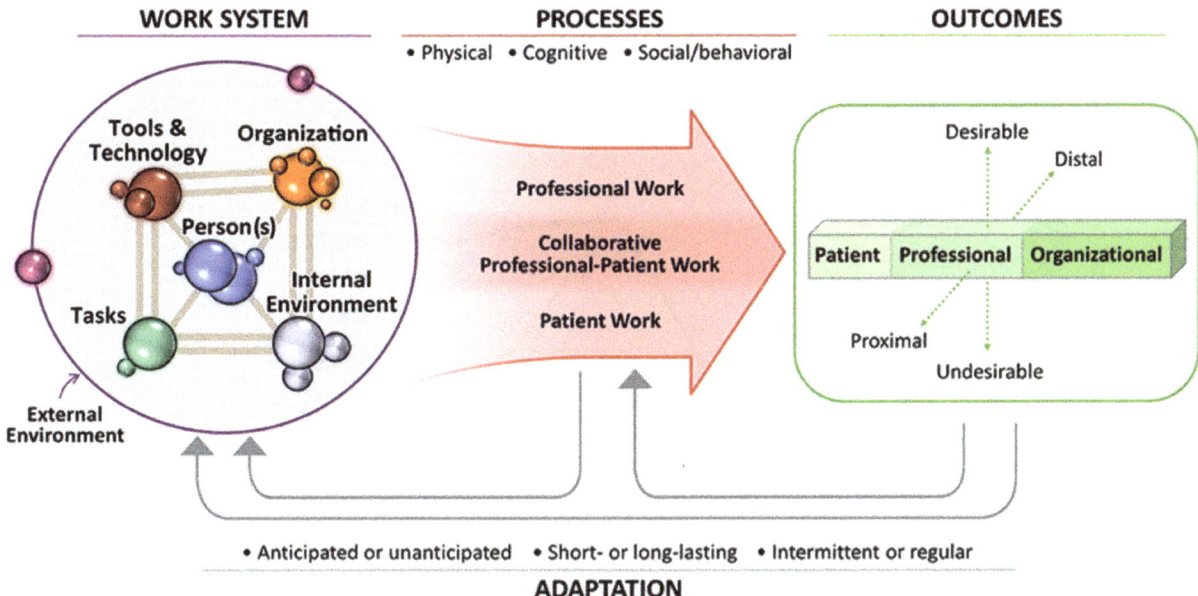

Figure 1.1 Systems Engineering Initiative for Patient Safety (SEIPS) 2.0: A model of work system and patient safety. (Reprinted from Holden RJ, Carayon P, Gurses AP et al. SEIPS 2.0: A human factors framework for studying and improving the work of healthcare professionals and patients. *Ergonomics.* 2013;56(11):1669–1686.)

memory, interruptions and distractions, overestimation of ability and overreliance on multi-tasking can make even the most seasoned healthcare providers commit medical errors. One of the first frameworks by which we can understand these complex interactions is the Systems Engineering Initiative for Patient Safety (SEIPS) (see Figure 1.1).

The SEIPS model provides a framework through which we can identify and addresses modifiable factors in the interaction of people and their environments with regard to patient safety events. For instance, the perfusionist (person) operating the cardiopulmonary bypass machine (tool) requires correct ergonomics, visual and auditory feedback. The complex machine the person operates should be situated in a location that provides short tubing length, is not at risk of being hit by opening OR doors and provides the perfusionist with clear lines of sight to the anesthesiologist, the surgeon and the monitor so that communication is unencumbered (environment).

Outcomes are not only affected by technical skill, but by the intersection of healthcare environment, team ethos, workload, team member morale, technology, effective communication and organizational variables. The SEIPS model contends that medical error can be a natural consequence of system wide breakdowns in the vast array of factors which influence

healthcare performance and outcomes. It celebrates measures which foster quality patient care and pinpoints interventions which can help healthcare organizations achieve and maintain surgical excellence. It is juxtaposed to individual-centered approaches which contend that human error is due to deficiencies on a personal level and remedies that are focused on disciplinary, punitive and litigious means.

Teamwork

Salas and coworkers have described teamwork as "a distinguishable set of two or more people who interact dynamically, interdependently, and adaptively towards a common and valued goal, who have each been assigned specific roles or functions to perform and who have a limited life-span membership." Teams share a common mission and must adapt to the dynamics and demands of various tasks in order to achieve their end goal. Teams collaborate, they synthesize and integrate information and coordinate among members to share responsibilities in a way that makes best use of the strengths of each individual. Successful teamwork is characterized by mutual trust, effective communication, realistic goal setting, fair division of tasks, desire to achieve a common goal and a shared passion for excellence.

3

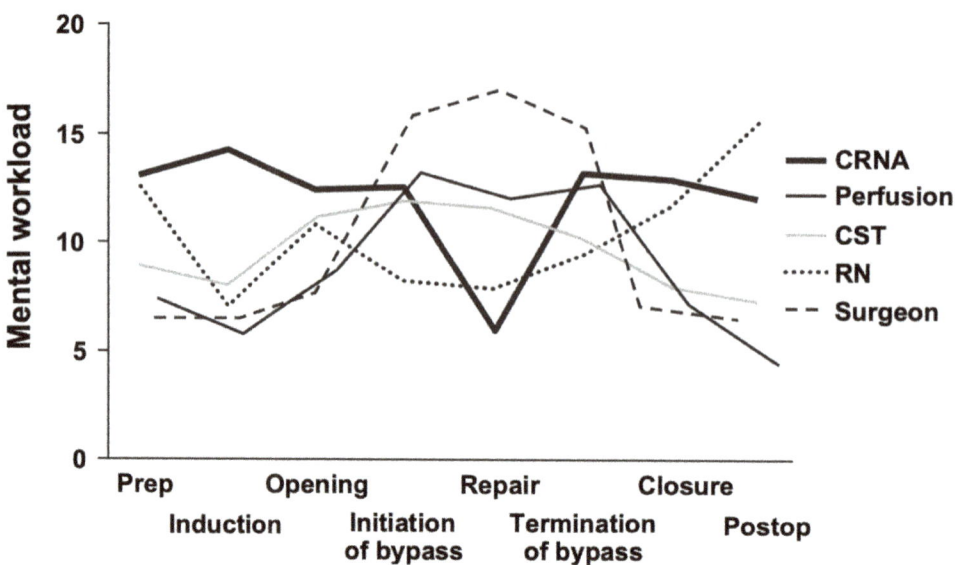

NASA-Task Load Index (NASA TLX) (n=30)

Legend:
- **CRNA**
- **Perfusion**
- **CST**
- **RN**
- **Surgeon**

X-axis: Prep, Induction, Opening, Initiation of bypass, Repair, Termination of bypass, Closure, Postop

Y-axis: Mental workload

Figure 1.2 Mental workload in the cardiac surgery operating room varies across the cardiac surgery procedure for individual providers depending on task complexity and responsibilities. CRNA indicates certified registered nurse anesthetist; CST, certified surgical technologist; NASA, National Aeronautics and Space Administration; Postop, postoperative; Prep, surgical preparation; RN, registered nurse; and TLX, Task Load Index. (Reprinted from *The Journal of Thoracic and Cardiovascular Surgery*, Volume 139, Issue 2, RK Wadhera et al., Is the "sterile cockpit" concept applicable to cardiovascular surgery critical intervals or critical events? The impact of protocol-driven communication during cardiopulmonary bypass, Pages 312–319. Copyright © 2010, with permission from Elsevier.)

The Joint Commission recognizes communication as one of the top three contributing factors to sentinel events. Broadly speaking, communication is "the exchange of information between a sender and a receiver." Effective communication is characterized by clarity, comprehensiveness and confirming that the message has been relayed effectively. It contributes to a shared mental awareness, clarifies what team members are worried about, identifies any issues that have arisen previously during similar moments and establishes an understanding of how to successfully navigate these scenarios. Fostering an environment which cultivates open, truthful, adaptable, succinct and constructive communication is critical to any successful team.

Clear communication is vital during times of stress. Critical situations don't need bystanders, they require the key team members to be in the room and rely on them adhering to their assigned roles. The "sterile cockpit" concept, widely in use in military and commercial aviation, describes the banning of non-essential communication during critical periods associated with high-risk and high mental workload. In aviation, chatting is not allowed below 10,000 feet

during takeoff and landing or in unusual or stressful situations. This principle is equally applicable to proceedings in the cardiac operating room – going on and coming off bypass, as an example, are treated similar to starting and landing. Some healthcare organizations have implemented the rule that when one member of the team spots trouble they call out "10,000 feet" to get attention and change the mood and focus in the room to problem-solving mode. Closed-loop communication or "call back," whereby the speaker's message is repeated or paraphrased by the receiver, is an effective way to reduce communication ambiguity, miscues, and non-verbalized critical actions.

We must recognize that at no point during a case is the mental workload the same for all providers (Figure 1.2). While the patient is on bypass the perfusionist is working hard while the anesthesiologist might have less to concentrate on; during the induction of anesthesia, the surgeon will usually be doing something unrelated; during the vitally important instrument count the scrub and circulating nurses are ensuring nothing will be left behind while the rest of the room is congratulating themselves on a job well done. Understanding when different members find themselves in a period of increased mental workload helps the entire team to identify the times where we can help our colleagues.

Transition of care is an especially high-risk period for communication breakdown. Handoff of a patient when OR staff change shift or from operating room to ICU staff are particularly vulnerable times. In the absence of standardized clinical practice guidelines, handoffs between providers may be highly variable and unstructured, missing important content items during transfer. Poor information transfers also lead to incomplete clinical tasks and disruptions in care. Standardized handoffs, such as the recently published AmSECT perfusion handoff tool or the Formula 1 type OR to ICU handoff tool proposed by Catchpole, greatly improve the accuracy of information transfer (see Figure 1.3).

Leadership

Leadership style in the cardiac operating room can have a significant impact on the function of the entire team. Transactional leaders focus more on individual tasks, responsibilities and blame. They rarely see the big picture and engage in unilateral communication which is not conducive to a team focused environment. Transformational leaders foster an environment of enthusiasm, learning, cooperation and a collective mission. Studies have shown a higher level of teamwork and information sharing with transformational leadership styles. Within a culture of excellence, there must also be a commitment to respect. Professionalism and courtesy are not negotiable. Effective leaders aim to flatten the hierarchy, create familiarity and foster an environment where everyone feels safe to speak up and participate. If there was an easy button for establishing a culture of excellence and effective leadership, we might not have a need for this chapter. Personal and institutional willingness to embrace tools such as Just Culture are important to tilt behavior toward personal accountability and adaptability.

Repair, Recovery and Resilience

Resilience alludes to the capacity of individuals and of teams to withstand and recover from pressures, stressors and challenges. Failure to recover from an unexpected event is a characteristic of poor performing perioperative programs. Resilient teams, on the other hand, overcome challenges in such a way that both performance and cohesion are at least sustained, if not improved, eventually leading to improved outcomes. The underpinnings of resilience are a shared vision and mission, healthy relationships and invested team members. Resilient teams

- support each other and encourage recovery after difficult situations,
- don't lay blame on individuals after such situations but engage in learning through effective communication and constructive criticism to facilitate a different outcome in the future.

A team which can band together during times of duress and lean on one another for support will invariably arise from challenging situations stronger and better equipped to deal with future problems. This is particularly true for the cardiac operating room.

Practical Solutions

Breakdown in teamwork is commonly attributed to a lack of role clarity among team members or ineffective communication. Proposals to improve communication and to reduce the possibility of error include, but are not limited to, standardized intraoperative communication, preoperative briefings, and postoperative debriefings.

Standardized Conversations

Standardizing communication practices facilitates stronger team communication and helps all team members "speak the same language." Communicating in a closed-loop, or read-back, fashion ensures that the entire team is aware of what is occurring and helps in retaining the shared mental model. Operating rooms can be chaotic places where background noise makes hearing difficult. Acknowledging comments and questions ensures that communications have been heard and understood. Repeating back essential information confirms that the sender's message has been received. It is important to foster an environment where closed-loop communication is encouraged and not looked at as disengagement (i.e. the individual repeating the message was not paying attention and hence needs clarification.) Knowing team members by name helps to make communications more direct and removes ambiguity as to who is being addressed.

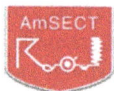

I PASS THE CLAMP OFF

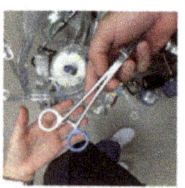

Patient Handoff Tool for Perfusionists

I	Isolation precautions	contact, droplet, airborne
P	Patient name/Procedure	surgical approach, cannulation, backup plan, target flows
A	Age/Allergies	medications, adverse reactions, associated risks
S	Stage of the procedure	preoperative, perioperative, postoperative, surgical status
S	Status of temperature	target temperatures, current temperatures, rewarming rate
T	Transfusion	blood type, targets, product use, availability
H	History	symptoms, risk factors, diagnosis, prior procedures, preoperative medications
E	Equipment condition	mechanical concerns or issues
C	Circuit	oxygenator, tubing size and coating, cardioplegia, shunts, hemoconcentrator, accessories
L	Lab values and targets	hematocrit, blood gasses, electrolytes, enzymes, targets
A	Anticoagulation	status, targets, heparin use, alternative anticoagulants, blood components
M	Medications	vasoconstrictors, vasodilators, cardioplegia, electrolytes, antiarrhythmics, colloids
P	Pump settings	FiO2, sweep, blood flow, vacuum, RPMs, timers, shunts
O	Other conditions or concerns	jehovah's witness, sickle cell anemia, pregnancy, sepsis, DIC
F	Fluid status	I/Os, crystalloid use, ultrafiltrate amount and rate, urine
F	Final thoughts	

Figure 1.3 AmSECT perfusionist handoff checklist. (Reproduced with kind permission of the AmSECT Safety Committee.)

Briefing and Debriefing

Briefings, both preoperative and postoperative, have been implemented to promote information exchange and team cohesion. They originated in the aviation and nuclear power industries to ensure that important information was communicated to every team member. Preoperative briefings are an opportunity for all operating room personnel to introduce themselves with name and role and identify any concerns. Introduction of team members encourages team familiarity which has been linked to improved teamwork. The operative plan needs to be discussed and anticipated difficulties are communicated to develop strategies as to how to deal with them. Any equipment requirements or lack of certain pieces of kit need to be highlighted. If everybody is on the same page the team is able to develop a shared mental model of the work ahead, creating a sense of teamwork and collaboration. Conducting team briefings before every case is especially important for newer surgical teams or for teams with new members who may not be aware of the unwritten or unspoken traditions. Open communication before the case establishes a road map for conducting the case and helps minimize disruptions during the surgery (i.e. leaving the room to obtain equipment and supplies).

The briefing, as described here, is distinct and separate from a "time-out." The "time-out" pause is intended to ensure the right patient, right side, and right operation.

Postoperative debriefings are equally critical as they provide an opportunity for the team to understand what went well during the case and identify areas for improvement in coming procedures. It is important to make postoperative briefings an arena for constructive feedback and not for blaming and finger-pointing. When executed effectively, debriefings improve teamwork, communication and unity. As teams gain experience together, debriefings will help solve problems encountered during the case, address "near misses" and hopefully prevent these issues from reoccurring in the future.

Creating the Team

Implementing formalized team training in the cardiac operating room is a vital measure in decreasing surgical morbidity and mortality. There are numerous organizations, nationally and internationally, providing recognized programs to integrate teamwork into clinical practice. Many of these programs have drawn on decades worth of evidence-based research pertaining to team building, culture change and teamwork in organizations such as the military, nuclear power and aviation. Their goal is to help improve teamwork and communication skills. They offer open and accessible training programs in communication, leadership, situation monitoring and mutual support (see Figure 1.4).

Providing this training to OR teams has been shown to improve teamwork, communication, reduce surgical mortality and morbidity, increase efficiency, and improve patient satisfaction. However, sustainability remains a challenge and often comes with the need for repeat training.

Non-Technical Skill Assessment Tools

Several non-technical skill (NTS) taxonomies aimed at rating behavior in the operating department have been reported in the literature. These instruments are designed to measure performance of multidisciplinary team interactions, such as decision-making, situational awareness, leadership, communication and teamwork. Several of the taxonomies have been previously adapted for the cardiac surgical arena and beyond, including NOTSS (Non-Technical Skills for Surgeons), Oxford Non-Technical Skills (NOTECHS), and ANTS (Anaesthetists' Non-Technical Skills). Rating systems assess individual practitioner's non-technical skills and team behavior. They should be used as a metric and an incentive for individuals as well as institutions to improve their performance. While conventional wisdom may suggest that enhancing NTS performance will confer significant improvements in the safety and the efficiency of patient care, the implementation across medical education and healthcare institutions is patchy. Unfortunately, there is no silver bullet to accomplishing perfect team-based performance. Change often starts small and propagates. Start small, build a well-functioning unit. Then, through good outcomes and happy staff, demonstrate what works for the broader organization. If you live and work in an organization whose leadership does not value these concepts, press on anyway. Create the culture you want, where you work. Change starts with you.

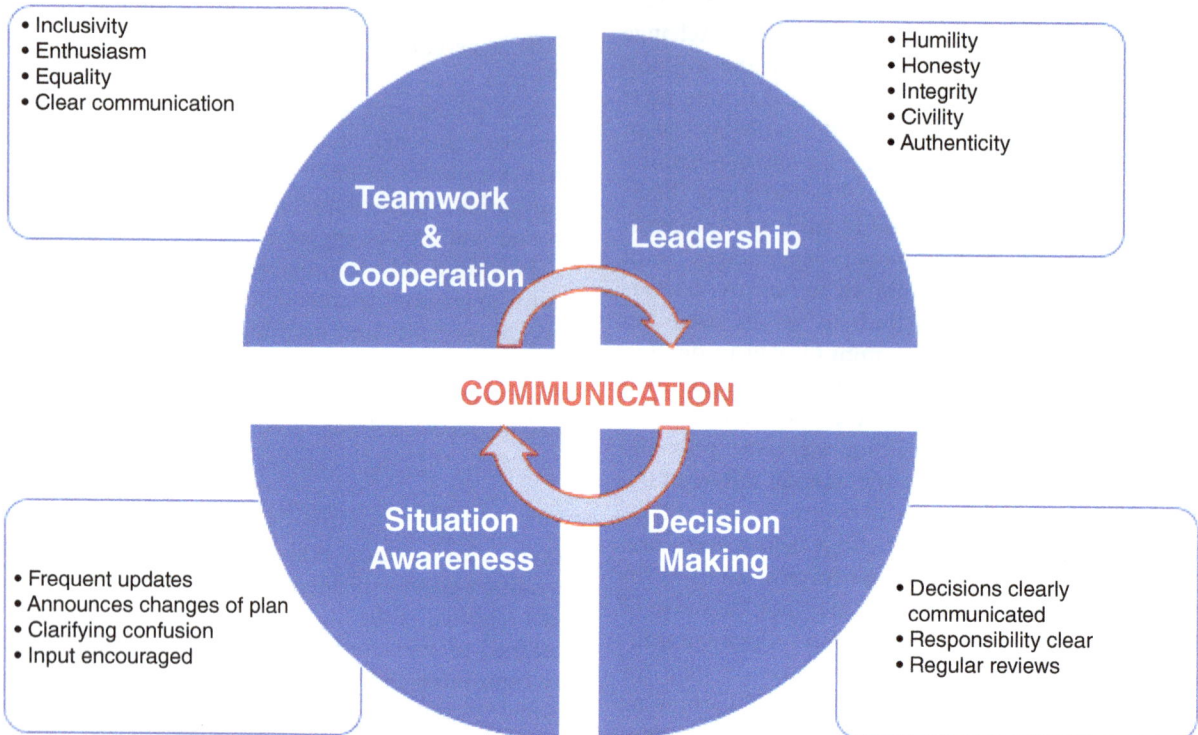

PROFESSIONAL TEAM BEHAVIOUR

- Inclusivity
- Enthusiasm
- Equality
- Clear communication

- Humility
- Honesty
- Integrity
- Civility
- Authenticity

Teamwork & Cooperation

Leadership

COMMUNICATION

Situation Awareness

Decision Making

- Frequent updates
- Announces changes of plan
- Clarifying confusion
- Input encouraged

- Decisions clearly communicated
- Responsibility clear
- Regular reviews

Figure 1.4 A visual model with the basic but critical concepts enabling teams to work together effectively. (Reproduced with kind permission from Atrainability, https://atrainability.co.uk)

Suggested Further Reading

1. Wiegmann DA, Eggman AA, Elbardissi AW, Parker SH, Sundt TM 3rd. Improving cardiac surgical care: A work systems approach. *Appl Ergon.* 2010;41(5):701–712.

2. Wahr JA, Abernathy JH. Improving patient safety in the cardiac operating room: Doing the right thing the right way, every time. *Curr Anesthesiol Rep. 2014;*4:113–123.

3. Wahr JA, Prager RL, Abernathy JH 3rd et al. On behalf of the American Heart Association Council on Cardiovascular Surgery and Anesthesia, Council on Cardiovascular and Stroke Nursing, and Council on Quality of Care and Outcomes Research. Patient safety in the cardiac operating room: Human factors and teamwork: A scientific statement from the American Heart Association. *Circulation.* 2013;128:1139–1169.

4. El Bardissi AW, Wiegmann DA, Dearani JA, Daly RC, Sundt TM 3rd. Application of the human factors analysis and classification system methodology to the cardiovascular surgery operating room. *Ann Thorac Surg.* 2007;83 (4):1412–1419.

5. Wadhera RK, Parker SH, Burkhart HM et al. Is the "sterile cockpit" concept applicable to cardiovascular surgery critical intervals or critical events? The impact of protocol-driven communication during cardiopulmonary bypass. *J Thorac Cardiovasc Surg.* 2010;139 (2):312–319.

6. Mazzocco K, Petitti DB, Fong KT et al. Surgical team behaviors and patient outcomes. *Am J Surg.* 2009;197(5):678–685.

7. Neily J, Mills PD, Young-Xu Y et al. Association between implementation of a medical team training program and surgical mortality. *JAMA.* 2010;304 (15):1693–1700.

8. Jung JJ, Yule S, Boet S, Szasz P, Schulthess P, Grantcharov T. Nontechnical skills assessment of the collective surgical team using the Non-Technical Skills for Surgeons (NOTSS) system. *Ann Surg.* February 21, 2019.

9. Gillespie BM, Harbeck E, Kang E, Steel C, Fairweather N, Chaboyer W. Correlates of non-technical skills in surgery: A prospective study. *BMJ Open.* 2017;7(1):e014480.

10. Flin R, Patey R, Glavin R, Maran N. Anaesthetists' non-technical skills. *Br J Anaesth.* 2010;105(1):38–44.

Equipment for Cardiopulmonary Bypass

Simon Anderson and Amanda Crosby

Cardiopulmonary bypass (CPB) provides optimum conditions for cardiothoracic surgery by combining a pump to substitute for the function of the heart and a gas exchange device, the "oxygenator," to act as an artificial lung. CPB therefore allows the heart and lungs to be temporarily suspended, to facilitate cardiac, vascular or thoracic surgery in a safe, still, bloodless and controlled environment.

History

The first successful open procedures were performed in 1954 by Dr. Clarence Walton Lillehei using a cross-circulation technique, acting as an extracorporeal circuit. This approach worked by circulating the parent's arterial blood into the recipient and controlling the amount of venous blood being returned, giving the surgeon up to an hour to perform cardiac surgery. The concept of the heart lung machine (HLM) and cardiopulmonary bypass circuit arose from this technique of "cross-circulation."

The development of the heart lung machine in 1953 was preceded by a number of perfusion pumps. The design of the first such pump originated in 1935 by Charles Lindbergh in collaboration with Dr. Alex Carrel. The pump was used to keep organs functioning outside of the body with a solution developed by Carrel to perfuse organs, only limited by the eventual failure of the organ itself or the breakdown of the constituents in the perfusate. In 1953 Dr. John Gibbon used the first total CPB system. Gibbon operated on four patients with congenital heart disease with only one survivor, and considered this series of work a failure, however his efforts were an inspiration to researchers around the world. The emergence of the DeWall-Lillehei helix reservoir with a bubble oxygenator in 1955 was the first disposable, efficient, and inexpensive bypass circuit, this innovation fueled the rapid expansion into open-heart surgery after 1956.

The heart lung machine and circuitry used in procedures today has advanced significantly since the advent of extracorporeal circulation and the first attempts at its use. The basic principles, however, remain the same to this day:

- Venous blood is drained by gravity or assistance into a reservoir via a cannula placed in a large vein, most typically the right atrium or vena cava.
- Blood is then pumped through the oxygenating device and an arterial filter. Transit through the oxygenator reduces the partial pressure of carbon dioxide in the blood and raises oxygen content. Current models have the oxygenator, heat exchanger and filter incorporated in one component (Figure 2.1 a and b)
- It is next returned into the patient's arterial system through a cannula in a large artery, most typically the aorta.

Older technology and bypass circuits consisted of large components that required manual cleaning, were reused after sterilization, and were primed with up to 14 units of blood. Due to the advances in technology and techniques, CPB circuits today are more reliable, have more safety devices and are disposable.

Tubing

The cardiopulmonary bypass circuit is created with tubing connected to the various components required to support the circulatory system and allow close monitoring. Table 2.1 provides an overview of the main components of a HLM. Different types of tubing may be used throughout the circuit depending on what function it serves, for example, tubing used to monitor pressure is different to tubing for the actual circulatory support. Tubing should be positioned in an orientation that avoids kinks and allows for smooth curves to limit areas of high velocity or

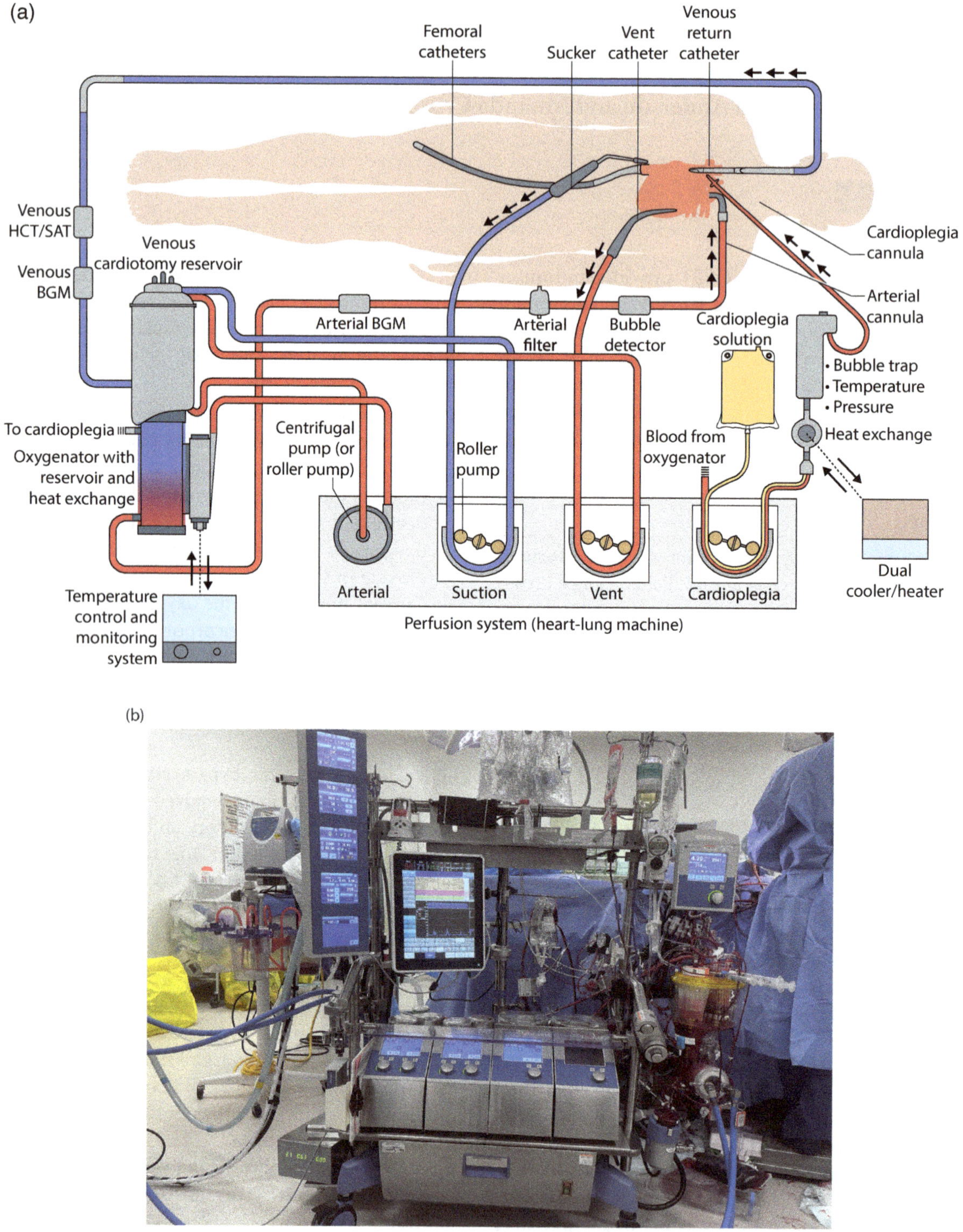

(a)

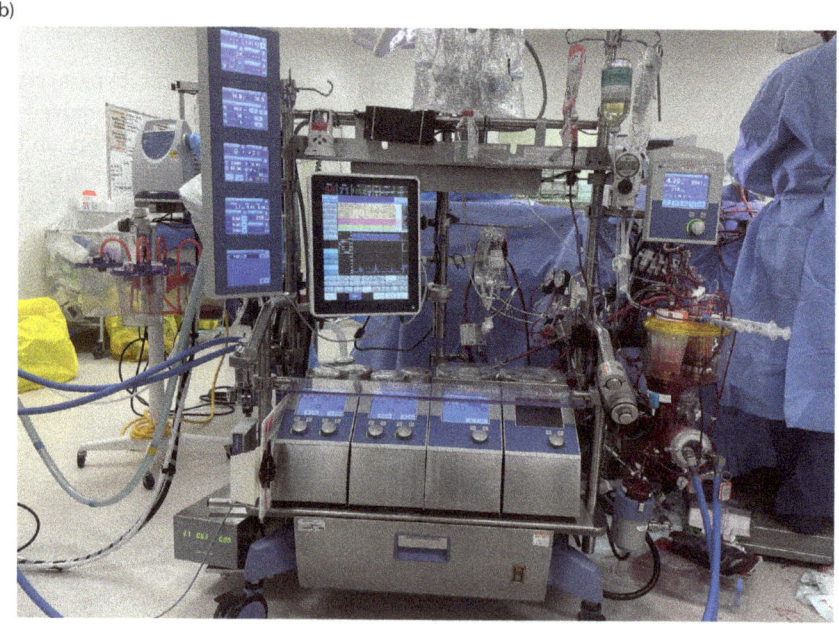

Femoral
catheters

Sucker

Vent
catheter

Venous
return
catheter

Venous
HCT/SAT

Venous
cardiotomy reservoir

Venous
BGM

Arterial BGM

Arterial
filter

Bubble
detector

Cardioplegia
solution

Cardioplegia
cannula

Arterial
cannula

• Bubble trap
• Temperature
• Pressure

To cardioplegia

Oxygenator with
reservoir and
heat exchange

Centrifugal
pump (or
roller pump)

Roller
pump

Blood from
oxygenator

Heat exchange

Temperature
control and
monitoring
system

Arterial

Suction

Vent

Cardioplegia

Dual
cooler/heater

Perfusion system (heart-lung machine)

(b)

Figure 2.1 (a) Typical configuration of a basic cardiopulmonary bypass circuit. BGM = blood gas monitor; SAT = oxygen saturation. (b) Full HLM in use.

Table 2.1. Components of the CPB machine and the extracorporeal circuit

Equipment	Function
Oxygenator system, venous reservoir, oxygenator, heat exchanger	Oxygenate, remove carbon dioxide and cool/rewarm blood
Gas line and FiO$_2$ blender	Delivers fresh gas to the oxygenator in a controlled mixture
Arterial pump	Pumps blood at a set flow rate to the patient
Cardiotomy suckers and vents	Scavenges blood from the operative field and vents the heart
Arterial line filter	Removes microaggregates and particulate matter >40 μm
Cardioplegia systems	Deliver high-dose potassium solutions to arrest the heart and preserve the myocardium
Cannulae	Connect the patient to the extracorporeal circuit

Table 2.2. Commonly used biocompatible tubing coatings

Manufacturer and Coating	Description of Coating Properties
Gore – Carmeda	Covalent bonding of heparin molecules
Baxter - Duraflo II	Heparin ionically joined with ammonium and attached to surface
Terumo – Xcoating	Biopassive polymer creates hydrophobic and hydrophilic properties without heparin
Maquet – Bioline	Heparin and albumin attached to polypeptides on tubing surface
LivaNova – P.H.I.S.O. Coating	Phosphorylcholine
Medtronic – Cortiva BioActive Surface	Endpoint-attached heparin coating

stagnation. Any junctions or connections between components have to be secured tightly to prevent leaks or air ingress. Clinicians must consider the intended use of the tubing when choosing materials to create the circuit.

Polyvinylchloride (PVC) is the predominant tubing material used today in cardiopulmonary bypass, but latex rubber and silicone rubber are other options. PVC is made up of polymer chains with polar carbon-chloride (C-Cl) bonds. These bonds result in considerable intermolecular attraction between the polymer chains, making PVC a fairly strong material. On its own, PVC is a rigid plastic, but plasticizers are added to the type of tubing used in a circuit, which make it malleable and easier to manipulate.

Silicone rubber is a semi organic synthetic. Its structure consists of a chain of silicon and oxygen atoms rather than carbon and hydrogen atoms, as is the case with other types of rubber. The molecular structure of silicone rubber results in a very flexible but weak chain. Silicone produces less hemolysis than

PVC when the tubing is occluded but can release more particles. Silicone rubber is sometimes utilized in the arterial pump roller head as an alternative to commonly used PVC tubing.

Tubing used during CPB is subject to repeated compression in pump roller heads. This intermittent compression can degrade the integrity of the walls of the tubing and may cause plastic micro particles to be released, this is called spallation.

Tubing can be made with a biocompatible coating (see Table 2.2), which may help reduce the inflammatory response to foreign material. Sequelae from the inflammatory response include platelet activation, initiation of the coagulation cascade, decreased levels of circulating coagulation factors, activation of endothelial cells and leukocytes, releasing mediators that may contribute to capillary leakage and tissue edema. This is discussed in more detail in Chapter 17.

There are a number of surface coatings available on the market today. One type of circuit coating uses both hydrophobic and hydrophilic properties to form a new layer on top of the tubing that reduces protein denaturation and platelet adhesion. Since this coating is made from a non-heparin-based biopassive polymer Poly(2-methoxyethylacrylate) (PMEA), this tubing can be used on heparin sensitive or intolerant patients. Another type of biocompatible tubing is

11

Table 2.3. Tubing sizes commonly used in different parts of the extracorporeal circuit (adults only)

Tubing size	Prime volume (cc/ft/ml/ 30cm)	Max flow (l/min) (To keep pressure gradient <10 mmH*)	Max flow (l/ min) (To keep Reynolds number <1000*)	Function
3/16" (4.5 mm)	5.4 /4.7	0.2	1.8	Cardioplegia section of the blood cardioplegia delivery system
1/4" (6.0 mm)	9.84/8.5	0.9	2.1	Suction tubing, blood section of the blood cardioplegia delivery system
3/8" (9.0 mm)	21.6 /19.1	4.0	3.7	Arterial pump line for flow rates <6.7 l/ minute, majority of the arterial tubing in the extracorporeal circuit
1/2" (12.0 mm)	42/33.9	7.0	5.0	Venous line, larger tubing is required to gravity drain blood from the patient

* Source: Hessel EA II, Hill AG in Gravlee GP et al.: *Cardiopulmonary Bypass: Principles and Practice.* Lippincott Williams & Wilkins, 2000, Table 5.4

made from phosphorylcholine that mimics the natural endothelium to reduce platelet activation and cell adhesion to the tubing surface. Some tubing contains heparin, which should be noted when providing care to a heparin intolerant patient. Some institutions maintain a small stock of non-coated circuits for these patients. Regardless of the type or manufacturer selected, biocompatible tubing can improve platelet preservation and reduce the inflammatory response to foreign surfaces.

Selecting the appropriate tubing size is based on the application. Larger bore tubing requires less pump head revolutions needed to displace the same amount of volume as smaller tubing, meaning less mechanical stress from repeated compression. The internal diameter as well as the length should be carefully considered as both will affect the priming volume. While a larger internal diameter allows for greater flow at lower pressures, it has a higher prime volume, increased contact activation, less resistance, and a larger pressure gradient. There are many factors to consider when selecting the best fit for the application required (see Table 2.3). When deciding upon the size of arterial and venous tubing, the patient's body surface area (BSA) and calculated cardiac index can help guide the appropriate size of tubing. Tubing for cardioplegia administration is based on the solution being used, the ratio of blood

to crystalloid needed, and the type of delivery device. When choosing tubing for scavenging blood from the surgical field and venting of the heart or aorta, the decision is usually based on institutional protocol, but will take into account the volume of the tubing length and the displacement per revolution of the pump head.

Arterial Cannulae

The arterial cannula is used to deliver oxygenated, pressurized blood from the HLM directly into the patient's arterial system. The size of the vessel that is being cannulated and the patient's required blood flow are considered in selecting the appropriately sized cannula.

The ascending aorta is most used as the site of arterial cannulation for routine cardiovascular surgery allowing antegrade flow to the cerebral and body circulation. The asceding aorta is large caliber, has a low associated incidence of aortic dissection (0.01–0.09%), and is easy access when using a median sternotomy approach. After sternotomy and exposure, the surgeon can assess the size of the aorta before choosing the most appropriate caliber cannula (see Figure 2.2).

Developments in cannula design allow the use of thin wall cannulae. By having a larger effective

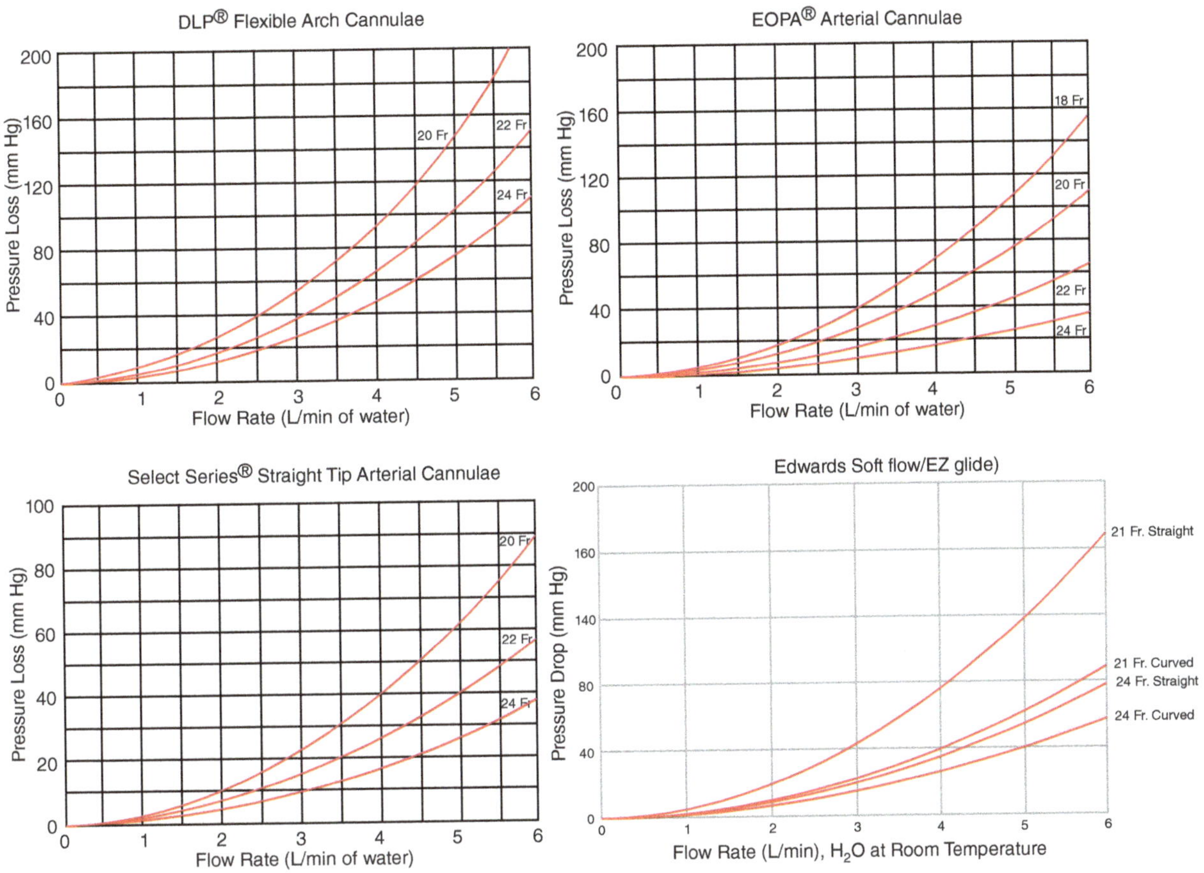

DLP® Flexible Arch Cannulae

(Graph: Pressure Loss (mm Hg) on y-axis, 0 to 200; Flow Rate (L/min of water) on x-axis, 0 to 6. Curves labeled 20 Fr, 22 Fr, 24 Fr)

EOPA® Arterial Cannulae

(Graph: Pressure Loss (mm Hg) on y-axis, 0 to 200; Flow Rate (L/min of water) on x-axis, 0 to 6. Curves labeled 18 Fr, 20 Fr, 22 Fr, 24 Fr)

Select Series® Straight Tip Arterial Cannulae

(Graph: Pressure Loss (mm Hg) on y-axis, 0 to 100; Flow Rate (L/min of water) on x-axis, 0 to 6. Curves labeled 20 Fr, 22 Fr, 24 Fr)

Edwards Soft flow/EZ glide)

(Graph: Pressure Drop (mm Hg) on y-axis, 0 to 200; Flow Rate (L/min), H₂O at Room Temperature on x-axis, 0 to 6. Curves labeled 21 Fr. Straight, 21 Fr. Curved, 24 Fr. Straight, 24 Fr. Curved)

Figure 2.2 Cannula flow profiles.

internal diameter, they achieve lower resistance to flow. Subsequently, within the extracorporeal circuit, this leads to a reduction in arterial line pressure and allows an increase in blood flow. Further developments come in the form of angled tip arterial cannulae. These manipulate the flow characteristics of blood leaving the cannula to produce a spray effect, dispersing blood into the aorta. This design not only minimizes damage to the vessel wall by directing blood flow toward the aortic arch rather than toward the vessel wall, but also reduces the pressure drop at the tip of the cannula. Figure 2.3 shows several designs of aortic cannulae.

Axillary, subclavian and femoral arteries are examples of alternative arterial peripheral cannulation sites, typically during complex or redo surgery. The femoral cannulae are longer than conventional ones and incorporate a spirally wound wire within their wall to prevent "kinking" (see Figure 2.4). X-ray

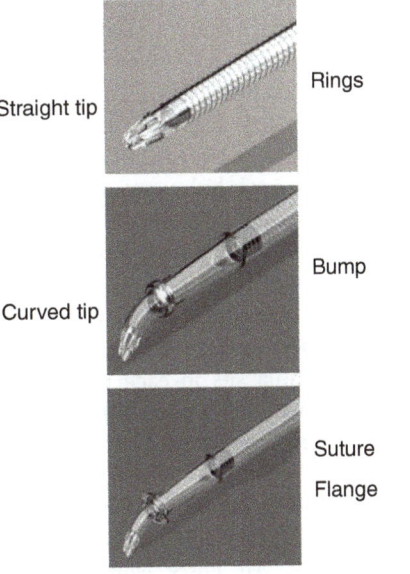

Straight tip — Rings

Curved tip — Bump

Suture Flange

Figure 2.3 Commonly used arterial cannulae. (Reproduced with kind permission from Edwards Lifesciences.)

13

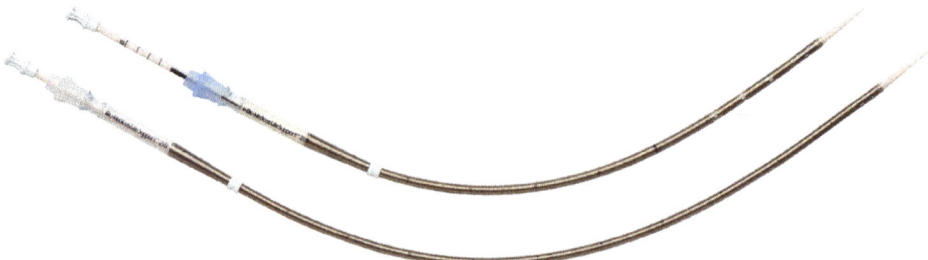

Figure 2.4 Femoral reinforced cannula. Biomedicus Life Support™ 21Fr. (Reproduced with ©2020 Medtronic. All rights reserved. Used with the permission of Medtronic.)

imaging or transesophageal echocardiography (TEE) is used to confirm correct cannula position. Axillary and subclavian cannulation is most commonly achieved by suturing a dacron graft end-to-side onto the vessel and a 3/8 × 3/8 inch connector to connect to the HLM arterial line.

Venous Cannulae

Venous cannulation provides the means to drain deoxygenated blood from the patient's venous system into the extracorporeal circuit. It is important to use appropriately sized cannulae in order to obtain maximum venous drainage from the patient so that full flow can be achieved when CPB is commenced. The type of venous cannulation used depends on the operation being undertaken. For cardiac surgery not involving opening chambers of the right heart, for example, coronary artery bypass grafts (CABG) or aortic valve replacement (AVR), a two-stage venous cannula is often used. The tip of this type of cannula sits in the inferior vena cava (IVC) and drains blood from the IVC through holes around the tip; a second series of holes a few centimeters above the tip is sited in the right atrium to drain venous blood from the superior vena cava (SVC).

During procedures that require the right atrium (RA) to be opened, bicaval cannulation, where a single-stage cannula sits in each of the inferior and superior vena cava, is necessary. The two single-stage cannulae are connected to the venous line of the CPB circuit using a Y-connector. This approach avoids air entry into the CPB circuit from the distal series of holes of a two-stage cannula, as they would be sitting in the open RA. Air entry would impede venous drainage – or stop it completely in case of an "air lock" – leading to the patient's calculated full flow becoming unachievable in addition to not providing

a bloodless field for the surgeon. Figure 2.5 shows commonly used venous cannulae.

Femoral cannulation can be utilized for more complex surgery. In this instance, a long cannula, which is in essence an elongated single-stage cannula, is typically passed over a guide wire up the femoral vein into the IVC and RA to achieve venous drainage. These cannulae are generally placed under TEE guidance. As with arterial cannulation sites, the size and length of the venous cannulae are patient specific and are determined by body surface area (BSA), required full flow and vessel size. In an average height adult (170 cm, 80 kg), a 25 Fr/55 cm cannula provides sufficient venous drainage from the IVC. However, in smaller patients, a 38cm length cannula may be a better option to ensure the cannula is short enough to be positioned in the IVC and not too long to potentially perforate the right atrium or SVC during cannulation.

Perfusion Pumps

Perfusion pumps, in the arterial position, propel blood forward through the circuit. There are two main types: positive displacement roller pumps and the impeller centrifugal pumps.

Roller Pumps

A peristaltic pump or "roller pump" is a positive displacement pump used for moving fluid. Initial HLM technology in the 1950s used a similar peristaltic pump, and the technology has not greatly changed from its inception. The raceway or the pump header accepts a length of tubing, the rotor and roller combination inside the middle of the pump housing rotate in a clockwise or counterclockwise direction. Typically, there will be two or more rollers that compress the tubing and a clutch mechanism to set the

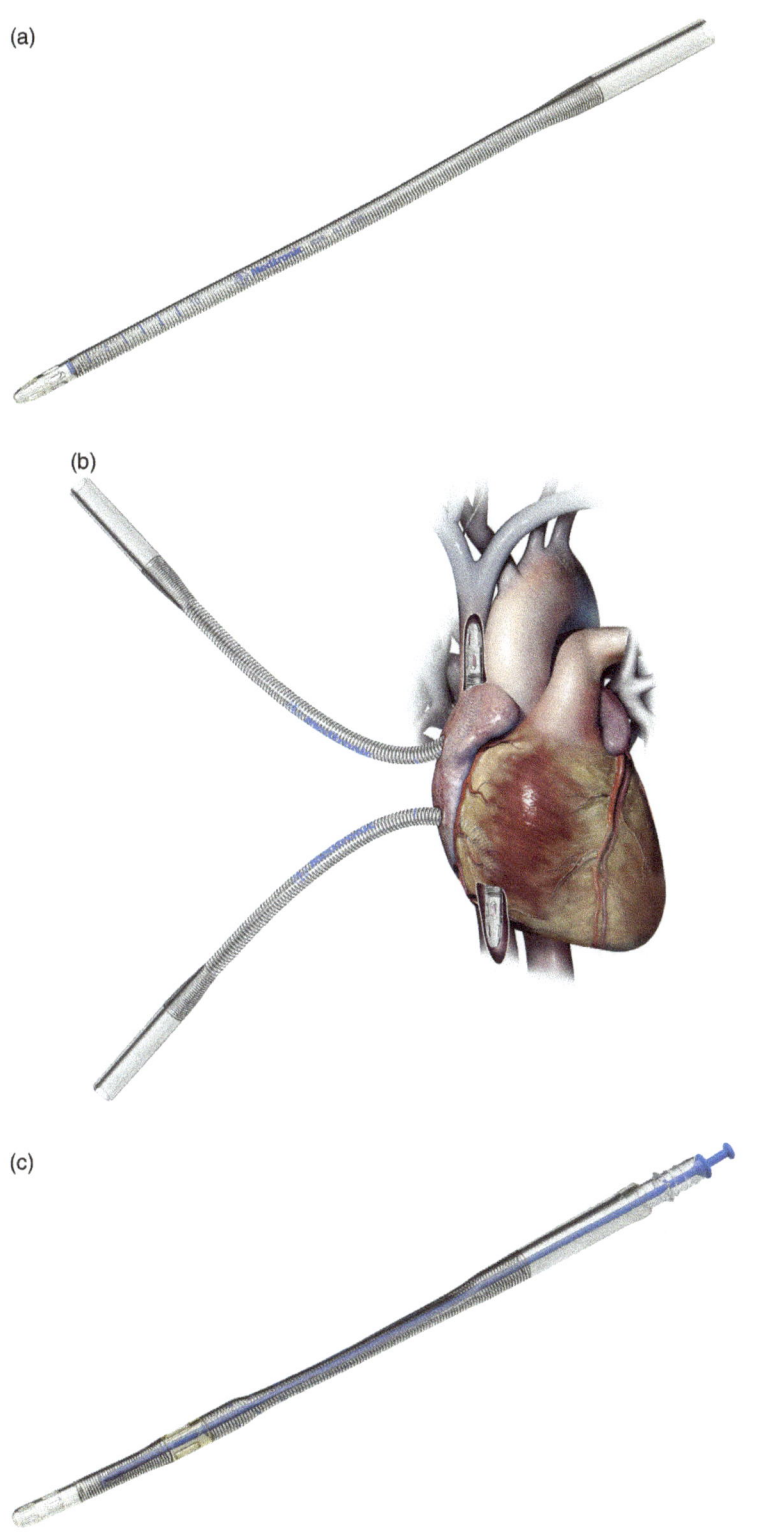

Figure 2.5 Commonly used venous cannulae (a) DLP™ single-stage cannula (b) Bi-caval cannulation technique (c) MC2™ two-stage cannula.
(Reproduced with ©2020 Medtronic. All rights reserved. Used with the permission of Medtronic.)

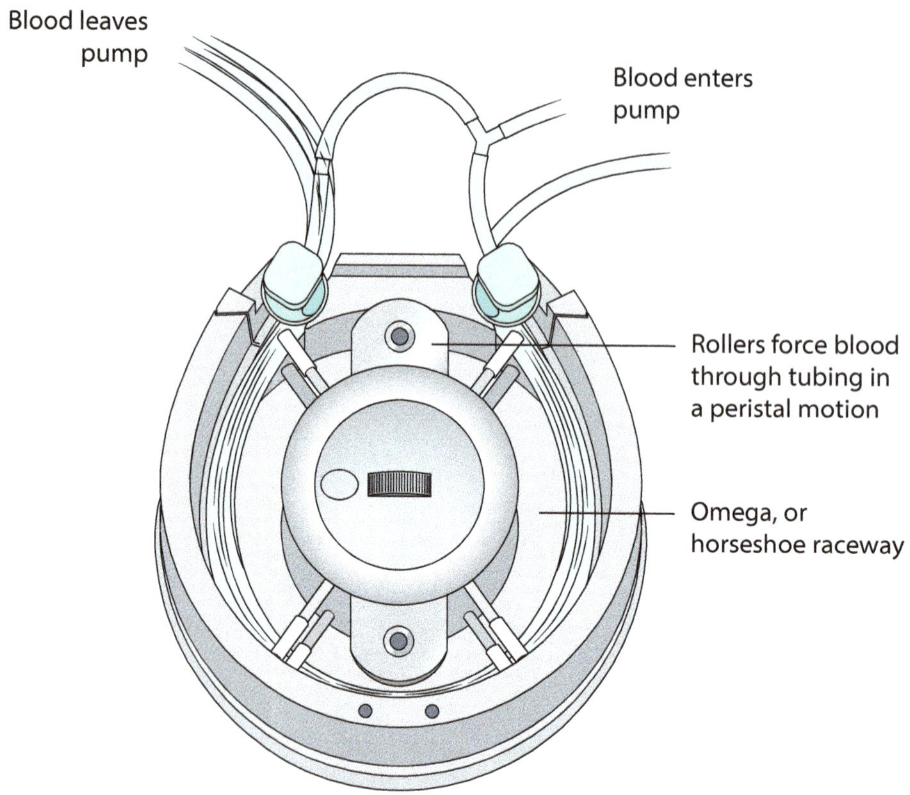

Blood leaves
pump

Blood enters
pump

Figure 2.6 Line drawing of a
roller pump.

Rollers force blood
through tubing in
a peristal motion

Omega, or
horseshoe raceway

degree of tubing occlusion, regulating the amount of compression applied to the tubing. Under-occlusive, or too loose, tubing may result in retrograde flow or inaccurate flow calculations, while over-occlusion, or too tight, may increase hemolysis, spallation, and inaccurate flow calculations. The roller head occlusion should be measured before each case to ensure it has the desired setting for the operation. The methods to test occlusions are described in detail in Chapter 4.

As the rollers compress and occlude the tubing, the fluid is moved in the corresponding direction(see Figure 2.6). The tubing inside the raceway is held in a fixed position by brackets or a locking mechanism and returns to its natural state once the roller passes over it. This intermittent occlusion creates positive and negative pressures on either side of the occlusion point, which is the driving force for the movement of fluid. Positive pressure created by the roller propels fluid and the recoil of the tubing creates negative pressure refilling the tube.

Roller pumps can be used in any position. They can be belt driven or have direct drive systems and are not affected by circuit resistance or hydrostatic

pressure. As they operate independently of resistance or pressure, pressures within the circuit must be monitored. It is essential to limit the pump flow if system pressure becomes excessive. Sudden occlusion of the inlet of the roller head can create extreme negative pressure to the point where the tubing may cavitate and create air bubbles in the circuit.

Very similar to the heart, output of a roller pump is determined by the internal diameter of the tubing (= stroke volume) and the number of revolutions of the pump head (= beats per minute). The larger the tubing in the raceway, the less rpms are needed to maintain the same output of smaller tubing. Note that reading or recording blood flow directly from the arterial roller head does not account for any shunts that may be present downstream in the circuit, and thus the actual flow reaching the patient may be less.

Centrifugal Pumps

Centrifugal pumps are non-occlusive pumps and utilize a magnet and impeller combination to propel blood

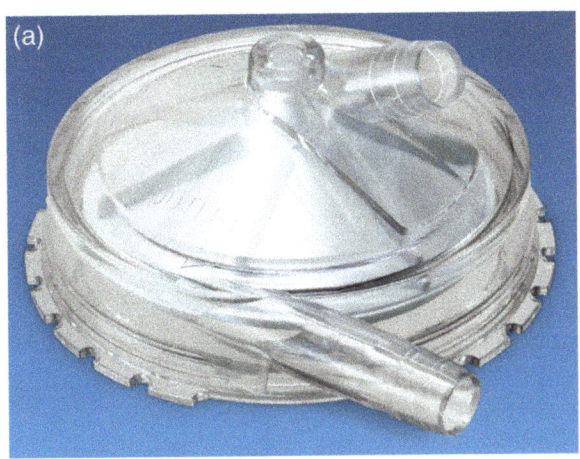

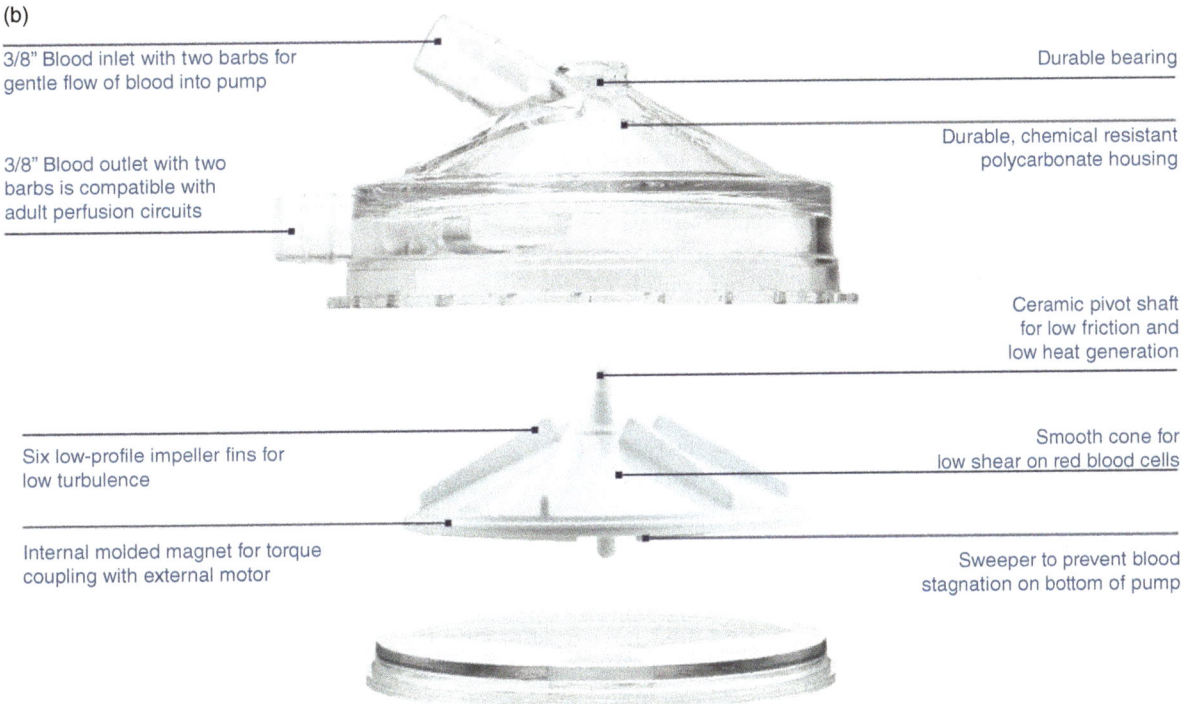

Figure 2.7 Centrifugal pump head (a) Medtronic Affinity™. (b) Schematic cut through of Affinity™ centrifugal pump. (Reproduced with ©2020 Medtronic. All rights reserved. Used with the permission of Medtronic.)

through the CPB circuit. The pump consists of a hard outer shell which incorporates an impeller design coupled magnetically with an electric motor and shaft or pin. When the console is turned on and the rpms are increased, the cones or fins spin rapidly, creating positive pressure that propels fluid forward (see Figure 2.7).

Centrifugal pumps, much like the heart, are afterload sensitive. If the post-pump resistance increases, the amount of forward flow will decrease, unless the rpms are altered to counter this. For this reason, centrifugal pumps have the potential to allow retrograde flow, however most flow meters will alert the user if this occurs. Unlike roller pumps whose flow is calculated based on tubing diameter and rpm (stroke volume and beats per minute), centrifugal heads require ultrasonic or electromagnetic meters to accurately determine blood flow. Unlike rollers, centrifugal pumps do not need to be pressure regulated because they will not be able to generate forward flow if the tubing is kinked, clamped, or suddenly occluded. When used for CPB, a special centrifugal head motor that can be manually operated must be available as backup.

The perceived benefits of the centrifugal pump are its low prime volume and, because of its non-occlusive nature, less hemolysis. Despite extensive research, there is little clinical evidence to show any benefit of CPB with centrifugal over CPB with roller pumps. Centrifugal pumps may produce less hemolysis and platelet activation than roller pumps, but this does not correlate with any difference in clinical outcome. Centrifugal pumps are less likely to create air embolism situations because as air is introduced to the cone, the pump will deprime and cease forward flow. Clinicians should remain vigilant, though, as there have been reports of air ingress into circuits using centrifugal pumps. Centrifugal pumpheads are expensive, adding a signficant additional cost to the CPB circuit. Clinicians favoring centrifugal systems have argued that the ability to create smaller circuits due to remote drive capabilities, allows the circuit to be closer to the surgical field unlike the fixed console based roller head position. The new generation roller pumps have largely overcome this issue and tubing length has decreased significantly in recent years. The decision to use centrifugal pumps or roller pumps for CPB is largely determined by institutional factors rather than clinical indication. Table 2.4 summarizes commonly used adult centrifugal pump heads.

Centrifugal head technology is not only used in cardiopulmonary bypass cases but also in extracorporeal membrane oxygenation (ECMO) and ventricular assist devices (VADs). Certain models possess fins or channels to help avoid areas of stagnation, while others have magnetically levitated bearingless motors to reduce heat generation. Each has a set rpm needed to generate forward flow, this minimum number will be different with blood viscosity (hemoglobin) and patients' vascular resistance pressure.

Reservoirs

Cardiotomy reservoirs may be hardshell or softshell (collapsible). Hardshell reservoirs usually comprise of a durable polycarbonate housing, a high-efficiency polyester depth filter and a polyurethane defoamer (see Figure 2.8).

Table 2.4. Common centrifugal heads, adult sizes

Manufacturer	Centrifugal Head	Brief Description
LivaNova	Revolution	Open impeller design, with impregnated nylon magnet and seal-less low friction bearings – 57 ml prime volume
Terumo	CAPIOX SP	Polycarbonate housing, impeller design, lip seal – 45 ml prime volume
Medtronic	Affinity CP	Low profile fins, ceramic pivot bearings, no stasis zones – 40 ml prime volume
Abbott - Thoratec	Centrimag	Free-floating magnetically levitated rotor, has no bearings or seals creating minimal stasis zones – 31 ml prime volume
Gettinge - Maquet	Rotaflow RF-32	Peg-top, one-point sapphire bearing – 32 ml prime volume

The reservoir acts as a chamber for the venous blood to drain into before it is pumped through the oxygenator and permits ready access for the addition of fluids and drugs. To reduce the risk of perfusion accidents, the level of fluid is monitored for the duration of CPB to prevent the reservoir from emptying and air entering the circuit. Each manufacturer details the minimum safe fluid level necessary to achieve the rated flow of their device. Low level alarms (see also Chapter 3), often coupled to automatic cessation of pump flow when triggered, add additional safety. Gross air embolism incidents can still occur if arterial flow exceeds venous drainage, subsequently emptying the reservoir.

Vacuum-assisted venous drainage may be used to optimize venous drainage during CPB. Using vacuum assistance can reduce hemodilution and subsequent transfusion requirements because improved drainage requires fewer "top-ups" with crystalloids or colloids. With the top of the cardiotomy reservoir positioned

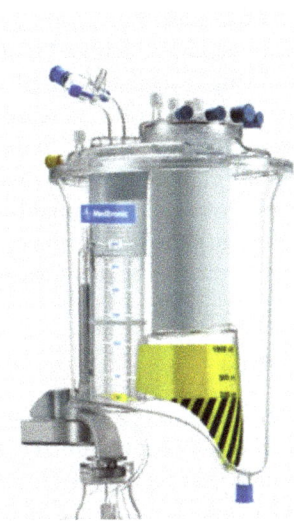

at the level of the patient's atrium, a negative pressure of approximately −60 mmHg is applied when maximal gravity drainage is reached. The negative pressure can be increased by small amounts during CPB, when the fluid in the reservoir decreases to the safety limit level. For weaning from bypass, the negative pressure is gradually decreased to zero, the reservoir is opened, and the venous line progressively closed.

Blood scavenged from the operative field via suckers is also returned to the reservoir. Suction relies on the "Venturi" effect, which is the change in pressure and fluid velocity through a narrowing in a tube. Suctioning blood from the operative field causes damage to blood cells and also results in concomitant entrainment of high volumes of air. The salvaged blood may contain tissue and other debris and is highly activated with inflammatory cells. It is vital that this blood is filtered through the reservoir before being pumped to the patient. Advances in technology have seen a more widespread use of reservoirs containing separate chambers for venous blood and cardiotomy suction, allowing the suction blood only to be added into the circuit when required. Segregating suction blood that way has the advantage that it can be passed through a specific filter that absorbs lipid cells, which have been shown to impair oxygenator effectiveness. The reservoir is constantly vented to prevent the entrained air causing a pressure buildup,

which can occur if the suckers are left running at a high level for prolonged periods. The blood returned from the intracardiac "vent" suckers is also returned to the reservoir.

Collapsible reservoirs are used mainly for pediatric or mini bypass cases and are dicussed in more detail in Chapters 8 and 15.

Oxygenators

The evolution of the oxygenator has been critical to the success of cardiac surgery and advanced patient care. Oxygenators are most often described as artificial lungs as they provide an alveolar capillary system for gas transfer. The general design goals are efficient gas exchange, low prime volume, minimized trauma to blood and efficient cooling and heating capabilities.

There are two main types of oxygenators commonly used in adult cases today, microporous polypropylene (PPL) and non-porous polymethylpentene (PMP). Both are hollow fiber membrane oxygenators, which are named for the membrane that separates the gas and blood phases. The main difference is their duration of use – the PMP type oxygenators typically maintain gas exchange longer. While PPL oxygenators are more common, extended use can cause plasma leaks across the membrane from the blood phase into the gas phase, resulting in decreased gas exchange efficiency. The non-porous fibers of the PMP oxygenator make them more durable than PPL, and they are typically used for longer term applications such as ECMO. The lack of pores does not allow exchange of volatile anesthetics, making PMP oxygenators unsuitable for use with CPB.

Oxygenators are regulated by federal guidelines, allowing their use for periods of time usually up to six hours. While using them longer is designated as off label, it is a widespread and acceptable application of the technology to facilitate bridging to recovery or transplantation when other advanced treatments have failed.

Once entering the device, blood first passes over the integrated heat exchanger before moving into the oxygenator compartment, where gas exchange takes place (see Figure 2.9). O_2 concentration and flow of the sweep gas, which drives gas exchange, are regulated with a gas blender and a flow meter integrated into the HLM. The sweep is piped into the oxygenator inlet port, its distribution throughout the membrane's capillary system varies with the oxygenator used and the patient's size. Typically the flow is 2–4 l/min for adults, depending on blood flow and the desired CO_2 removal rate. Volatile anesthetics can be added depending on oxygenator type and HLM in use.

Gas scavenging can be attached to the exhaust port. Gas sampling to determine O_2 consumption and end-tidal CO_2 can be attached at this point as well.

Integrating the heat exchanger and arterial line filter into the oxygenator has decreased circuit size and reduced prime volume. The heat exchanger is separated from the blood phase by a highly thermal conductive material and is biologically inert. An external heater cooler is connected with thick water lines, usually made of antimicrobial-coated tubing. Fine control of the water bath temperature allows precise regulation of the patient temperature.

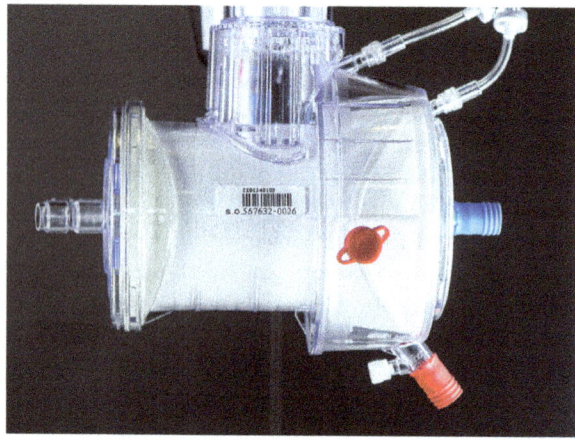

Figure 2.9 Fusion™ oxygenator combined with and a heat exchanger in a single unit. (Reproduced with ©2020 Jose Canamares. All rights reserved. Used with the permission of Jose Canamares.)

Cooling the blood, and thus cooling the patient, results in a lower metabolic demand that helps ensure all tissues are being adequately perfused while on bypass. Chapters 9 and 10 discuss temperature management and rewarming strategies in more detail.

Intended duration of use, requirement for volatile anesthetics, prime volume, biocompatible coating, gas exchange capacity, and the heat exchanger's efficiency are the main determinants that inform the choice of oxygenator used for a case.

Gas Supply System

The gas supply is connected to the blender, which mixes oxygen and air to provide the desired FiO_2 and to a flow meter to regulate sweep gas flow (see Figure 2.10). CO_2 may be added to the sweep when pH-stat blood gas management is desired during hypothermia or cases requiring deep hypothermic circulatory arrest (DHCA, see Chapter 9). Blending units and flow meters may be mechanical, but are now mostly digitally controlled via the HLM. Continuous inspired O_2 analysis is mandatory to prevent the inadvertent administration of a hypoxic mixture.

Filters and Bubble Traps

Air entrainment through the venous return line, fluid, drug and blood administration through the cardiotomy reservoir, as well as ingress of air and particulate matter from cardiotomy suckers and vents, all contribute to the embolic load patients may be exposed to. While it is not possible to eliminate the embolic load in its entirety, the use of arterial filters and

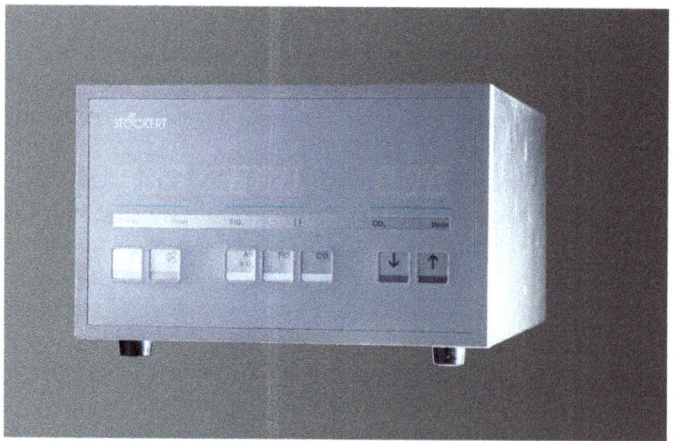

Figure 2.10 LivaNova S5® Electronic Gas Blender, courtesy of LivaNova PLC. (Reproduced with kind permission from LivaNova.) Photograph by *Jose Canamares used with permission.*

Table 2.5. Filtration devices used within the cardiopulmonary bypass circuit

Filter type	Application and specification
Gas line	Removes 99.999% of bacteria found in the gas stream minimizing cross-contamination between the patient and the equipment
Pre-CPB	0.2 μm filter is used during the priming and recirculation phase. It is designed for the removal of inadvertent particulate debris and microbial contaminants and their associated endotoxins
Arterial line	Designed to remove microemboli >20 μm in size from the perfusate during extracorporeal circulation. This includes gas emboli, fat emboli and aggregates composed of platelets, red blood cells and other debris. Pore size depends on manufacturer
Venous reservoir	Designed to remove debris and gross air, some models may contain a defoamer to reduce bubbles from incoming suction or ports
Cardioplegia	Blood cardioplegia: >40 μm filter. Crystalloid cardioplegia: >0.2 μm filter. Low priming volume filter for cell-free solutions. Removes inadvertent particulate debris and microbial contaminants and their associated endotoxins
Leukodepletion	Reduces the levels of leukocytes, either from the arterial line or cardioplegia system, and excludes microemboli >40 μm
Blood transfusion	Designed to reduce the levels of leukocytes and microaggregates from one unit of packed red blood cells or whole blood, used when giving blood products to the patient
Cell salvage	Designed for the filtration of salvaged blood, to remove potentially harmful microaggregates, leukocytes and lipid particles

bubble traps can reduce this significantly. Table 2.5 gives an overview of the filters most commonly used in CPB circuits.

Depth filters create a tortuous path between fibers and retain particles mechanically. Screen filters are the most common type and are typically made of a woven polyester mesh. They are usually pleated to allow for a larger surface area in a confined space and trap particulates or emboli that are larger than their particular pore size. Filters come in a size range from 0.2 μm for gas line filters to 40 μm for arterial line filters.

0.2 μm pre-bypass filters are meant to capture any particles left from the manufacturing process and are removed after priming and before initiating bypass.

Separate arterial line filters are indicated for use in all CPB procedures where the oxygenator does not have an integrated filter. The main goal of an arterial filter, whether integrated into the oxygenator or not, is to stop gaseous macro-emboli from entering the circulation, although there is some debate about their effectiveness. Several arterial filters with varying characteristics are commercially available (see Table 2.6).

The US Food and Drug Administration (FDA) have outlined key areas of importance pertaining to arterial line filters (FDA, 2000). The following list sets forth the risks to health associated with this device that were identified in the proposed classification ruling (dated February 26, 1979), as well as additional adverse event reporting since the classification ruling:

- Amount of damage to formed blood elements, clotting and hemolysis
- Degree of pressure drop resulting in inadequate blood flow, damage to the device or structural integrity and damage to the arterial line
- Structural integrity of the product
- Excessive pressure gradients, for example, blood damage and inadequate blood flow
- Filtration efficiency and gas emboli-handling capacities
- User error
- Blood incompatibility and the requirements of ISO 10993: Biological Evaluation of Medical Devices
- Compatibility of the product when exposed to circulating blood and infections
- Shelf life

These stringent criteria aim to ensure the production of high-quality arterial line filters that will not have any deleterious effects on the CPB circuit or patient.

Table 2.6. Different commercially available arterial line filters, both external and integrated

Manufacturer	Filter type	Fiber material	Filter size (μm)
LivaNova	Screen, External	Phosphorylcholine-coated polyester net	27, 40, 120
	Screen, Integrated	Phosphorylcholine-coated polyester net	38
Medtronic	Screen, External	Cortiva Bioactive surface coating or uncoated	20 or 38
	Screen, Integrated	Cortiva Bioactive surface coating or uncoated	25
Terumo	Screen, External	Polyester, X-coating	37
	Screen, Integrated	Polyester, X-coating	32
Pall	Screen, External	Heparin-coated polyester	40
Lifeline-Delhi	Screen, External	Polyester	40, 20
Membrane solutions	Screen, External	Woven Polyester	40

Suckers and Vents

The suckers allow spilled blood from the operative field to be returned to the circuit via the reservoir, but they can also be used to help salvage emergency situations. In case of life-threatening, excessive bleeding before venous cannulation has been established, the suckers can be used to scavenge blood to the venous reservoir and subsequently be transfused back into the patient via the arterial line. This is commonly known as "sucker bypass" and grants the surgeon time to attempt to fix the problem at least temporarily.

"Vent" suckers are used to drain blood from the left ventricular cavity, typically via these sites:

- Aortic root
- Right superior pulmonary vein
- Left atrium or pulmonary artery
- Left ventricle
- Left ventricular apex

The main reasons for venting the heart during CPB are to:

- prevent distension of the heart
- evacuate air from the cardiac chambers during the de-airing phase of the procedure
- improve surgical exposure
- reduce myocardial rewarming
- create a dry surgical field.

There are complications associated with all sites used for venting, most commonly relating to injury to tissues at the site. Venting via the left ventricular (LV) apex can be associated with particularly serious consequences including:

- LV wall rupture if inadequately closed
- Damage to the LV wall due to excessive suction
- Embolization through air entrained into the LV through the vent site.

Cardioplegia Delivery Systems

One of the major concerns during cardiac surgery is protection of the myocardium during procedures. Cardioplegia solution is administered to maintain controlled and protected electrical arrest of the myocardium during the ischemic period. Chapter 11 is dedicated to myocardial protection techniques.

Regardless of the type of cardioplegia delivery device, monitoring of temperature, appropriate delivery pressure, and time intervals between doses are critical to the success of the operation.

Cardioplegia delivery systems typically include a line for pressure monitoring, an over-pressure relief valve, and a recirculation line for easy priming or de-airing. Pressure monitoring is essential when delivering cardioplegia into small vessels and the coronary sinus to prevent damage. An air detection device is often added to the infusion line for additional protection against microemboli. Most cardioplegia delivery systems today have their own dedicated integrated heat exchanger. This heat exchanger and accompanying water lines are separate from the oxygenator since cardioplegia is typically delivered at temperatures much colder than the patient's core temperature.

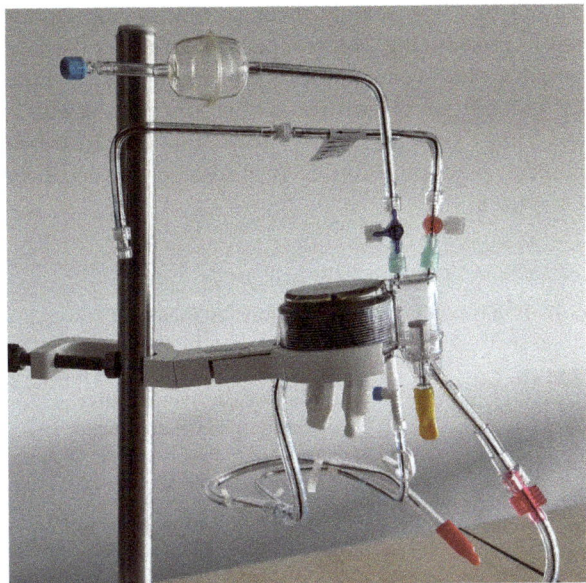

Figure 2.11 Cardioplegia delivery system allows mixing of blood and cardioplegia solution and warming or cooling of solution by Myotherm™. (Reproduced with ©2020 Jose Canamares. All rights reserved. Used with the permission of Jose Canamares.) Photograph by *Jose Canamares used with permission.*

Table 2.7. Cardioplegia delivery systems

Manufacturer	Integrated Heat Exchanger	Air Trap	Delivery System
LivaNova	Yes	Yes	Dual roller head or dual shims adapter for two sizes of tubing for different ratio options
Medtronic	Yes	Yes	Blood cardioplegia 4:1 ratio via roller pump (can also be used with a syringe driver for the potassium solutions)
Getinge	Yes	Yes	Blood or crystalloid cardioplegia ratio via roller pump depending on tubing set
Quest Medical	Yes	Yes	Piston pump for microplegia or compatible for numerous ratios including all crystalloid

Cardioplegia delivery systems vary from simple to complex. Administration in early procedures was accomplished by either using a pressure bag at the head of the surgical field or elevating glass bottles to the operating theater ceiling via a pulley system and a needle inserted directly into the cross-clamped aorta. More complex microplegia systems require hardware to be added to the heart lung machine and deliver specific aliquot measurements of medications to arrest and protect the myocardium. Standard blood cardioplegia delivery systems use roller pumps and specific tubing sizes to deliver a set ratio of blood to clear cardioplegic solutions (see Figure 2.11).

Table 2.7 summarizes the characteristics of some of the most commonly used cardioplegia systems. While many designs are available, every system should be capable of changing the ratio of blood to crystalloid, control flow to administer through different routes of the heart, and be temperature controlled to allow cold, warm, or tepid doses of cardioplegia.

Hemofilters

Ultrafilters or hemoconcentrators contain semipermeable, hollow fiber membranes that permit passage of water and electrolytes out of the blood. They are normally connected to the CPB circuit at the arterial side (high pressure port) and returned to the venous side (low pressure port) to provide a driving force for blood through the membrane.

Hemofilters are used to concentrate blood in order to maintain or increase hematocrit (HCT) levels in the presence of excess fluid and can to a degree help avoid blood transfusion. They may also be used to manage electrolyte or acid/base derangements.

The rate of filtration is dependent on the transmembrane pressure and the surface area of the filter and is typically 30–50 ml/minute. The Sieving coefficient denotes whether a substance will be retained or passed through the membrane to be filtered out. Sieving coefficients are based on molecular weight and the pore size on the filter. Depending on the membrane used, molecules of up to 50,000 Daltons are removed. It is important to note that molecules like heparin or sodium bicarbonate are partially filtered and their level should be monitored when using a hemoconcentrator.

Miniaturized Extracorporeal Circulation (MiECC)

There has been increasing interest in miniaturized bypass circuits. Their aim is to decrease the trauma caused by CPB, mainly through minimizing circuit size, introducing biocompatible surfaces where possible and reducing prime volume to as little as 500 ml. As promising as the concept sounds, it has not yet found its way into mainstream clinical practice. MiECC is discussed in detail in Chapter 8.

Suggested Further Reading

1. Gourlay T. Biomaterial development for cardiopulmonary bypass. *Perfusion*. 2001 September; 16(5): 381–90.

2. Kim WG, Yoon CJ. Roller pump induced tubing wear of polyvinylchloride and silicone rubber tubing: Phase contrast and scanning electron microscopic studies. *Artif Organs*. 1998 October; 22(10): 892–897.

3. Rodney F Patterson, Silicones. in Handbook of Thermoset Plastics (Second Edition), 1998.

4. Denton A Cooley and O H Frazier. The Past 50 Years of Cardiovascular Surgery.

   Circulation. 2000;102: Iv-87–Iv-930

5. Black S, Bolman RM III. C. Walton Lillehei and the birth of open heart surgery. *J Card Surg* 2006; **21**: 205–208.

6. Johagen D, Appelblad M, Svenmarker S. Can the oxygenator screen filter reduce gaseous microemboli? *The Journal of Extra-corporeal Technology* 2014; **46**: 60–66.

7. Saczkowski R, Maklin M, Mesana T, Boodhwani M, Ruel M. Centrifugal pump and roller pump in adult cardiac surgery: A meta-analysis of randomized controlled trials. *Artificial Organs* 2012; **36**: 668–676.

8. Dickinson TA, Riley JB, Crowley JC, Zabetakis PM. In vitro evaluation of the air separation ability of four cardiovascular manufacturer extracorporeal circuit designs. *Journal of Extra Corporeal Technology* 2006; **38**: 206–213.

9. Durandy Y. Vacuum-assisted venous drainage, angel or demon: PRO? *Journal of Extra Corporeal Technology* 2013; **45**: 122–127.

10. Potger KC, McMillan D, Ambrose M. Microbubble generation and transmission of Medtronic's affinity hardshell venous reservoir and collapsible venous reservoir bag: An in-vitro comparison. *Journal of Extra Corporeal Technology* 2011; **43**: 115–122.

Monitoring during Cardiopulmonary Bypass

Richard F Newland and Pascal Starinieri

A fundamental area of responsibility for the perfusionist during cardiopulmonary bypass (CPB) is to monitor, respond to, and document heart lung machine (HLM) parameters as well as physiological variables obtained from the anesthetic monitor and other physiological monitoring devices. The heart lung machine typically provides monitoring of blood flow and circuit pressures (e.g., arterial, cardioplegia), temperatures (e.g., arterial, venous, cardioplegia, oxygenator inflow and outflow), oxygen and air supply and timers (e.g., CPB time, myocardial ischemia, circulatory arrest). Patient physiological parameters are monitored via the anesthetic monitor (e.g., arterial and central venous blood pressure, heart rate and ECG, core body temperature, oxygen saturation, capnography). Blood gas parameters may be monitored using devices that provide continuous measurements and/or intermittently using point of care or laboratory blood gas analyzers. Non-invasive methods may be used for cerebral monitoring, such as regional cerebral tissue oxygenation and electroencephalography (EEG) based depth of anesthesia. Anticoagulation is monitored using point of care devices that measure the activated clotting time. These parameters together with procedural events and CPB interventions should be accurately recorded to provide documentation of the CPB period. CPB monitoring recommendations published in the 2019 EACTS/EACTA/EBCP guidelines on cardiopulmonary bypass in adult cardiac surgery are summarized in Table 3.1. Combined recommendations of the Society of Clinical Perfusion Scientists of Great Britain and Ireland for Standards of Monitoring and Safety during CPB and the American Society of ExtraCorporeal Technology Standards and Guidelines for Perfusion Practice are summarized in Table 3.2.

Heart Lung Machine

The complexity and extreme invasiveness of CPB demands that strict attention is paid to all aspects of extracorporeal flow, with importance placed on providing a safe environment for both the patient and personnel. Technological advancements, together with an increased understanding of the pathophysiological effects of extracorporeal flow, have made the conduct of CPB both safe and reliable. An essential part of this success has been the development of monitoring devices that measure the combination of both physiological and mechanical functions that are unique to CPB.

Blood and Gas Flow

The HLM typically measures systemic blood flow continuously and in real time either via

- the rpm of a roller pump and with knowledge of the tubing size placed through the raceway or
- an ultrasonic flow probe.

Blood flow may also be monitored using continuous blood gas monitoring systems (see below). A measurement of blood flow distal to any circuit shunts is important to provide an accurate understanding of actual blood flow to the patient.

A continuous supply of oxygen and air is delivered to the oxygenator during CPB while some specialist procedures might require adding CO_2 into the gas mix. Modern heart lung machines are equipped with digital flowmeters rather than the older style rotameters. Electronic gas blenders are generally controlled from the HLM work panel, while manual blenders have a ball or cylinder rotameter which is read against a scale and therefore cannot be continuously monitored electronically. Monitoring gas

Table 3.1. Summary of Class I recommendations CPB monitoring parameters from the 2019 EACTS/EACTA/EBCP guidelines

It is recommended that pressure monitoring devices are used on the arterial line and cardioplegia delivery systems during CPB.

A bubble detector is recommended during CPB procedures on all inflow lines.

It is recommended to use a level sensor during CPB procedures utilizing a (hard-shell) reservoir.

Continuous arterial line pressure monitoring (preoxygenator and postoxygenator) in the CPB circuit is recommended.

Continuous oxygenator arterial outlet temperature monitoring is recommended.

It is recommended to continuously monitor SvO2 and HCT levels during CPB.

Monitoring of blood gas analyses through regular intervals or continuous observation is recommended during CPB.

It is recommended to objectively report, adequately record and properly analyse all adverse events related to CPB practice in an efficient and timely manner.

It is recommended that the perfusionist collect data concerning the conduct of perfusion via a clinical registry or database and use such data to actively participate in institutional and departmental quality assurance and improvement programmes.

It is recommended that the venous line pressure be monitored when using assisted venous drainage.

Table 3.2. Recommended extracorporeal circuit parameters for Standards of Monitoring and Safety during CPB by the Society of Clinical Perfusion Scientists of Great Britain and Ireland and the American Society of ExtraCorporeal Technology Standards and Guidelines for Perfusion Practice.

Oxygen saturation of the blood in the arterial line

Oxygen saturation of the blood in the venous return line

The flow of the blood to the patient (best measured after shunt lines with a separate flow meter)

Arterial line pressure (preferably before AND after the oxygenator)

Gas flow and oxygen fraction to the oxygenator

Venous occlusion percentage

Oxygen concentration in the gas to the oxygenator

Level sensor during CPB procedures utilizing (hard-shell) reservoir

Cardioplegia dose, delivery method, line pressure (antegrade), coronary sinus pressure (retrograde), and ischemic intervals

Blood temperature at the arterial outlet and venous inlet of the oxygenator

Water temperature in the heater-cooler system

Anticoagulation – Activated Clotting Time (ACT)

Arterial blood gases (regularly or continuously) containing the following measurements:

pH

pCO_2

pO_2

SaO_2

HCO_3

Base excess

Haemoglobin (Hb)

Haematocrit (HCT)

Potassium

Sodium

Glucose (or other point-of-care device)

Lactate

supply and exchange, together with an oxygen analyzer to display the O_2 concentration delivered at any point in time, is mandatory. Volatile anesthetics may also be used via the heart lung machine gas delivery system during CPB to maintain anesthesia and/or as an adjunct to blood pressure control. A scavenging system for waste anesthetic gases is recommended as being mandatory in many countries, as volatile anesthetic agent waste is a risk to staff. The end-tidal anesthetic gas concentration can be monitored at the oxygenator exhaust port.

Temperature

The purpose of using hypothermia is to provide a degree of organ protection and safety margin during cardiopulmonary bypass. As a general rule, metabolic rate and oxygen consumption reduce by 50% for every 7°C of temperature drop.

Core temperature monitoring sites include naso-pharynx, tympanic membrane, bladder, esophagus, rectum, pulmonary artery, jugular bulb, arterial inflow, and venous return. Nasopharyngeal, jugular bulb and arterial inflow temperature give an estimate of cerebral temperature. Due to its invasive nature and cumbersome placement, jugular bulb probes are rarely used and the oxygenator arterial outlet blood temperature is recommended as the surrogate for cerebral temperature. Oxygenator inlet and outlet temperatures are measured using thermistors. Monitoring the temperature of the arterial blood delivered to the body and of venous return blood helps to protect sensitive organs such as the brain and to confirm adequacy of cooling and rewarming.

A temperature gradient of less than 10°C between arterial outlet and venous inlet is recommended during cooling to avoid cerebral injury, generation of gaseous emboli or outgassing when blood is returned to the patient. Maintaining a low gradient between inflow and outflow temperature is equally important during rewarming from hypothermia as a fast temperature rise is associated with poor neurological outcomes. The perfusate temperature to the body should not exceed 37°C.

The measurement accuracy of the thermistors is affected by their immersion depth. The recommendations with regard to temperature monitoring during CPB published in the 2015 STS/SCA/AMSECT Clinical Practice Guidelines are summarized in Table 3.3.

Pressure

Adequate blood pressure is one of the factors necessary for adequate perfusion of vital organs. It is generally agreed that in most cases a mean systemic arterial pressure (MAP) of 50–80 mmHg provides sufficient end-organ perfusion while cerebral autoregulation is preserved.

Circuit pressures are monitored primarily for safety reasons, in order to avoid over-pressurization and the potential for circuit disconnection, cannula dislodgement or vascular and tissue injury. Monitoring of circuit line pressure can also provide an indication of adequate positioning of cannulae, in particular ensuring that the aortic cannula is correctly positioned to avoid dissection. Both pre- and post-oxygenator monitoring is recommended to detect changes in transmembrane pressure, as rises may indicate platelet deposition/aggregation within the oxygenator. Cardioplegia line pressure monitoring may avoid injury to the coronary

Table 3.3. 2015 STS/SCA/AmSect Clinical Practice Guidelines on temperature monitoring during CPB

CLASS I RECOMMENDATIONS

The oxygenator arterial outlet blood temperature is recommended to be utilized as a surrogate for cerebral temperature measurement during CPB. (Class I, Level C)

To monitor cerebral perfusate temperature during warming, it should be assumed that the oxygenator arterial outlet blood temperature under-estimates cerebral perfusate temperature. (Class I, Level C)

Surgical teams should limit arterial outlet blood temperature to <37°C to avoid cerebral hyperthermia. (Class 1, Level C)

Temperature gradients between the arterial outlet and venous inflow on the oxygenator during CPB cooling should not exceed 10°C to avoid generation of gaseous emboli. (Class 1, Level C)

CLASS IIa RECOMMENDATIONS

Pulmonary artery or nasopharyngeal temperature recording is reasonable for weaning and immediate post-bypass temperature measurement. (Class IIa, Level C)

Rewarming when arterial blood outlet temperature ≥30°C:
i. To achieve the desired temperature for separation from bypass, it is reasonable to maintain a temperature gradient between arterial outlet temperature and the venous inflow of ≤4°C. (Class IIa, Level B)
ii. To achieve the desired temperature for separation from bypass, it is reasonable to maintain a rewarming rate of ≤0.5°C/min. (Class IIa, Level B)

Rewarming when arterial blood outlet temperature <30°C: To achieve the desired temperature for separation from bypass, it is reasonable to maintain a maximal gradient of 10°C between arterial outlet temperature and venous inflow. (Class IIa, Level C)

vasculature, coronary ostia or coronary sinus, depending on the route of delivery. The most commonly used mode of giving cardioplegia is antegrade, directly into the aortic root proximal to the aortic cross-clamp or into the coronary ostia at a line pressure of 80–150 mmHg. Retrograde cardioplegia is administered via a catheter in the coronary sinus, using a flow of 200–400 ml/min to a coronary sinus pressure of between 30 and 80 mmHg.

Servo regulation of pump flow rate coupled to pressure limits is an important safety feature of the

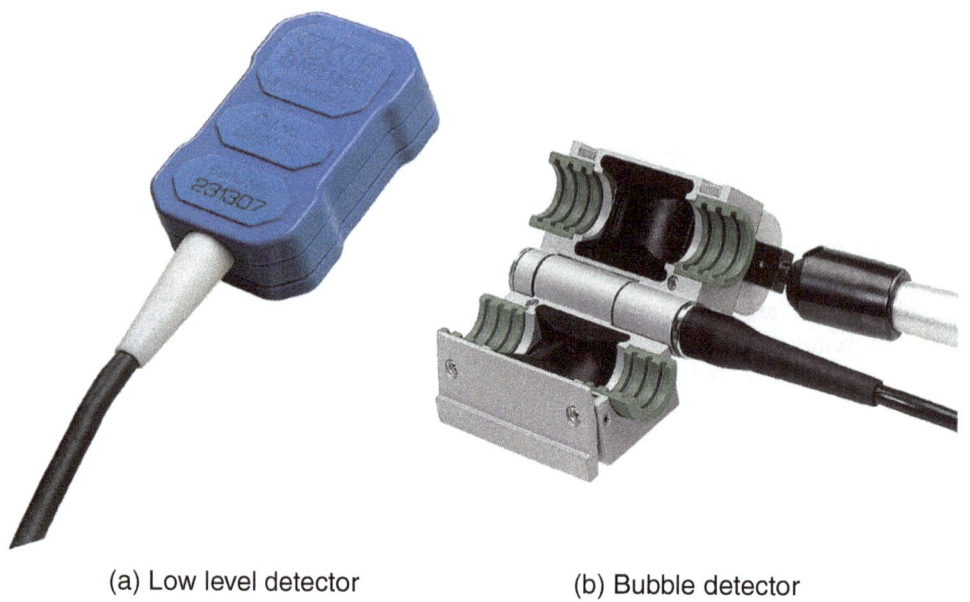

(a) Low level detector   (b) Bubble detector

Figure 3.1 Detectors for low reservoir blood level (a) and air emboli (b). (Livanova, UK.)

HLM. The higher limit has to be set in a way that stops the pump causing injury at the cannulation site, generally at <250 mmHg. Cardioplegia pressure is typically limited at lower pressures, depending on the route of delivery (<150 mmHg antegrade and <80 mmHg retrograde).

The negative pressure inside the venous reservoir is monitored when either vacuum-assisted venous drainage (VAVD) or kinetic-assisted venous drainage (KAVD) is used. The vacuum is typically adjusted in a way that the negative pressure does not exceed 30mmHg in order to reduce hemolysis and the risk of air entrainment into the venous line or across the membrane oxygenator. The latter can potentially lead to serious harm to the patient through gaseous arterial micro emboli or massive arterial embolization. Negative pressure in the venous line during kinetic-assisted venous drainage should not exceed –80 mmHg to avoid cavitation and hemolysis. Other circuit pressures monitored may include antegrade or retrograde cerebral perfusion with servo regulation limits around 150 mmHg for antegrade and 80 mmHg retrograde.

Circuit pressures are usually monitored using reusable electronic transducers, where the fluid is isolated from the transducer by a dedicated disposable circuit component.

Low Level and Air Bubble Detection

Heart lung machines have alarm systems embedded within monitoring on the display panel of the HLM. Alarms either provide an audible and/or visual indication to the perfusionist or, more critically, can adjust or entirely stop pump flow if necessary when servo-regulated. Checking alarm levels and functionality is part of the pre CPB checklist; alarms must be engaged prior to the initiation of CPB.

The low level alarm is a critical safety feature on the HLM. A sensor on the venous reservoir is placed at a level below which there is the danger of emptying the reservoir and entraining air into the arterial circulation (see Figure 3.1a). If triggered, the servo regulation will stop or significantly reduce the flow rate of the arterial pump in addition to sounding an acoustic alarm. The pump will only resume flow once the fluid level is above the sensor again. Ultrasonic air bubble detectors on the arterial side of the HLM operate in the same way to protect against gross air embolism (see Figure 3.1b). Both alarm systems received a Class I recommendation in the 2019 EACTS/EACTA/EBCP guidelines.

Bubble detectors may also be used in the cardioplegia line, and the venous line in minimized CPB circuits. Although contemporary equipment, technology, and perfusion techniques have reduced the potential for massive air embolism, arterial gaseous microemboli still remain a concern. Integrated air bubble detectors can provide quantification of microbubbles during CPB, yet the values they report have been found to be less reliable than those generated by specifically designed microemboli detectors. This suggests that that microbubble counts from air bubble detectors integrated in the circuit should not be reported. However, any events where the low level and/or air bubble alarms have been triggered should be included in the perfusion record.

Calibration of Heart Lung Machine Monitoring Systems

All monitors and alarms used should be calibrated and maintained regularly according to the manufacturer's instructions and the recommended service schedule. All equipment must be checked before use (see Chapter 4 for more detail).

Gas Exchange

The primary function of the respiratory system is to take in oxygen and eliminate carbon dioxide. Inhaled oxygen enters the lungs and reaches the alveoli where it passes through the air-blood barrier and into the blood in the capillaries. Similarly, carbon dioxide passes from the blood into the alveoli and is then exhaled. Oxygenators on the HLM function using exactly the same principle.

In-line Blood Gas Analysis, Venous Saturation and Hematocrit Monitors

The theoretical advantages of using continuous in-line blood gas and electrolyte monitoring during CPB are well established; however, the clinical impact remains controversial. The available devices may be divided into those using electrochemical electrodes and cuvettes, which are placed in the circuit, and those that use light absorbance or reflectance, which require sensors placed external to the circuit tubing.

The Terumo CDI550 in-line blood gas analyzer (Terumo Cardiovascular Systems Corp., Ann Arbor, MI) is an optical fluorescence and reflectance based in-line system that continuously monitors 12 key blood gas parameters. Fluorescence sensors measure pH, pCO_2, pO_2 on both the arterial and the venous

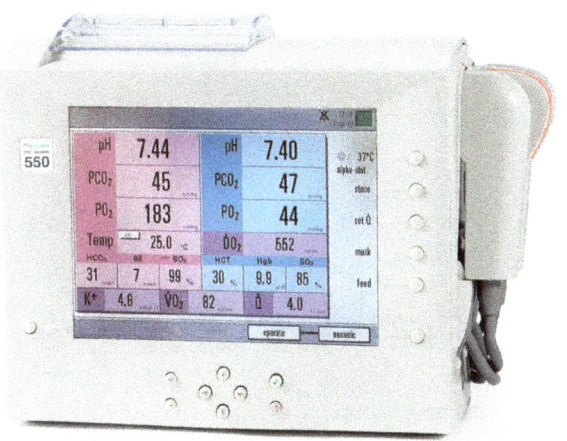

Figure 3.2 Terumo CDI550 in-line blood gas analyzer. (Terumo Cardiovascular Systems Corp., Ann Arbor, MI.)

limb and HCO_3 and K+ using direct blood contact, while SO_2, Hct and Hb are measured using optical reflectance (see Figure 3.2). The cost of the disposable sensors associated with this technology has led to the CDI technology not always being routinely adopted. In some centers it is used for complex or prolonged cases – such as when blood gas management strategy is changed from α-stat to pH-stat during cooling or rewarming in procedures involving deep hypothermic circulatory arrest (DHCA).

The System M (Spectrum Medical, Gloucester, UK) is an example of a diagnostic monitor which provides continuous non-invasive measurement of blood gases (pCO_2, pO_2), SO_2, flow and bubble/emboli detection and ventilation parameters (sweep, oxygenator inlet O_2 and outlet CO_2) as well as Hb, however no electrolyte measurements are provided. The reusable sensors are attached to the circuit, negating the requirement of ongoing disposable costs (see Figure 3.3).

The 95% limits of agreement both devices have with laboratory or point of care blood gas analysis do not allow complete substitution and they should be considered as trending devices only. The few randomized studies that have evaluated the efficacy of these devices found that they lead to improved adherence to institutional perfusion protocols, which did not translate into improved patient outcomes.

More basic forms of in-line monitoring, using absorbance or reflectance of infrared light signals, are commonly used to continuously monitor venous and arterial blood oxygen saturations during CPB.

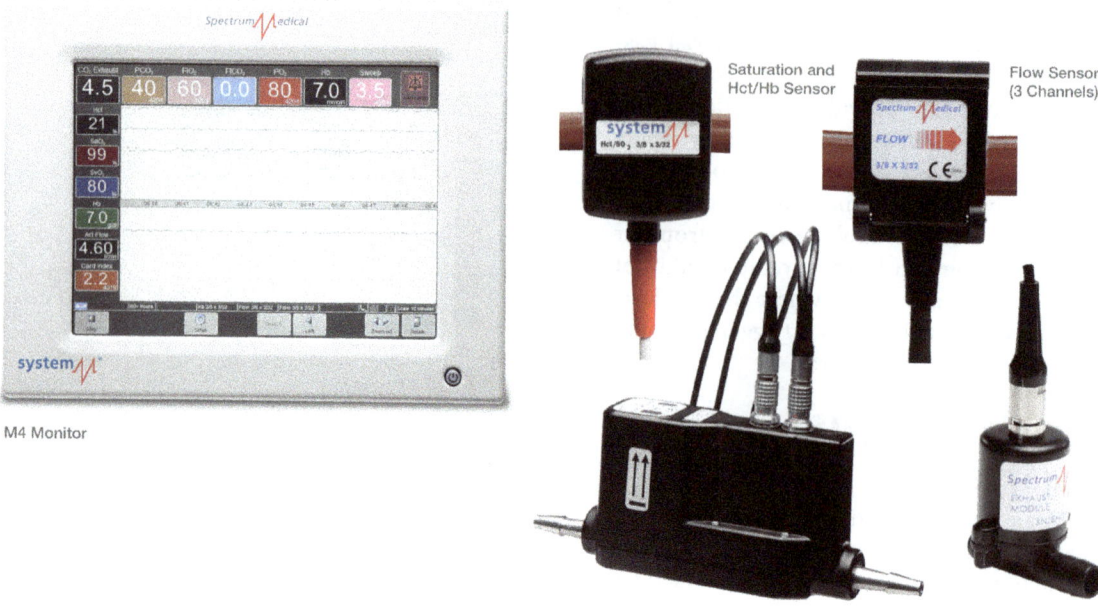

Figure 3.3 M4 monitor. (Spectrum Medical, UK.)

Similar to the more advanced devices above, they lack in accuracy but are valuable tools for observing and recording trends.

As a minimum, it is recommended to continuously monitor SvO_2 and Hct and perform full blood gas analyses at regular intervals throughout the duration of CPB (Class I recommendation, 2019 EACTS/EACTA/EBCP guidelines).

Cerebral Oxygen Saturation

Adverse cerebral outcomes after cardiac surgery are associated with increased mortality, prolonged ICU and hospital stay and the use of additional healthcare resources. Continuous monitoring of cerebral oxygen saturation may provide a tool to detect an imbalance between cerebral oxygen demand and supply and may decrease the likelihood of intraoperative cerebral injury.

Near-infrared spectroscopy (NIRS) can be used to monitor cerebral oxygen saturation during cardiac surgery. Self-adhesive sensors containing the infrared light source and detectors are placed on one or both sides of the forehead. Cerebral desaturation is defined as a 20% reduction from baseline values or an absolute decrease below 50% taking the duration of desaturation into account.

The evidence regarding its clinical benefit is however contradictory. Although early studies showed improved neurocognitive function in patients undergoing NIRS based algorithms to improve oxygen supply/demand ratio, recent randomized trials and a recently published meta-analysis and systematic review showed no clinical benefit. Cerebral saturation monitoring is discussed in more detail in Chapter 18 and its clinical application in Chapter 9.

Oxygen Delivery and Carbon Dioxide Extraction

Oxygen delivery (DO_2) is determined by hemoglobin, arterial blood flow, oxygen saturation and PaO_2. Many current HLM monitors are able to continuously calculate and display DO_2 during CPB. Alternatively it can be calculated manually from reference charts. Evidence from a randomized trial and multicenter registry data shows that a goal-directed perfusion strategy to maintain oxygen delivery index (DO_2i) during CPB > 280 mL/min/m^2 reduces the incidence of acute kidney injury following cardiac surgery.

Anticoagulation Monitoring

Systemic heparinization is required for CPB to avoid coagulation due to contact activation and stasis in the reservoir or the operating field. Safe anticoagulation is ascertained by measuring the activated clotting time (ACT), which is generally done in the operating theater. The ACT is a highly unspecific whole blood coagulation assay and is influenced by factors such as temperature, hematocrit, fibrinogen level and platelet count or function. The majority of centers around the world target ACT values between 450 and 550 seconds. The ACT is typically measured every 20–30 minutes and recorded in the perfusion record.

The 2018 STS/SCA/AMSECT Clinical Practice Guidelines recommend as Class 1 evidence that *"a functional whole blood test of anticoagulation, in the form of a clotting time, should be measured and should demonstrate adequate anticoagulation before initiation of, and at regular intervals during cardiopulmonary bypass. (Level of Evidence C)"*

Furthermore, a Class IIa recommendation in the same publication states *"it is reasonable to maintain activated clotting time above 480 seconds during CPB. However, this minimum threshold value is an approximation and may vary based upon the bias of the instrument being used. For instruments using 'maximal activation' of whole blood or microcuvette technology, values above 400 seconds are frequently considered therapeutic. (Level of Evidence C)"*

It is important to note that ACT devices from different manufacturers must not be used interchangeably. Anticoagulation during cardiopulmonary bypass is discussed in detail in Chapter 6.

Hemodynamic Monitoring

Assessment of myocardial function is important both pre CPB and during separation from CPB. Hemodynamic monitoring includes the electrocardiogram (ECG), pulmonary artery catheter (PAC) and transesophageal echocardiography (TEE).

Electrocardiogram – ECG monitoring is one of the minimum monitoring requirements during anesthesia. Although native cardiac function is unnecessary during CPB, the ECG can provide important clues to

- efficacy of initial cardioplegia delivery by broadening QRS complexes and the appearance of towering T waves,
- adequacy of myocardial protection by showing signs of electrical activity,
- early signs of ischemia (ST segment changes or ventricular tachyarrhythmias) after cross-clamp removal or before weaning off CPB and

- need for temporary atrial or ventricular pacing.

Pulmonary artery catheter – although not used routinely in many parts of the world, the PAC may be used to provide assessments of cardiac output and pulmonary artery pressure, which may help guide inotropic support during separation from CPB.

Transesophageal echocardiography – TEE is widely used in cardiac surgery. Recent guidelines by the American Society of Anesthesiologists and the Society of Cardiovascular Anesthesiologists recommend that, in the absence of contraindications, intraoperative TEE be performed in all cardiac valve and thoracic aortic procedures (Class 1) and is reasonable for CABG operations (Class IIa). The advantages in the use of TEE prior to CPB include

- confirming the preoperative diagnosis,
- detecting undiagnosed pathologies,
- confirming the success of surgical intervention, particularly in valve repairs and replacements,
- confirming appropriate de-airing after open chamber surgery and
- guiding inotrope management by continuous assessment of left and right ventricular function.

Documentation of Intraoperative Monitoring Data: The Cardiopulmonary Bypass Record

The CPB or perfusion record is a legal record and should therefore be accurate and legible. Historically, the perfusion record had been handwritten, with the perfusionist documenting physiological parameters and heart lung machine values. Typically, this happened every 5–10 minutes, when changes occurred or when events or interventions (e.g., drug administration) required documentation. A manual record will always be a snapshot of what occurs during bypass and may be incomplete or inaccurate, with errors able to be introduced in a number of ways. These inadequacies include missing data, biased recording, transcription error and subjectivity of observation. There are a number of systems that are able to generate an electronic record with the aid of data collection software. They provide automatic data acquisition and integrate data from the HLM and other monitoring systems in the operating room, most importantly the anesthetic, hemodynamic monitoring (Figure 3.4). As the number of monitors

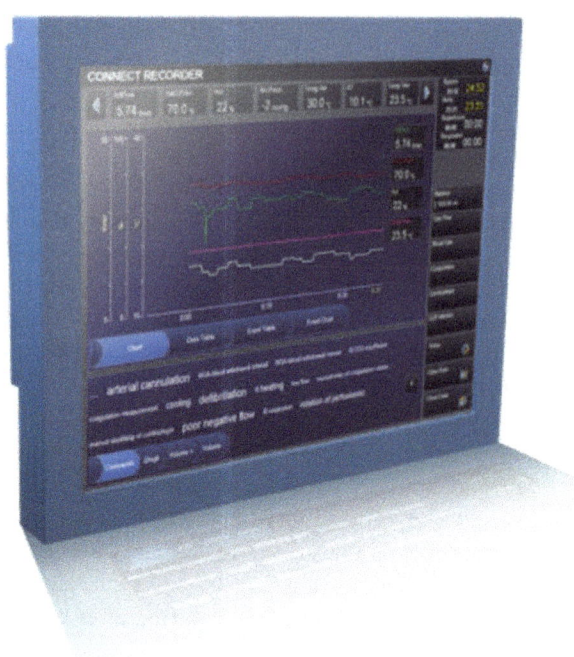

(a) Connect Datapad

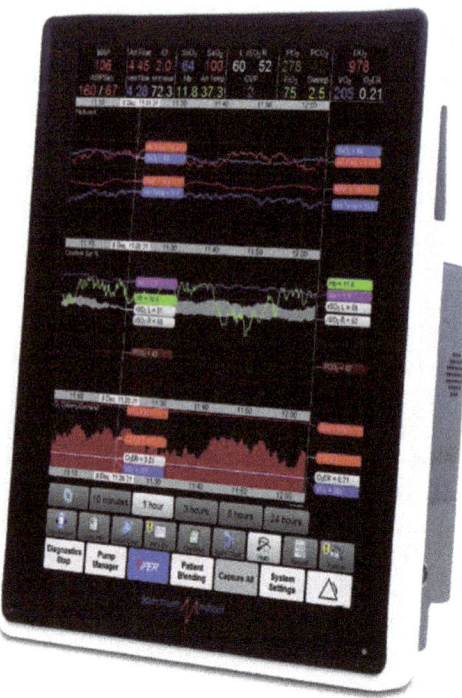

(b) Quantum Workstation

Figure 3.4 Examples of automatic data acquisition and monitoring systems for cardiopulmonary bypass; (a) Connect Datapad (Livanova, UK), (b) Quantum Workstation. (Spectrum Medical, UK.)

in the operating room increases, the operating team needs to observe, record, and respond to more and more data. Where this is recorded automatically, the perfusionist and the anesthesiologist are less distracted and more able to concentrate on the patient rather than on documenting the procedure. The integrity of the data from automatic data acquisition removes the bias that is inherent in the manual record.

Apart from creating a record of the patient and heart lung machine physiological parameters, these products provide documentation of CPB equipment, priming solutions, fluid balance, coagulation and blood gas values, cardioplegia and drug administration. Electronic perfusion data collection, including the ability to produce a printout, is a general recommendation of the Society of Clinical Perfusion

Scientists of Great Britain and Ireland for Standards of Monitoring and Safety during CPB and is a Class IIa recommendation in the 2019 EACTS/EACTA/EBCP guidelines. Comprehensive records also provide individual departments with the ability to define CPB quality metrics based on institutional guidelines.

Application of Electronic Perfusion Data

Generating an accurate perfusion record is only one component of the value that can be gained from automated electronic perfusion data collection systems. The data provide an enormous resource for ongoing research activities and quality management. The importance and benefits of quality assurance and quality improvement in healthcare delivery are well recognized. The collected data can be used to monitor and improve quality of care processes and to report practices at an individual or institutional level, or to facilitate multicenter reporting through participation in a CPB registry.

Registry

Some examples of CPB registries include the Northern New England Cardiovascular Disease Study Group, the Australian and New Zealand Collaborative Perfusion Registry (ANZCPR) and the PERFORM registry (USA), which is an integral part of the Michigan Society of Thoracic and Cardiovascular Surgeon Quality Collaborative's program. Electronic data collection meets the needs of registry endeavors because it provides a method of transferring de-identified data from multiple sites, integration of this data into a central database, and a means to generate calculated CPB parameters and perform complex data analysis. The ANZCPR has a defined process of core metrics and uses these to calculate benchmarks for the management of blood glucose, arterial outlet temperature, and blood gas management during CPB utilizing electronic data. These benchmarks provide a baseline for the implementation of multicenter continuous quality improvement processes for perfusion practice. By examining CPB data and related outcomes, registries have been able to define risk factors associated with adverse outcomes.

One of the problems inherent in determining relationships between CPB parameters and the clinical measures of outcomes is the low rate of adverse events, resulting in the requirement of large cohorts to achieve adequate and statistically well powered studies. Amalgamation of collected data provides a means to increase cohort size and therefore reduce the confounding effects of variations in patient risk factors and practice changes over time. Registry data also play an important role in confirming the generalizability of results of clinical studies and in recommending them for implementation into clinical practice.

Suggested Further Reading

1. Puis L, Milojevic M, Boer C et al. 2019. 2019 EACTS/EACTA/EBCP Guidelines on cardiopulmonary bypass in adult cardiac surgery. *Interact Cardiovasc Thorac Surg.* February 1, 2020;30(2):161–202.

2. Recommendations for Standards of Monitoring during Cardiopulmonary Bypass. The Society of Clinical Perfusion Scientists of Great Britain and Ireland, Association of Cardiothoracic Anaesthetists, Society for Cardiothoracic Surgery in Great Britain and Ireland, August 2016.

3. Report from AmSECT's International Consortium for Evidence-Based Perfusion: American Society of ExtraCorporeal Technology Standards and Guidelines for Perfusion Practice: 2013. Baker RA, Bronson SL, Dickinson TA et al, on behalf of the International Consortium for Evidence-Based Perfusion for the American Society of ExtraCorporeal Technology. JECT. 2013;45:156–166.

4. Engelman, R, Baker, RA, Likosky DS et al. The Society of Thoracic Surgeons, The Society of Cardiovascular Anesthesiologists, and The American Society of ExtraCorporeal Technology: Clinical practice guidelines for cardiopulmonary bypass – Temperature management during cardiopulmonary bypass. JECT. 2015;47:145–154.

5. Shore-Lesserson L, Baker RA, Ferraris V et al. STS/SCA/AmSECT Clinical practice guidelines: Anticoagulation during cardiopulmonary bypass. *J Extra Corpor Technol.* 2018;50:1–14.

6. Ranucci M, Johnson I, Willcox T et al. Goal-directed perfusion to reduce acute kidney injury: A randomized trial. *J Thorac Cardiovasc Surg.* November, 2018;156(5):1918–1927.

7. Newland RF, Baker RA, Woodman RJ et al. Australian and New Zealand Collaborative Perfusion Registry. Predictive capacity of oxygen delivery during cardiopulmonary bypass on acute kidney injury. *Ann Thorac Surg.* June 22, 2019.

8. Ottens J, Tuble SC, Sanderson AJ et al. Improving cardiopulmonary bypass: Does continuous blood gas monitoring have a role to play? *J Extra Corpor Technol.* September, 2010;42(3):191–198.

Chapter

4

Cardiopulmonary Bypass Circuit Setup and Safety Checks

Victoria Molyneux and Shahna Helmick

Introduction

Assembling the cardiopulmonary bypass (CPB) circuit and checking the heart lung machine (HLM) for faults prior to clinical use is an essential and integral part of the provision of clinical perfusion. This chapter describes the procedure for setting up the extracorporeal circuit and the safety checks that should be undertaken before embarking on a case.

The evolution of CPB has been marked on one side by sophistication and complexity and on the other side by an increased requirement for safety. The death of a pediatric cardiac surgical patient and the subsequent Gritten Report of 2007 marked a turning point for perfusion safety. This led to the implementation of minimum standards and practice recommendations within the United Kingdom. The medical communities in many countries have issued recommendations concerning the training of clinical perfusionists and the use of monitoring and safety devices for CPB. Although studies have not established a cause-to-effect relationship, the decrease in CPB-related mortality may be partly attributed to these measures. Vigilance is paramount to the safety of CPB. Modern perfusion systems are designed to optimize safety. Technological advances have seen the incorporation of automatic, servo-regulated alarms and fail-safe devices; however, the clinical perfusionist's attention to detail, as well as performance of pre-CPB checklists and protocols, underpins safe practice. Investigations around the world have repeatedly pointed to medical errors that could have been prevented as an important cause of morbidity and mortality; human error is a far greater cause of accidents than mechanical mishap.

Preparing the CPB circuit and HLM, attending to the patient's clinical details and to the surgical requirements for the procedure all form part of the process of safe provision of CPB. By necessity, the preparation of the HLM and assembly of the CPB circuit components should ritualistically follow a routine dictated by institutional protocols and the process confirmed by following a recognized, institutionally agreed pre-CPB checklist.

CPB Machine Preparation and Setup

CPB Components

Cardiopulmonary bypass circuits are comprised of a number of disposable components supported by the HLM. We consider four essential elements of the CPB system that remain the same, despite different manufacturers and different component designs. Principally these are as follows:

- Membrane oxygenator and venous reservoir
- Cardioplegia system
- Custom tubing pack
- Arterial line filter (unless integrated in oxygenator/reservoir).

CPB Setup

These components can be assembled in a myriad of configurations, depending on institutional and clinician preference and specific patient requirements. Although there is no universally agreed or commonly used sequence for setting up and priming a standard CPB system, the following list provides a general routine to ensure a safe setup:

- All components are checked for sterility, cleanliness, integrity, and expiration date.
- The heat exchanger on both the oxygenator and the cardioplegia delivery system (if present) must be leak-tested either upon opening the sterile packaging or once the CPB circuit has been set up but prior to the initiation of priming. In practice this is usually done once the CPB circuit has been set up dry. The integrity of the heat exchanger may be tested using a pressure occlusion device

and ensuring there is no pressure drop once set to 250 mmHg or by attaching the water lines to the heat exchanger and leaving them to run for 10 minutes prior to priming. This ensures that the barrier between the blood side and the water side of the devices is intact.

- Occlusions are set on the main arterial roller pump, the suction pumps, and the cardioplegia pumps. Pump occlusions may be set using one of two methods: pressure drop or fluid drop. Many institutional protocols state that pumps should be set to fully occlusive at 240 mmHg. "Fully occlusive" is defined as a pressure fall of no more than 1mmHg per minute. Alternatively, the occlusion may be set using the fluid method – HLM manufacturer Sorin recommends adjusting the occlusion to a one-inch fall per minute in a 30-inch column of fluid. Suction occlusion, direction and function of pressure relief valves are all checked prior to the initiation of CPB.

- Speed controls and pump direction are checked to be operational and correct. The flow rates and tubing size calibrations are set for each individual case and the rollers on the pumps are checked to make sure that they rotate freely. The pump head rotation should be smooth and quiet, and servo-regulated connections should be tested prior to the initiation of CPB.

- Electrical power cord connections are checked to be secure, and HLM batteries are checked to ensure that they are fully charged and operational. It is essential that the HLM is connected to an uninterrupted power supply (UPS) in the operating room. The HLM should be temporarily disconnected from the power source, ascertaining the power failure alarm and battery backup unit are all functional.

- Oxygen and air gas lines are secured to the gas source and checked for functionality.

- A gas scavenging system may be used, either directly as part of the CPB circuit or as a wider operating room air flow management system. Scavenging is mandatory in the majority of countries if a volatile anesthetic vaporizer is part of the HLM. The gas exhaust from the oxygenator has to be unobstructed.

- The integrated oxygenator and venous reservoir is placed on its secure holder and oriented in a way that allows the perfusionist to have it in full view

for the duration of the procedure. The gas line, the oxygen/air blender, and the exhaust scavenging system (where used) are attached to the appropriate ports on the base of the oxygenator. Ensuring safe attachment of all connections is essential. Tubing should be pushed over the connector to at least the second barb. The sampling port manifold is positioned with taps secured. The arterial line tubing is then put in place and connected to the venous reservoir outlet and oxygenator inlet. Many providers now supply fully preconnected circuits. When using these it is essential to visually check that the entire circuit has been assembled in the correct order. Similarly, if "quick-connect" fittings are used anywhere in the circuit, their integrity must be checked.

- The cardioplegia circuit is usually positioned on the HLM. A number of different configurations are in common use:

  1. The cardioplegia pump may accommodate two segments of tubing with varying diameters within it so that blood and cardioplegia solution mix in the desired ratio – for example, a 4:1 blood to high-strength cardioplegia solution when using Harefield or St. Thomas' solution or 1:4 when using Del Nido cardioplegia.

  2. The cardioplegia system may comprise of two separate mini pumps that may be used to independently deliver the mix of blood and high strength cardioplegia in the desired ratio.

  3. The microplegia technique delivers blood and additives for cardioplegia with minimal crystalloid. A number of external devices – such as the Quest MPS2 – offer specific, variable cardioplegia delivery, allowing different ratios (4:1, 8:1, 1:4) or extended arrest protocols with a single dose strategy.

- The arteriovenous (AV) loop is connected to the venous reservoir inlet and oxygenator outlet. The arterial line filter, arterial line pressure transducer and the arterial line bubble detector are all attached to the arterial line tubing. The bubble detector and the pressure transducer are both coupled to the HLM and are servo-regulated. This ensures that if air is detected in the arterial line, or the pressure exceeds preset limits, an alarmed automatic cutout facility is activated. Once handed out onto the operating table, the surgeon will divide the AV loop prior to aortic cannulation and connect the respective ends to the arterial and venous cannulas.

- Suction and venting tubing should be color coded to aid communication between the surgeon and the perfusionist during setting up for the procedure. They are fixed into the various roller head pump assemblies. To ensure that they are in the right orientation, suckers and vents should be water tested by the perfusionist and the scrub nurse prior to the initiation of CPB. This water test was introduced as a mandatory minimum standard in the United Kingdom in 2016 to ensure that the suction tubing has been placed in the pump head in the correct orientation and that there is no chance of blowing air into the heart instead of sucking air or blood into the venous reservoir. Alternatively, checklists to ensure the safety of suction and venting tubing are used in some jurisdictions to ensure safety. These tests need to be completed prior to the initiation of CPB.
- The CPB circuit may be flushed with carbon dioxide (CO_2) prior to priming. CO_2 is nearly 30 times more soluble in blood than nitrogen and flushing the dry circuit is thought to decrease the number of gaseous emboli compared to a conventional circuit once primed. At present, this is not a universally accepted practice and is subject to institutional preference. If a standalone arterial line filter is being utilized, this filter should now be clamped off and isolated; the arterial line should also be clamped if there is a recirculation shunt line distal to the arterial line filter. This step is not required if an integrated arterial line filter is being utilized (as is more commonplace nowadays).

This is the final stage of setting up the CPB circuit, after which the perfusionist can move onto the priming stage.

CPB Priming

The method for priming varies according to institutional protocol. Different centers use different fluids, different volumes, and different drug combinations based on their institutional preferences (see also Chapter 5 for more detail).

Pre-bypass filtration is considered mandatory for contemporary perfusion practice. Filtration of crystalloid CPB priming solutions with a pre-bypass filter with a pore size of 0.2 micron has been found to effectively reduce the number of microemboli and endotoxin contamination that may potentially occur in infusion solutions. The prime volume is added to the venous reservoir. The main arterial pump is roughly occluded before turning it on. The perfusionist observes the filling of the pump tubing, the oxygenator, and any ancillary lines. These must be closed or clamped after priming while fluid is recirculated via the arterial recirculation line back into the venous reservoir. The arterial pressure dome – or monitor isolator – is primed and secured to the arterial pressure line transducer. The arterial line filter is primed according to the manufacturer's instructions, and its bypass line is clamped. The main recirculation line can then be clamped and priming fluid diverted through the AV loop. Once the loop is filled, the pump can be left recirculating and the tubing inspected for air bubbles. Once the main circuit has been primed, the cardioplegia circuit is primed. The occlusions on the main arterial pump, cardioplegia pumps, and the suction pumps can be set, and tubing direction should also be checked at this point. Institutional protocol will determine whether the pump is left to recirculate or whether it is stopped, and the circuit is left pressurized prior to initiation of CPB. Both methods are safe and acceptable practice.

Centrifugal pumps are often used in adult practice. These pumps are non-occlusive and should be gravity filled to ensure that they are fully de-aired. Centrifugal pump consoles have integrated flow probes and are unidirectional. As they are afterload sensitive, pump speed must be set to produce forward flow before initiating CPB. A one-way valve or an electronic, servo-regulated clamp can be placed in the circuit to prevent retrograde flow.

Final monitoring checks should be undertaken once circuit setup and priming have been completed. Arterial and venous circuit temperature probes should be in place, and pressure transducers should be calibrated and set to appropriate scales. The fluid-level sensor of the reservoir has to be set at an appropriate level for the case being undertaken. This is generally determined by the flow as predicted by the patient's cardiac index and the manufacturer's instructions for use. The oxygen analyzer should also be calibrated and operational. Backup equipment, including hand cranks, duplicate components, emergency lighting, an oxygen cylinder, and ice, should be available for the duration of the procedure. Drugs should be drawn up, in conjunction with the Drugs and Fluid Treaty and any Patient Specific Directions, and properly labeled. At this point all alarms must be operational, audible and engaged, and all parameters should now be set in preparation for the initiating CPB. The final setup checklist should be completed at this time.

Human Factors

Healthcare will always involve risks, particularly when very complex systems and procedures are involved. In 2012, the UK National Patient Safety Agency estimated that around 10% of patients admitted to National Health Service (NHS) hospitals had experienced a patient safety incident and up to half of those incidents could have been prevented, providing a similar message to the earlier US Institute of Medicine report "To Err is Human: Building a Safer Health System."

The practice of cardiac surgery demands daily interface with sophisticated technologies including the HLM. For many decades the safety checklist concept has been an integral part of industries facing high-complexity tasks. Aviation has been at the forefront of utilization of the safety checklist, and the understanding of the importance of human factor effects on safety.

The evolution of CPB over the past half-century has mostly been characterized by modifications of component parts. Investigating human factors in cardiac surgery in general and perfusion in particular has been a relatively recent addition to the quest for safety (see Chapter 1 for more detail).

In 2007, in response to the investigation of a fatal pump-related incident in the United Kingdom, the NHS published the Gritten Report. The report presented an independent review of current perfusion practice in the United Kingdom and identified the system-wide failure of perfusion as a profession to take adequate safety precautions. Gritten highlighted a series of events that led to the death of a pediatric cardiac surgery patient. The report concluded that the incident was caused by inadvertent human error, perfusion systems failures at national and local levels and local system problems. The Society of Clinical Perfusion Scientists of Great Britain and Ireland responded to the Gritten Report by adopting a new code of practice and instructing their member organizations to place the highest priority on perfusion safety. This was to be the biggest shake-up of perfusion minimum standards and recommendations in recent years. Perfusion communities throughout the world have responded by either initiating the development of standards of practice or, as the American Society of Extracorporeal Technology (AmSECT) has done, revising and continuously updating their Standards and Guidelines to ensure they remain contemporary.

The Pre-CPB Checklist

The World Health Organization (WHO) developed and evaluated a simple checklist in 2007, which has formed the basis for several iterations specific to cardiac surgery. Figure 4.1 shows a typical example of a cardiac surgical safety checklist. The introduction of this extra step has dropped the rate of major inpatient complications from 11% to 7% and that of the inpatient death following major operations from 1.5% to 0.8%.

Specialist checklists are likely to reduce morbidity and mortality more effectively than the available generic general surgical checklists. This idea is represented in the cardiac surgical safety checklist with regard to perfusion. The time-out phase states that "there should be a perfusionist check and briefing to ensure that the perfusionist is fully aware of the plan for CPB or any special requirements that are needed." Perfusion strategies including patient specific target cooling temperature, cannulation technique and size and special equipment are all discussed as part of the cardiac surgical safety checklist at the multidisciplinary preoperative briefing.

The UK Department of Health states that there should be a clear requirement to check each component of the CPB circuit before its operation and that a standard checklist is signed off by the perfusionist. The format of the checklist may be handwritten or part of the electronic patient records. Double checking of the CPB circuitry by two perfusionists has in many institutions become minimum standard, as has the availability of a second perfusionist for all CPB cases. Figure 4.2 illustrates the thorough and comprehensive pre-CPB checklist published by American Society of ExtraCorporeal Technology (www.amsect.org).

37

Society for Cardiothoracic Surgery in Great Britain & Ireland

CARDIAC SURGICAL SAFETY CHECKLIST

SIGN IN
Before Induction of Anaesthesia

- ☐ IDENTITY CONFIRMED
  Has the patient confirmed their identity, site, procedure and consent.
- ☐ SITE MARKED (or not applicable)
- ☐ CONSENT FORM CORRECT & SIGNED
  Implants to be used confirmed
- ☐ WARD PREPARATION COMPLETE
  (Fasting, Shower/Hair removal, Glycaemia, Blood)
- ☐ MRSA/MSSA STATUS KNOWN
  Positive? - YES / NO
- ☐ ANAESTHESIA MACHINE, MONITORING & MEDICATION CHECKS
  Perfusion regime & prescriptions agreed
- ☐ KNOWN ALLERGIES? YES/NO
- ☐ DIFFICULT AIRWAY/ASPIRATION RISK? YES (equipment available)/ NO
- ☐ RISK OF EXCESSIVE BLOOD LOSS?
  YES / NO If YES preparations and plan agreed
- ☐ PROCEDURE BRIEFING WITH ANAESTHESIA TEAM COMPLETE
- ☐ SPECIAL EQUIPMENT IDENTIFIED

TIME OUT
Before start of Surgery

- ☐ TEAM MEMBERS INTRODUCED (Name & Role)
- ☐ PATIENT AND PROCEDURE CONFIRMED
  Surgeon, Anaesthetist and Registered Practitioner verbally confirm procedure, site and position
  Surgical Incision/Access agreed.
- ☐ THEATRE TEAM BRIEFING COMPLETE
  Critical or Unexpected events planned for.
  Special equipment requirements ready.
- ☐ INSTRUMENT STERILITY CONFIRMED
- ☐ THROMBOPROPHYLAXIS Yes/Not applicable
- ☐ EQUIPMENT/STAFFING CONCERNS IDENTIFIED
- ☐ PERFUSIONIST CHECKS & BRIEFING COMPLETE Myocardial protection strategy agreed
- ☐ SURGICAL SITE INFECTION BUNDLE GIVEN
  Prophylactic IV antibiotics within 60 minutes, Idophor impregnated drapes, Patient warming, Hair removal, Glycaemic control
- ☐ IMAGING DISPLAYED AND/OR REVIEWED

Patient Label

S.C. CLARK February 2010 Version 6.0 for the SCTS.
Approved by the National Patient Safety Agency

SIGN OUT
Before patient leaves theatre

- ☐ INSTRUMENTS, SHARPS & SWAB CONFIRMED AS CORRECT
- ☐ DEBRIEFING PERFORMED
  Equipment or procedural problems identified and addressed
- ☐ OPERATION NOTE DONE
- ☐ CONCERNS FOR RECOVERY/ POST OPERATIVE CARE DISCUSSED & RECORDED
  Pacing Box Mode & Thresholds checked
- ☐ ICU & DRUG CHARTS CHECKED CORRECT AND FILED

Checklist Signed Complete and Correct

Surgeon ____________

Anaesthetist ____________

Scrub Nurse ____________

DATE ____________

Figure 4.1 Cardiac Surgical Safety Checklist. (Reproduced by kind permission of The Society for Cardiovascular Surgery in Great Britain and Ireland www.scts.org.)

Checklists have been clearly demonstrated to facilitate multi-step processes to improve team dynamics and minimize error. Multiple international organizations including the World Health Organization, the Society of Thoracic Surgery and the National Patient Safety Agency support their use in surgery. Checklists are now accepted to be an integral part of surgery as a whole and, more specifically, in cardiac surgery and CPB.

Safety Concerns prior to Commencing CPB

Before embarking on a case, the perfusionist undertakes a comprehensive review of the patient's notes. In addition to the information required by the checklist the following details are important:

- Significant co-morbidities, such as renal dysfunction, diabetes, genetic conditions affecting CPB.
- Metabolic or hematological abnormalities, such as anemia, sickle cell anemia, thrombocytopenia, or hyperkalemia.
- The patient's height and weight are essential to calculate:
  - Dose of heparin required (usually 300–500 IU/kg)
  - Body Surface Area (BSA) in metres^2, which is required to determine the calculated flow rate at normothermia (BSA × Cardiac Index) and therefore select appropriate CPB circuitry as well as arterial and venous cannula and
  - Predicted hematocrit on initiation of CPB.

Safety issues relating to the pre-operative information the perfusionist needs to know about are summarized in Table 4.1.

Additional checklists may of course be used at different stages of the operation, for example, perfusion handover checklists or prior to weaning from CPB. The latter is discussed in further detail in Chapter 12.

Patient
Patient identity confirmed
Procedure confirmed
Blood type, antibodies confirmed
Allergies checked
Blood bank number confirmed
Medical record number confirmed
Chart reviewed

Sterility and Cleanliness
Components checked for package integrity
Equipment Clean
Heat exchanger leak tested

Pump
Occlusions set
Speed controls operational
Flow meter in correct direction & calibrated
Flow rate indicator correct for patent/tubing size
Rollers rotate freely
Pump head rotation smooth and quiet
Holders secure
Servo regulated connections tested

Electrical
Power cord connections secure
Servo regulated connections secure
Batteries charged and operational

Cardioplegia
System debubbled and operational
System leak-free after pressurisation
Solution checked

Monitoring
Circuit/patient temperature probes placed
Pressure transducers calibrated/proper scale
Inline sensors calibrated
Oxygen analyser calibrated

Anticoagulation
Heparin time & dose confirmed
Anticoagulation tested & reported

Temperature Control
Water source connected & operational
Temperature range tested & operational
Water lines unobstructed

Signature:

Gas Supply
Gas line & filter connections secure
Gas exhaust unobstructed
Source & connections of gas confirmed
Flow metre/gas blender operational
Hoses leak free
Anaesthetic gas scavenge line operational

Components
System debubbled
Connections/stopcocks/caps secure
Appropriate lines clamped/shunts closed
Tubing direction traced & correct
Patency of arterial line/cannula confirmed
No tubing kinks noted
One-way valve in correct direction
Leak-free after pressurisation

Safety Mechanisms
Alarms operational, audible & engaged
Arterial filter/bubble trap debubbled
Cardiotomy/hardshell venous reservoir vented
Vents tested
Venous line occlude calibrated & tested
Devices securely attached to console

Assisted Venous Return
Cardiotomy positive-pressure relief valve present
Negative-pressure relief valve unobstructed
Vacuum regulator operational

Supplies
Tubing clamps available
Drugs available & properly labelled
Solutions available
Blood products available
Sampling syringes available
Anaesthetic vaporiser correct
Vaporiser operational & filled

Backup
Hand cranks available
Duplicate components/hardware available
Emergency lighting/torch available
Backup full oxygen cylinder available
Ice available

Date & Time:

Figure 4.2 Pre-Cardiopulmonary Bypass Checklist. (Reproduced by kind permission of The American Society of ExtraCorporeal Technology.) AmSECT promotes the use of pre-CPB checklists, or a reasonable equivalent, in clinical perfusion practice. AmSECT encourages perfusionists to use this checklist as a guide and modify the checklist to accommodate differences in circuit design and variations in institutional clinical practice. AmSECT can accept no liability whatsoever for the adoption and practice of this suggested checklist.

Table 4.1. Pre-CPB Safety Concerns

Heparin administration	○ Activated Clotting Time (ACT) >400 seconds or > 3x baseline (depending on institutional protocol)
Arterial cannulation	○ Pulsatile swing on an aneroid pressure gauge connected to a side arm of the arterial line
	○ Pump volume transfuses well with no rapid rise in arterial line pressure
Venous reservoir fluid level	○ Additional fluid available and attached to the circuit
	○ Low-level alarm placed at appropriate level for the case and activated
Oxygen analyzer	○ Functional and alarm activated
Sweep rate & FiO$_2$	○ Appropriate settings for case after review of notes
Venous cannula	○ De-aired
CPB shunt lines	○ Clamped
Clamps on surgical side	○ Off
Alarm overrides	○ Deactivated
Drugs and fluids	○ Available, prepared, labeled
Pre-CPB checklist	○ Complete

Minimal Extracorporeal Circulation Safety Features

Minimally invasive extracorporeal circulation (MiECC) is the term given to describe a multidisciplinary strategy focused on the reduction of the adverse effects of CPB. For MiECC, the safety briefing is conducted similar to conventional CPB cases, however the team also needs to agree when and how to convert to conventional bypass, should MiECC not be adequate.

The safety devices recommended for MiECC are:

- Pulmonary artery and aortic root vent bubble trap.
- Air Protection System (APS) – this is required because MiECC does not include an open

reservoir for air removal, therefore it is essential that a safety device is in place to prevent air from entering either the centrifugal pump or the venous bag. The APS device is activated:

- ○ when air is detected in the venous line, allowing it to be purged before possible entrainment into the circuit, or
- ○ by a level sensor if there is a reduction in the amount of blood in the bubble trap due to displacement by entrained air. The level sensor is servo-regulated and, once activated, the automatic arterial clamp is closed to temporarily stop flow, allowing the perfusionist to remove the air.

- Bubble sensor post APS system – if the venous bubble trap fails to eliminate sufficient air, the pump may de-prime. If air passes toward the pump, the auto clamp is triggered, and the pump will stop, allowing the air to be displaced into the soft-shell bag.
- Electronic Venous Line Occluder (EVO) – can be used in a manual or automatic mode for clamping the venous line.

MiECC is discussed in detail in Chapter 8.

In summary, the many technological developments concerning HLM hardware and related components have made it possible to reduce the incidence of complications and problems during CPB. The likelihood of death or severe injury from CPB-related incidents has been declining from 1: 1,400–3,200 in the early 2000s to currently 1: 4,450–4,850 patients, which is testament to the safety culture in perfusion.

The use of checklists is well established in medicine, specifically surgery, as well as other industries. It has been proven that their use saves lives, time and money as well as reducing the rate of complications. It therefore appears logical to assume that the use of pre-CPB checklists will have similar effects, particularly with regard to complications during CPB. Checklists should be used in an appropriate, diligent, and professional manner. They need to be adapted to the specific working environments as well as emerging technologies, and they should be revised regularly.

Suggested Further Reading

1. Department of Health. Guide to Good Practice in Clinical Perfusion, London, 2009.

2. Society of Clinical Perfusion Scientists of Great Britain and Ireland, Association of Cardiothoracic Anaesthetists and Society of Cardiothoracic Surgeons in Great Britain and Ireland. *Recommendations for Standards of Monitoring during Cardiopulmonary Bypass.* 2016.

3. National Patient Safety Agency (NPSA). Seven Steps to Patient Safety. An Overview Guide for NHS Staff 2004. www.npsa.nhs.uk/ sevensteps

4. Weigmann D, Suther T, Neal J et al. A human factors analysis of cardiopulmonary bypass machines. *Journal of Extracorporeal Technology* 2009; 41(2):57–63.

5. Gritten M. *The independent root cause analysis report into the adverse incident that led to the death of a paediatric cardiac surgery patient at United Bristol Healthcare NHS Trust on 27th May 2005.* NHS Publication 2007.

6. NHS England. Decade of improved outcomes for patients thanks to surgical safety checklist 2019 www.england.nhs .uk/2019/01/surgical-safety- checklist/

7. Clark SC, Dunning J, Ottavio RA et al. EACTS guidelines for the use of patient safety checklists. *European Journal of Cardiothoracic Surgery* 2012; 41: 993–1004.

8. Charriere JM, Pelissie J, Verd C et al. Retrospective survey on monitoring/safety devices and incidents of cardiopulmonary bypass for cardiac surgery in France. *Journal of ExtraCorporeal Technology* 2007; 39:142–57.

9. Wahba A, Milojevic M, Boer C De et al. EACTS/EACTA/EBCP Guidelines on cardiopulmonary bypass in adult cardiac surgery. *European Journal of Cardiothoracic Surgery* 2019; 00: 1–42. https://doi:10.1093/ejcts/ ezz267

Priming Solutions for Cardiopulmonary Bypass Circuits

Filip De Somer and Robert Young

The composition of the fluid used to prime cardiopulmonary bypass (CPB) circuits has been a source of great interest and debate ever since the inception of cardiopulmonary bypass in 1953. There has been significant progress in our understanding, but the ideal priming solution has still to be agreed upon and practice continues to vary widely between cardiac units.

The volume of contemporary bypass circuits varies enormously from less than 400 ml to over 2000 ml for adult circuits and from as little as 120 ml for pediatric CPB. Circuits must be carefully de-aired with a compatible priming solution in order to prevent gas emboli from passing into the patient's circulation at the commencement of CPB. In the early days, circuits were primed with allogeneic whole blood. This practice proved to be unsustainable due to issues of availability and cost and the growing appreciation of the potential risks, such as infection, immunosuppression and various forms of transfusion reactions, associated with its use. The use of a non-hemic priming solution was first reported in 1958. Crystalloid and colloid priming solutions are now commonplace.

The partial or total replacement of blood in the prime with other fluids inevitably leads to changes in the characteristics of the circulating blood as soon as CPB is commenced. The impact of these changes can be thought of as being both quantitative and qualitative. The quantitative changes depend on the volume of the non-blood prime and the effects of hemodilution. The qualitative changes depend on the constitution of the prime, which may affect electrolyte concentrations, acid-base balance and osmolarity among other things.

Hemodilution

Hemodilution with commencement of CPB has a number of positive effects but also some less desirable effects.

Blood Flow

Delivery of oxygen to tissues depends on blood flow and oxygen content. Blood flow is inversely related to both vascular resistance and viscosity. Hemodilution with crystalloid or colloid prime leads to a reduction in overall viscosity, resulting in improved tissue oxygen delivery with reduced risk of organ ischemia during CPB. The optimal average hematocrit for the microcirculation is 30% (Hb 10 g/dL) but this value varies from organ to organ. For example, the kidney needs higher hematocrit values compared to the heart. As some aspects of cardiac surgery and CPB increase blood viscosity (see Table 5.1), prime hemodilution can be helpful to counterbalance this.

Under normothermic conditions hematocrit values below 24% should be avoided. However, oxygen supply to the tissues depends not only on the carrying capacity of the blood (hemoglobin) but also on convective transport. Hemodilution decreases hemoglobin concentration and thus oxygen carrying capacity. For this reason hemodilution might require an increase of blood flow to maintain the desired oxygen delivery to the organs. To illustrate this, to maintain the same oxygen delivery before and after a decrease in hemoglobin concentration from 10 g/dL to 8 g/dL, an increase in blood flow by 20% is required. During normothermia an oxygen delivery of at least 274 mL/min/m² should be maintained to preserve renal function.

Cardiac surgery carries increased morbidity and mortality when the decrease in hemoglobin concentration is not compensated by higher blood flow. This is not surprising as adequacy of tissue oxygenation depends on multiple other factors such as temperature, blood flow, duration of CPB and preoperative organ function. In a healthy patient under physiological conditions, a decrease in hemoglobin is compensated for by an increase in cardiac output. Until recently most centers did not adapt blood flow on

Table 5.1. Factors increasing blood viscosity

Hypothermia	A fall of 1°C increases viscosity by 2%
Flow rates	Low flow rates lead to aggregation of blood cells (shear rate <10/s)
Red cell deformability	Turbulent flow and hypothermia cause reduced deformability of the cell membrane
Coagulation	Activation of clotting cascades leads to platelet aggregation, and interaction with plasma proteins

Table 5.2. Factors affecting hematocrit prior to the initiation of CPB

Patient size

Starting hematocrit

Blood loss pre bypass

Intravenous fluids pre CPB

Urine output pre CPB

Volume and nature of circuit prime

Transfusion policy

CPB in the presence of pronounced hemodilution, thus potentially jeopardizing tissue oxygen delivery. Recent research has shown that individualized goal directed tissue perfusion based on calculated oxygen delivery reduces morbidity post CPB. This is discussed in more detail in Chapter 10.

Clotting Factors

A further potential complication of hemodilution is the relative reduction in concentrations of clotting factors such as fibrinogen, which can contribute to the coagulopathy associated with CPB (see also Chapter 16).

Drug Bioavailability

Hemodilution results in a change in the pharmacokinetic behaviour of administered drugs. The plasma drug concentration before hemodilution depends on its plasma protein binding, its original distribution volume and the equilibration between tissue and plasma concentration. Hemodilution, by decreasing plasma protein concentration, decreases the ratio of bound to free drug. With less drug bound, bioavailability increases as only unbound compounds can diffuse into tissues. Conversely, changes in viscosity and availability of free drugs may impact their renal and hepatic clearance. Chapter 10 provides more detail about drug management during CPB.

Controlling Hemodilution

A number of factors will affect the hematocrit on CPB (see Table 5.2). The perfusionist can influence the hematocrit by modifying the extent of hemodilution in several ways:

- Choice of circuit – minimization of prime volume by circuit volume reduction is widely practiced. It is primarily achieved by shortening the length of circuit tubing and removing the venous reservoir, which can reduce priming volume to as low as 400 ml. Over the last decade the quest to reduce circuit size has led to the evolution of minimal invasive extracorporeal circulation (MiECC) systems, incorporating circuit and clinical practice optimization to reduce priming volume. This promising approach is not yet in widespread use. MiECC is discussed in detail in Chapter 8.

- Autologous Prime – is done once the patient has been cannulated but prior to establishing CPB and Blood is passively drained into the circuit, displacing the prime into a removeable reservoir. This can take the form of Retrograde Autologous Prime (RAP), where the patient's blood is drained retrogradely through the aortic cannula, or of Venous Autologous Prime (VAP), where blood is drained antegradely through the venous cannula. The extent of autologous circuit priming is limited by the hypotension caused by loss of the patient's intravascular blood volume. This can be ameliorated to some extent by the administration of vasopressors. Autologous prime volumes may vary from as little as 150 ml to in excess of 1500 ml. The decision to use autologous priming can be based on the predicted hematocrit during CPB calculated from the patient's estimated total blood volume (TBV), intraoperative fluid balance and starting hematocrit. The total blood volume may be estimated using the Allen formula (see Figure 5.1). Not every patient might be suitable for RAP or VAP and the clinical team needs to make a careful decision on a case by case basis.

- Adding blood to the prime – this is commonly done in pediatric cardiac surgery to achieve a target hematocrit where, even with the use of

43

Table 5.3. Typical characteristics of common crystalloid priming solutions

	Human Plasma	5% glucose	0.9% saline	Ringer's lactate	Normosol R	Plasmalyte 148
[Na⁺] mmol/l	135–145		154	131	140	140
[K⁺] mmol/l	3.5–5.0			5.4	5	5
[Ca²⁺] mmol/l	2.2–2.6			1.8		
[Mg²⁺] mmol/l	0.7–1.0				3	1.5
[Cl⁻] mmol/l	98–106		154	112	98	98
Glucose g/l	4–6	50				
Acetate mmol/l					27	27
Lactate mmol/l	0.7–1.8			28		
Gluconate mmol/l					23	23
pH	7.4	3.5–6.5		5–7	4–8	6.5–8.0
Osmolarity mOsm/l	275–295	278	308	277	294	295

$$\text{TBV males} = \{0.000417 \times \text{height (cm)}^3\} + \{45.0 \times \text{weight (kg)}\} - 30.$$
$$\text{females} = \{0.000414 \times \text{height (cm)}^3\} + \{32.8 \times \text{weight (kg)}\} - 30.$$

$$\text{Hct post dilution} = \frac{\text{TBV} \times \text{predilution Hct}}{\text{TBV} + \text{PV} + \text{CV} + \text{intravenous fluids - urine output}}$$

PV = priming fluid volume, CV = cardioplegia fluid volume, TBV = total blood volume.

Figure 5.1 The Allen Formula.

minimum volume circuits, the fall in hematocrit associated with pure crystalloid/colloid primes would be excessive. The use of non-blood primes in neonatal and infant surgery is generally not possible. The specific requirements for pediatric bypass are discussed in more detail in Chapter 15.

Priming Solutions

The ideal priming solution should not cause any physiological disturbance when added to the patient's circulation. In reality, however, choice of fluids for circuit prime will affect oncotic pressure, acid-base balance, glucose homeostasis, osmolarity and individual electrolyte concentrations. For clinicians there are a number of considerations to take into account. A first one is the choice of whether to use a crystalloid, a colloid or combined crystalloid colloid priming solution.

Crystalloid Solutions

Medically used crystalloids are aqueous solutions of various electrolytes with or without glucose. The most commonly used crystalloids are summarized in Table 5.3. These solutions are cheap, widely available and have long shelf lives. When an isosmolar crystalloid solution is administered intravenously, it will distribute throughout the extracellular space. Only 25% of the administered volume will remain in the intravascular space while 75% passes into the interstitium. The hemodilution crystalloids cause leads to a further reduction in the concentration of the oncotically active components in the blood, primarily albumin, allowing further movement of fluid into the interstitial space. Excessive volumes of interstitial fluid cause tissue edema with the potential for reduced perfusion and organ dysfunction in the postoperative period.

Table 5.4. The properties of colloids currently in clinical use

	Albumin 4%	Gelofusine	Haemaccel	HES	HES balanced
[Na$^+$] mmol/l	140	150	145	154	137
[K$^+$] mmol/l		5	5.1		4
[Ca^{2+}] mmol/l			12.5		
[Cl-] mmol/l	128	100	145	154	110
Lactate mmol/l		30			
Acetate mmol/l					34
Molecular weight (Daltons)	69,000	30,000	35,000	130,000	130,000
Half-life	21 days	8 hours	5 hours	12.1 hours	12.1 hours
pH	6.7–7.3	5.8–7.0	7.3	4–5.5	5.7–6.5

In patients with a large blood volume, the use of balanced crystalloid electrolyte solutions for priming is often the first choice as the impact of hemodilution will be comparatively small. However, in small patients or in patients where it is anticipated that a large volume of crystalloid cardioplegia will be used, a drastic reduction of colloid oncotic pressure by dilution of plasma proteins can be expected and therefore colloids or a mixture of colloids with crystalloids might be the better choice.

Colloid Solutions

Colloid solutions are essentially made up of large organic molecules dispersed in water. Colloids remain within the intravascular space to a much larger extent than crystalloids, thereby maintaining oncotic pressure. The amount of time this oncotic effect lasts differs between solutions and depends on endothelial integrity. Their use in CPB prime has been advocated to reduce the sudden fall in oncotic pressure associated with crystalloid priming solutions. Colloids are most commonly used as an addition to a crystalloid prime rather than as the sole fluid. Available colloids include human albumin solution, gelatins and hydroxyethyl starches and are summarized in Table 5.4.

Electrolyte Management

Electrolyte disturbances are common following cardiac surgery. Causes include changes in temperature, acid-base status, catecholamine levels, diuresis and the administration of intravenous fluids, including cardioplegia and citrate-containing blood products. The extent of these changes is difficult to predict. A sensible approach with regard to formulation of the circuit prime is to maintain levels of key electrolytes such as sodium, potassium, calcium and magnesium at physiologically normal concentrations.

Independent of the choice of colloid or crystalloid, a pH balanced solution with an appropriate concentration of electrolytes is recommended. This will prevent significant biochemical changes when going on bypass.

Sodium

Solutions with a high chloride concentration, such as 0.9% saline, will create a hyperchloremic acidosis. The resulting fall in pH will shift the hemoglobin dissociation curve to the right and improve oxygen delivery. However, this potential benefit is outweighed by the adverse effects on coagulation, myocardial contractility and adrenoceptor function.

Rapid decreases in plasma sodium concentration are associated with altered mental status, seizures and coma, and values of <130 mEq/L are predictive for stroke. For this reason electrolyte solutions containing low sodium such as Lactate-Ringer (130 mEq/L) should be replaced by one containing a higher sodium concentration such as Plasma-Lyte (140 mEq/L) in patients with a low preoperative plasma sodium concentration.

Hyponatremia is one of the most common electrolyte disturbances in cardiac patients, particularly if

45

they have been on long-term diuretic treatment. A modified priming solution needs to be used in cases where an operation cannot be delayed, and the baseline sodium is low enough to suggest that standard CPB prime might cause severe harm (generally <125 mmol/l). The sodium level in the CBP prime can be adjusted to a level that is similar to that of the patient's serum sodium level by using a mixture of sodium lactate (Hartmann's solution) and 5% glucose:

1. Determine the patient's serum sodium level pre-CPB
2. Volume (ml) of fluid to remove from 1l Hartmann's bag and to be replaced with 5% Glucose $= 1000 - \left(\frac{pre-CPB\ Na}{131} \times 1000\right)$, i.e. the fluid volume in the bag remains 1l.

In addition, autologous priming should be considered to decrease the volume of crystalloids and the use of mannitol should be avoided as it is hyperosmolar and can worsen cerebral dehydration.

Potassium

Potassium levels will inevitably rise after the administration of cardioplegia solution. To the contrary, hypokalemia is most commonly observed in the post-operative period due to increased renal excretion as part of the surgical stress response and diuretic use. None of the fluids in routine use for circuit priming contain supraphysiological levels of potassium. Exacerbation of cardioplegia-induced hyperkalemia during CPB tends to occur because of hyperglycemia, acidemia or the administration of large volumes of homologous blood, particularly blood with a longer storage time. Intraoperative hyperkalemia can be corrected by using an insulin-glucose infusion, increased diuresis or ultrafiltration.

Calcium

Mild intraoperative hypocalcemia is common. This may occur due to hemodilution, calcium binding to citrate in transfused blood or hypomagnesemia. Hypocalcemia adversely affects coagulation and can induce arrhythmias and depress myocardial function. Calcium is contained in Ringer's lactate and in urea-linked gelatin-based colloids. Calcium levels are generally monitored intraoperatively as part of standard blood gas analyses; supplemental calcium is administered via the bypass circuit as appropriate.

Magnesium

Hypomagnesemia following cardiac surgery is also common. It can cause arrhythmias, hypertension and coronary vasoconstriction. A number of studies have identified a link between hypomagnesemia and post-operative atrial fibrillation. There may also be a link with short-term cognitive dysfunction. Magnesium is contained in Plasmalyte and Normosol. Point of care magnesium assays exist but are not in widespread use. Magnesium supplementation is often empirical, and the benefit remains subject to debate.

Osmolarity and pH

The electrolyte concentration in the prime will define its osmolarity. Hyperosmolarity, >320 mOsm/L, may cause renal failure and brain damage. Osmolarity (in the absence of mannitol) can be estimated using the formula in Figure 5.2.

pH balanced solutions should be used to prevent haemodilution acidosis. These solutions contain buffers such as acetate and lactate. Both of these are precursors of bicarbonate (HCO_3) and are converted within 10 min through the citric acid cycle to H_2O and CO_2. In patients with liver disease, acetate is preferred as its metabolism is less dependant on liver function than is that of lactate.

Glucose

Maintaining glucose concentration below 180 mg/dL (10 mmol/L) is recommended during CPB and

$$Osm = (Na \times 2) + \left(\frac{blood\ glucose}{18}\right) + 15$$

Where Na (mEq/L), blood glucose (mg/dL), Osm = predicted osmolarity

Figure 5.2 Formula for the estimation of Osmolarity.

postoperatively by the recent STS and EACTS/EACTA/EBCP guidelines. Hyperglycemia during CPB is associated with an increased risk of wound infection, cardiac dysfunction, neurological injury and increased overall mortality. The use of glucose containing priming solutions in both diabetic and non-diabetic patients is not recommended as this can exacerbate the hyperglycemia – caused by surgical stress response, hypothermia, hyperoxia and heparin administration – regularly seen during CPB. Hyperglycemia increases plasma osmolarity, causing movement of water from the intracellular to the extracellular space and with a subsequent reduction in electrolyte concentrations by dilution. A metabolic acidosis may occur due to the dilution of plasma bicarbonate. Insulin may be required to obtain a satisfactory glucose concentration.

Prime Additives

The fluid prime can be used as a carrier of additional substances thought to be of clinical benefit. Commonly used additives include sodium bicarbonate, mannitol and heparin. Corticosteroids are also used by some centers, however, their use as part of CPB prime is subject to much debate.

Sodium Bicarbonate (NaHCO₃)

$NaHCO_3$ can be added as a buffer to unbalanced crystalloid and colloid primes. This will prevent a fall in bicarbonate levels caused by dilution and ameliorate the metabolic acidosis associated with the use of unbalanced solutions. In order to prevent this non-perfusion related acidosis from building up, it is common to add 2.5 mEq $NaHCO_3$ for every 100 mL of non-buffered solutions in the circuit. Sodium bicarbonate should not be given too liberally because the addition of large volumes can cause hypernatremia. The use of sodium bicarbonate to treat acidosis caused by transient tissue hypoxia, as may occur with deep hypothermic circulatory arrest, is controversial.

Mannitol

Mannitol is a hypertonic crystalloid solution that acts as an intravascular volume expander and osmotic diuretic. It is metabolically inert. Doses of 0.25–0.5 g/kg body weight added to the prime are common, but the evidence of benefit is weak. In theory, its diuretic properties are useful for the prevention of excessive fluid accumulation and post-operative interstitial edema. It was thought to have a protective effect on renal function, possibly by increasing renal blood flow. More recent studies, however, have indicated that while increasing urine output, mannitol does not protect renal function and may even have a detrimental effect on it. It cannot currently be recommended as a prophylactic agent to reduce the incidence of acute kidney injury following cardiac surgery.

Heparin

Heparin is added to circuit priming solutions either dosed according to patient weight or as a fixed dose. The rationale behind adding this, in addition to the systemic heparin given before aortic cannulation, is to provide additional safety at initiation of bypass and in the event of emergency CPB. Doses between 2.500 and 5.000 IU of heparin are common as an additive to the prime of an adult CPB circuit.

Corticosteroids

A small number of institutions routinely add corticosteroids to the prime. Several studies have examined the various theoretical benefits of steroids used this way. None found any clinical benefit in reducing the inflammatory response, the rate of post-operative atrial fibrillation or of renal failure. To the contrary, adding steroids to the pump prime has been shown to regularly lead to severe post-operative hyperglycemia, which can be difficult to manage. Steroids as additives to CPB prime are currently not recommended.

The constitution of cardiopulmonary bypass prime has a significant impact on the perioperative care of patients undergoing cardiac surgery. Minimizing the volume of prime has become a key goal. Although the use of crystalloid and colloid fluids is now standard practice, the specific constitution of priming solutions varies widely between centers. The challenge remains to formulate a circuit prime that leads to an optimum level of hemodilution while minimizing any detrimental physical and biochemical changes when mixed with patients' blood.

Suggested Further Reading

1. Miles L, Coulson T, Galhardo C et al. Pump priming practices and anticoagulation in cardiac surgery: Results from the Global Cardiopulmonary Bypass Survey. *Anesth Analg* 2017; 125(6): 1871–1877.

2. Ranucci M, Conti D, Castelvecchio S et al. Haematocrit on cardiopulmonary bypass and outcome after cardiopulmonary surgery in nontransfused patients. *Ann Thorac Surg* 2010; 89: 11–18.

3. Ranucci M, Johnson I, Willcox T et al. Goal-directed perfusion to reduce acute kidney injury: A randomized trial. *J Thorac Cardiovasc Surg*; 2018: 156: 1918–1927.e2.

4. Kunst G, Milojevic M, Boer C et al. 2019 EACTS/EACTA/EBCP guidelines on cardiopulmonary bypass in adult cardiac surgery. *Br J Anaesth* 2019; 123 (6): 713–757.

5. Najmaii S, Redford D, Larson D. Hyperglycemia as an effect of cardiopulmonary bypass: Intra-operative glucose management. *J Extra Corpor Technol* 2006: 38(2); 168–173.

6. Munoz E, Briggs H, Tolpin D et al. Low serum sodium during cardiopulmonary bypass predicts increased risk of postoperative stroke after coronary artery bypass graft surgery. *J Thorac Cardiovasc Surg* 2014; 147: 1351–1355.

7. Polderman K, Girbes R. Severe electrolyte disorders following cardiac surgery: A prospective controlled observational study. *Crit Care* 2004; 8: 459–466.

8. Waskowski J, Pfortmueller A, Erdoes G et al. Mannitol for the prevention of peri-operative acute kidney injury: A systematic review. *Eur J Vasc Endovasc Surg* 2019; 58(1): 130–140.

9. Whitlock R, Devereaux J, Teoh K et al. Methylprednisolone in patients undergoing cardiopulmonary bypass (SIRS): A randomised, double-blind, placebo-controlled trial. *Lancet* 2015; 386: 1243–1253.

10. Canaday S, Rompala J, Rowles J et al. Chronic severe hyponatremia and cardiopulmonary bypass: Avoiding osmotic demyelination syndrome. *J Extra Corpor Technol.* 2015;47(4): 228–230.

Anticoagulation for Cardiopulmonary Bypass

Martin Besser and Linda Shore-Lesserson

Anticoagulation is mandatory for any form of extra-corporeal circulation to prevent activation of the coagulation system through contact between blood and artificial surfaces and through blood stasis. The absence of sufficient anticoagulation is likely to result in clot formation within minutes of aortic cannulation and commencement of CPB, with detrimental consequences for the patient. Even microvascular clots can lead to death, in their lesser forms they can lead to organ dysfunction, manifesting mostly either as renal or neurological dysfunction.

The principles of anticoagulation for cardiopulmonary bypass have remained fundamentally unchanged in the past 45 years. The majority of practitioners still give doses of up to 500 IU/kg of unfractionated heparin (UFH) prior to CPB. The effect of heparin is monitored using the Activated Clotting Time (ACT). The development of improved biomaterials is likely to allow reduced intensity of anticoagulation. This technology and its application are currently subject to intense research efforts. Smaller heparin doses might help to reduce undesirable effects such as post-operative bleeding and heparin rebound. Although there are numerous approaches and protocols in place, there still is no universal agreement on how to best treat patients who cannot receive heparin but require surgery on CPB. This chapter briefly outlines the history of heparin before discussing its pharmacology, intraoperative hemostasis monitoring, the management of heparin resistance and Heparin Induced Thrombocytopenia (HIT) and the outlook for anticoagulation on CPB.

Heparin

In 1916 at Johns Hopkins University, Jay McLean isolated a phosphatide anticoagulant from canine liver which could anticoagulate blood in vitro and in vivo. In 1926 a similar compound was produced by an aquatic extraction. The early production process introduced impurities, and side effects included fever, shock and death in laboratory animals. By 1936 Charles and Scott had refined technology and were able to crystallize 'clean' heparin as a barium salt. The first episode of treating venous thromboembolism (VTE) is attributed to Lam and McLure in 1939 in Detroit. By this time the biosource had changed from canine liver to bovine lung and then porcine mucosa.

The original US pharmacopeia (USP) from the 1950s was based on the action of heparin sodium on sheep plasma. Unexpectedly, between 2007 and 2008, thousands of adverse reactions and more than 200 deaths occurred when Chinese suppliers contaminated their product with cartilage-derived oversulfated chondroitin sulphate to lower production costs. As a result, in 2009 the USP standardization was changed to match the European units. The standard now is based on a Factor IIa assay instead of the sheep plasma, which has reduced the potency of the US stock by about 10% after 2009.

Pharmacology

Heparin is a complex mixture of polysaccharides of different chain lengths and a molecular weight between 3,000 and 30,000 kDa. It has a number of unique characteristics that make it particularly suitable for use in CPB.

It naturally occurs in mast cells and basophils and fulfills a number of physiological functions, such as chemotaxis, leukocyte cell diapedesis, upregulation of overall inflammation, cellular repair, vessel growth and anti-cancer activity. In addition, heparin activates osteoclasts rather than osteoblasts and attenuates proliferation of vascular smooth muscle cells.

Heparin needs to bind to the enzyme inhibitor antithrombin III (AT III) which leads to a conformational change that inactivates thrombin (Factor II) and other proteases involved in clotting, namely

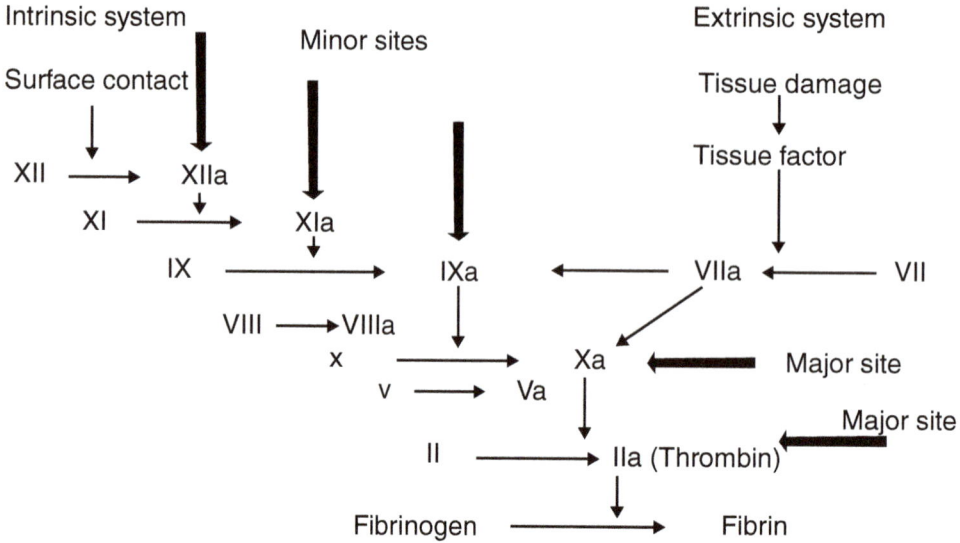

Figure 6.1 Major and minor sites of heparin action.

Factors IXa, Xa, XIa and XIIa. Thrombin inhibition also blocks activation of Factors V, VIII, XI and of platelets. Heparin increases the activity of heparin cofactor II (HC II), which additionally inhibits thrombin. Figure 6.1 gives an overview of the major and minor sites of heparin action.

The mode of action of heparin is determined by its chain length: only a third of molecules have the key pentasaccharide that interacts with antithrombin, while short heparin chains of <18 saccharides can only inactivate Factor Xa. In high doses (>1.0 U/ml) heparin will bind to HC II to interact with clotting factors independent of antithrombin; at doses >2.0 U/ml heparin prevents the generation of factor Xa independent of antithrombin via a charge-based interaction. At these concentrations the activity of fibrinogen-bound thrombin is also inhibited. Heparin activity can be measured by using the plasma anti-Xa assay. The target doses for heparin for VTE treatment is 0.3–0.7 anti-Xa IU/ml, whereas during CPB levels of >3 IU/ml are intended.

Heparin is eliminated by two mechanisms, both of which appear to follow non-linear kinetics: a rapid and saturable mechanism, likely due to internalization by endothelial cells and macrophages and a second, slower mechanism via renal clearance. After administration of smaller doses between 5,000 and 10,000 units, heparin is found in urine as an inactivated and desulphated molecule, while after larger doses it is eliminated intact with its anticoagulant activity preserved. These kinetics lead to the context-sensitive half-life based on the dose of heparin administered. At a dose of 100 U/kg its half-life is approximately 60 minutes, increasing to 126 minutes at a dose of 400 U/kg.

Heparin Monitoring

In 1953 Langdell described the Partial Thromboplastin Time (PTT) later modified to the activated PTT (aPTT), which has become the most commonly used laboratory test to monitor heparin outside the operating room. There is a confusing array of different platforms and technologies to test the adequacy of anticoagulation for CPB. The two general classes of heparin monitoring devices are functional assays and quantitative measures of the level of circulating heparin. If quantitative measures are used to maintain heparin concentration, a functional test must also be employed to assure adequacy of anticoagulation.

The first clotting time test, described in 1913, was the whole blood clotting time (WBCT), or the Lee–White WBCT, in which whole blood was placed in a glass tube and tilted until clotting visibly occurred. In the un-activated state this test took more than 30 minutes, and it was replaced by the activated clotting time (ACT). The ACT provides the basis on which most functional anticoagulation monitors are modeled. Initially an ACT prolongation of 300 seconds was considered the safe minimum level of heparinization; later Young et al. described fibrin strand formation during in vivo experiments in monkeys at ACT < 400 seconds. To this day there is great institutional variation in heparin dosing and even more so in ACT values considered safe to go on CPB. The majority of cardiac centers around the world prefer an ACT between 400 and 550 seconds.

Modern ACT devices are nearly all cartridge based, require less than 1 ml of blood to run the assay and tests can be done in the operating room by non-laboratory trained staff. They work on the principle of adding blood to an activator, however they differ in the method for clot detection. Clot formation can be detected using mechanical, optical or amperometric methods. The time taken to detect clot signals the end of the test and represents the "clotting time." Numerous ACT assays are in clinical use and many have been studied in clinical trials showing them to be safe for anticoagulation monitoring during CPB. Owing to their different analytical methods, these devices cannot be used interchangeably and need to be validated before use, particularly when switching manufacturer. The heterogeneity of the response to heparin by different ACT devices is so great that minimum therapeutic or safe values remain difficult to recommend.

Initiation of CPB

The recommended weight-based dose of unfractionated heparin to achieve safe anticoagulation for aortic cannulation and commencing CPB is 300–500 U/kg in adult patients. It makes sense to choose an initial heparin dose based upon a known institutional heparin formulation, as heparin preparations vary in potency, different ACT monitoring systems have a certain bias, and patient-specific conditions vary.

An alternative way to ascertain the dose of heparin needed to safely initiate CPB is to calculate a patient-specific dose-response curve. Such in vitro assays are available from different manufacturers. The concept is that a baseline ACT and an ACT with a known amount of heparin are measured. The dose-response relationship generated by connecting these two points on a line is then extrapolated to the desired ACT. An algorithm that incorporates the patient's baseline ACT, estimated blood volume, and heparin-response curve calculates the dose of heparin needed to achieve adequate anticoagulation. Unfortunately, different concentrations of various endogenous heparin-binding proteins such as vitronectin and Platelet Factor 4 (PF4) make the response to an intravenous bolus of heparin extremely unpredictable.

The large interpatient variation in heparin responsiveness and the potential for heparin resistance make using a functional monitor of heparin anticoagulation (with or without a measure of heparin concentration) critically important in all cardiac surgical patients. In vitro testing platforms that promote a heparin dose-response calculation are often inconsistent in their ability to accurately predict the heparin dose needed for safe CPB initiation. This is because in vitro heparin additives do not always mimic the in vivo response to a dose of heparin. These dose-response curves do, however, provide insight into patients' heparin sensitivity and can identify those who are heparin resistant.

Maintenance of Heparin Effect

Clinicians are able to reassure themselves about maintaining a safe level of anticoagulation throughout CPB by performing regular ACTs. Although it is a functional test and not a quantitative test, the ACT has several flaws. Its use has been criticized because of the extreme variability and the absence of a correlation with changes in plasma heparin levels. The variation in ACT values may represent true variability in a patient's coagulation status or it may be artifactual, reflecting altered sensitivity of the ACT to heparin or other factors influencing anticoagulation during CPB. Many factors commonly encountered during cardiac surgery can alter ACT readings. Hemodilution and relative hypofibrinogenemia caused by the pump prime may increase the ACT; hypothermia increases the ACT in a "dose-related" fashion; extremes of thrombocytopenia will prolong the ACT; patients treated with platelet inhibitors such as prostacyclin, aspirin or platelet-membrane-receptor antagonists have a prolonged heparinized ACT. Platelet lysis, however, significantly shortens the ACT because of the release of platelet membrane components and PF4 which neutralizes heparin. Anesthesia and surgery shorten the ACT and create a hypercoagulable state, possibly by creating a thromboplastic response or through activation of platelets.

Using the plasma anti-Xa activity level as the gold standard, it has been shown that the ACT does not correlate well with anti-Xa activity or with whole blood heparin concentration (see Figure 6.2).

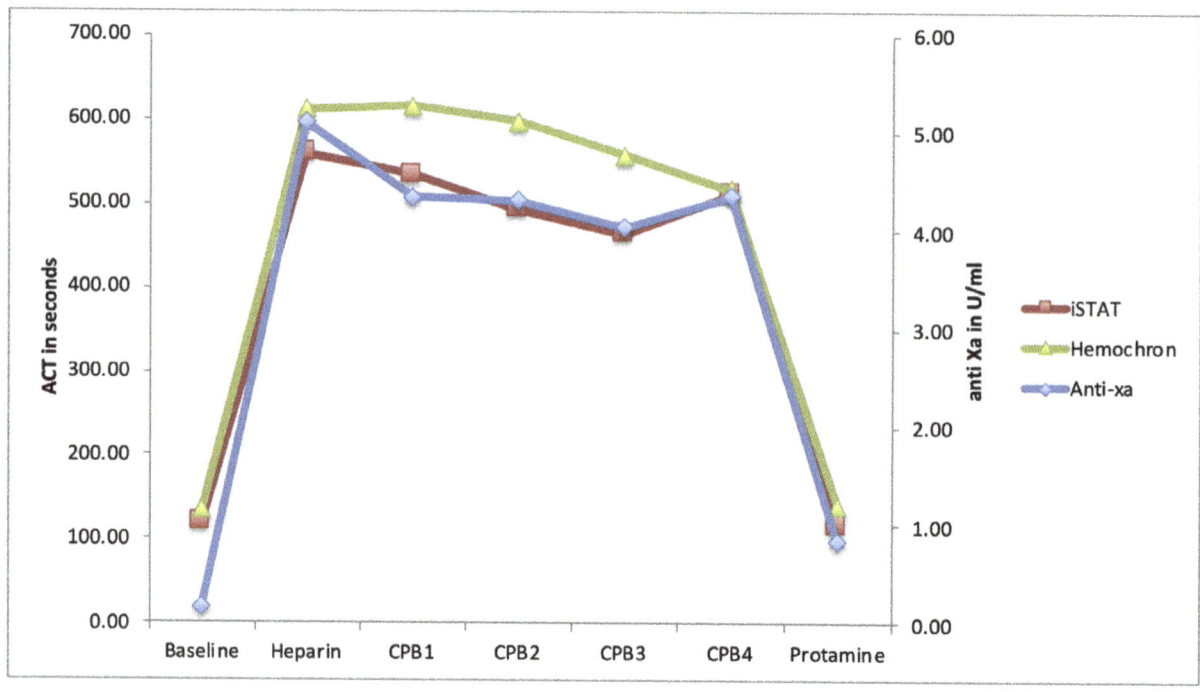

Figure 6.2 Activated clotting time as measured by i-STAT and Hemochron Signature and heparin activity as measured by anti-Xa at all time points. ACT, activated clotting time; CPB, cardiopulmonary bypass. (Reproduced from Falter F, MacDonald S, Matthews C et al. Evaluation of Point-of-Care ACT Coagulometers and Anti-Xa Activity During Cardiopulmonary Bypass. *J Cardiothorac Vasc Anesth.* November, 2020;34(11):2921–2927.)

Despite this, the ACT remains the most common test used to affirm safe initiation and maintenance of anticoagulation on CPB. The ACT is a functional test of anticoagulation which is supported as a Class 1 recommendation by the STS/SCA/AmSECT Guidelines for Best Practices in Anticoagulation for Cardiac Surgery.

Point of care heparin concentration measurement uses a protamine titration technique. Multiple chambers in a cartridge contain tissue thromboplastin and a series of known incremental protamine concentrations. When heparinized blood is added, the first channel to clot is the channel whose protamine concentration most accurately neutralizes the heparin without a heparin or protamine excess. Using known pharmacokinetics, the device then calculates the concentration of heparin in the blood sample. Attempting to maintain a stable derived heparin concentration will lead to the administration of larger doses of heparin than required. The device algorithm does not take into account factors such as hemodilution and hypothermia on CPB, which increase anticoagulation and do not require a stable heparin concentration. In comparison, ACT values typically *increase* when CPB is initiated even as the heparin concentration *decreases*. Although measuring heparin concentration on CPB has been shown to correlate more closely with anti-Xa activity than the ACT, the exclusive use of this test without an ACT is not acceptable for cardiac surgery anticoagulation monitoring. Clinical studies have attempted to validate heparin concentration monitoring as a blood sparing technique, but the variable reproducibility of benefits has resulted in a IIb recommendation only.

Clot formation in the bypass circuit and subsequent failure to provide sufficient oxygenation are inevitable if the safe level of anticoagulation is not maintained throughout CPB. Best practices for maintenance of anticoagulation during CPB include regular interval monitoring – usually every 20–30 minutes – of a functional test of anticoagulation, such as ACT. Bolus dosing to achieve a pre-specified heparin concentration or routine fixed interval dosing of heparin during CPB may be used to maintain anticoagulation, and both approaches are supported as a Class IIb recommendation in the STS/SCA/AmSECT Best Practices Guidelines.

Heparin Resistance

Heparin resistance is defined as an inadequate anticoagulant response to heparin despite an adequate plasma concentration. The clinical picture is one of failure to achieve anticoagulation adequate for CPB with heparin doses of up to 600 IU per kilogram of body weight. In many clinical situations, especially when heparin desensitization or the presence of a heparin inhibitor is suspected, heparin "resistance" can be treated by administering increased doses. If the ACT does increase in response to a higher dose, then a more accurate description of this condition would be heparin tachyphylaxis or "altered heparin responsiveness," which is regularly seen in cardiac surgical patients who have been on heparin prior to surgery. It is thought that their altered heparin responsiveness is due to a reduction of AT3 levels, although numerous other mechanisms have been proposed (see Table 6.1). The fact that the temporal course of ACT decrease and AT3 concentration do not mirror each other suggests that AT3 depletion may not be solely responsible. Other possible causes of a heparin resistant state include enhanced factor VIII activity and platelet effects. AT3 concentrate, available as a heat-treated human product or in recombinant form, is indicated as a Class I recommendation for treating patients with documented AT3 deficiency. Congenital AT3 deficiency must be recognized by the inability to increase the ACT even by 50–100% using escalating doses of heparin. In these patients, AT3 repletion should be carefully calculated and administered in close cooperation with a hematologist. In a patient whose ACT will not elevate beyond 350–400 seconds, who has been given additional large heparin doses to treat heparin resistance, to a total dose approaching 600 IU/kg, an empiric diagnosis of acquired AT3 deficiency is usually assumed. In this situation, the STS Blood Conservation Guideline recommendation is to administer AT3. Heparin Induced Thrombocytopenia (HIT, see below) should be considered in the differential diagnosis of intraoperative heparin resistance in patients receiving preoperative heparin therapy.

Heparin Neutralization

Heparin needs to be neutralized in order to avoid unnecessary bleeding after separation from CPB. To this day protamine is the only drug licensed for this indication. Protamine, a strong cation, forms a salt aggregate with heparin, a strong anion. This salt

Table 6.1. Common reasons for heparin resistance

Antithrombin mediated

- Reduced synthesis
- Accelerated clearance
  - o Nephropathy

- Accelerated consumption
  - o Pre-op heparin use
  - o Upregulated hemostatic system
    - DIC
    - Endocarditis
    - DVT/PE
  - o Mechanical
    - CPB
    - VAD
    - IABP
    - ECMO

Non-Antithrombin mediated

- Increased heparin binding
  - o Proteins
    - Chemokines
    - Extracellular matrix proteins
    - Growth factors
    - Enzymes
  - o Platelets
    - Nonspecific binding
    - Thrombophilia
    - Platelet activation
    - Nitroglycerin

aggregate is inactive, has no anticoagulant activity and is rapidly removed from the circulation.

Protamine, in the presence of heparin, has intrinsic anticoagulant properties if given at a higher than necessary dose. Ideally protamine is administered in a way that leaves neither free drug nor free heparin in circulation because non-neutralized heparin results in clinical bleeding and an excess of protamine may produce an undesired coagulopathy. Heparin undergoes metabolism and elimination during the time spent on CPB and it is difficult to estimate the required dose of protamine needed to neutralize the remaining heparin based upon the dose administered and the ACT alone. Doses of protamine in excess of a 1:1 ratio to the amount of heparin administered before and during CPB are not recommended as they may increase the incidence of protamine-related adverse effects.

Ideally the concentration of heparin in blood is measured so that a more accurate dose of protamine can be given. In recent years there has been renewed interest in this subject and several approaches to protamine dosing have been published. Pharmacokinetic models have been yielding promising results in reducing the dose of protamine administered without compromising hemostasis, but they are so far lacking the confirmatory evidence of randomized controlled trials. What all these approaches have in common is the reduction of the protamine dose by 30–50% compared to a 1:1 fixed dose and an associated reduction in post-operative blood loss from pleural and mediastinal drains.

Heparin rebound describes the re-establishment of a heparinized state after heparin has been neutralized. The mechanism behind this phenomenon is not fully understood, but the most common reasons given are:

i. a rapid distribution and clearance of protamine, leaving unbound heparin in circulation;
ii. residua of low molecular weight heparin fragments;
iii. release of heparin from tissue (endothelium, connective tissues) after protamine has been cleared.

Sensitive tests are able to detect low levels of residual heparin for up to six hours after reversal. Clinicians should always consider heparin rebound if there is sudden excessive bleeding after a period of stable hemostasis.

Successful heparin neutralization is usually confirmed by the ACT returning to within 10% of the baseline. It has to be borne in mind that the ACT is relatively insensitive to low levels of heparin and is inferior to aPTT, thrombin time, heparin concentration monitoring or viscoelastic whole blood assays. In case of doubt, one or a combination of these more sensitive tests should be employed to diagnose the cause for intra- or post-operative bleeding (see Chapter 16).

Heparin Induced Thrombocytopenia

Heparin induced thrombocytopenia (HIT) is an immunologic disorder marked by antibodies that bind to the heparin–PF4 complex on platelets. Binding of the antibody causes platelet activation, hyperaggregability, and moderate degrees of thrombocytopenia. It occurs mostly in response to UFH and less commonly to low molecular weight heparin (LMWH). The incidence is between 0.2 and 5% in patients exposed to heparin, with some reports suggesting an incidence as high as 15–20% in patients undergoing cardiac surgery. The increased platelet reactivity causes thrombosis marked by platelet (white) clots. It is often seen 5–14 days after heparin exposure and, if unrecognized, it is potentially life-threatening. Treatment requires immediate cessation of heparin and the institution of an alternate anticoagulant.

The antibodies associated with HIT often become undetectable several weeks after discontinuing heparin and the syndrome does not always reoccur on reexposure. This variability in clinical manifestation makes the management of patients with a history of HIT very complex. The safest option is to avoid further heparin exposure where possible. It is important to be aware that prothrombin complex concentrates and other clotting factor concentrates may contain heparin and may be contraindicated in patients known to have HIT.

Alternative Anticoagulants and Other Techniques in HIT

The choices when treating these patients are few but there are several options if there is no alternative to using heparin:

i. In non-emergency situations surgery has to be postponed until at least 90 days after the last heparin exposure. This allows the antibody to disappear and one short period of heparinization for CPB is generally tolerated without complications.
ii. There have been favorable reports of supplementing heparin administration with pharmacologic platelet inhibition using prostacyclin, iloprost, aspirin, tirofiban or dipyridamole.
iii. Plasmapheresis may be used to reduce antibody levels and immunoglobulin can be given additionally to block platelet activation in the presence of heparin.

The data to support these interventions indicate that they can be used safely, however the lack of randomized controlled trials has rendered them Class IIb recommendations.

The use of heparin can be avoided altogether through anticoagulation with direct thrombin inhibitors such as argatroban or bivalirudin. These thrombin inhibitors have become the standard of care in the management of patients with HIT. Bivalirudin has been studied in prospective multicenter trials in HIT patients undergoing cardiac surgery on CPB. Its use is supported in guidelines published by the Society of Thoracic Surgeons/Society of Cardiovascular Anesthesiologists/American Society of Extracorporeal Technology, where it receives a Class IIa recommendation, and by the American College of Chest Physicians (ACCP). Bivalirudin has a short half-life of 24 minutes and is auto-digested by thrombin, especially in static blood. For these reasons, bivalirudin bolus is accompanied by an infusion during CPB in order to maintain safe anticoagulation. Because of rapid elimination of the anticoagulant, the blood in the circuit must always be flowing, and conduits for parallel flow should be established in the event that the pump flow must be stopped for a period of time. Stasis of blood leads to thrombus formation because bivalirudin is eliminated. This must be taken into consideration when constructing a CPB circuit for use with bivalirudin. As there is no direct antidote to bivalirudin, cessation of its activity occurs by stopping the drug infusion. The infusion must be running until approximately 15–20 minutes before weaning from CPB, which facilitates continued anticoagulation yet allowing hemostasis after CPB to be achieved in a reasonable time frame. See Table 6.2 for the adaptations that need to be made in case a patient is anticoagulated with bivalirudin.

The Future of Anticoagulation for CPB

New anticoagulants that target contact factor activation such as the monoclonal antibody 3F7 to XIIa or a variety of aptamers show promise to either completely replace or reduce the need for co-treatment with heparin. The aptamer 11F7t alone or in combination with R9d-14t, or in its combined form as $RNA_{BA}4$, may be of particular benefit as heparin replacements. Others that target Factor XII (R4c-XII-1t), Kallikrein (Kall1-T4) or factor XI (FELIAP) also allow reduced anticoagulation in combination with conventional heparin or Xa inhibitors. Future CPB tubing is likely to use biomimetics such as covalently bonded heparin or direct thrombin inhibitors like argatroban. Passivation of circuits is currently being attempted using phosphorylcholine,

Table 6.2. Recommended adaptations for CPB with Bivalirudin

	Heparin Protocol	Bivalirudin Protocol
HLM Setup		
Prime	5.000–10.000 IU Heparin	50 mg Bivalirudin
Pressure monitoring on CPB	Post-membrane line pressure	Pre-and post-membrane pressure
Anticoagulation		
Monitoring	ACT	ACT, aPTTr
ACT on CPB	>400 sec, according to institutional practice	>2.5x baseline
aPTTr on CPB		>5x baseline
Conduct on CPB		
Avoiding stagnation	n/a	Recirculation through all closed shunts every 10–20 mins
Collection of blood from surgical field	n/a	Every 15–20 mins, all blood having sat stagnant for longer needs to be discarded or processed with cell salvage
Displacement of excess blood	Standard blood storage bag	Storage in CPCA-1 bag

Table 6.3. Strategies for circuit coating to reduce heparinization

Passivation	• Phosphrylchlorine • Albumin • 2-methoxyrthylacrylate (PMEA)
Biomimetics	• Heparin bonding • Argatroban bonding • N-diazeniumdiolates • RSNO conversions (Cu^{++})
Endothelialization	• Pre-endothelialization with patient stem cells

albumin or poly-2-methoxyethylacrylate (PMEA), which allow the reduction of systemic heparinization during CPB. Using nitric oxide (NO) releasing materials like N-Diazeniumdiolates in combination with a polymer-linked thrombin inhibitor like argatroban has shown promise.

An interesting future concept is the pre-endothelialisation of the circuit. This could either be done as pre-endothelialisation with patient stem cells prior to CPB or by in situ capture of patient stem cells. Currently these concepts are problematic and impractical as they require time to coat a patient circuit (see Table 6.3).

Suggested Further Reading

1. Wardrop D, Keeling D. The story of the discovery of heparin and warfarin. Br J Haematol. 2008;141 (6):757–763.

2. Garcia DA, Baglin TP, Weitz JI et al. Parenteral anticoagulants: Antithrombotic therapy and prevention of thrombosis, 9th ed: American College of Chest Physicians Evidence-Based Clinical Practice Guidelines. Chest. 2012;141 (2 Suppl):e24S–e43S.

3. Bull BS, Korpman RA, Huse WM et al. Heparin therapy during extracorporeal circulation. I. Problems inherent in existing heparin protocols. J Thorac Cardiovasc Surg. 1975;69 (5):674–684.

4. Welsby IJ, McDonnell E, El-Moalem H et al. Activated clotting time systems vary in precision and bias and are not interchangeable when following heparin management protocols during cardiopulmonary bypass. J Clin Monit Comput. 2002;17 (5):287–292.

5. Pappalardo F, Franco A, Crescenzi G et al. Anticoagulation management in patients undergoing open heart surgery by activated clotting time and whole blood heparin concentration. Perfusion. 2006;21(5):285–290.

6. Shore-Lesserson L, Baker RA, Ferraris VA et al. The Society of Thoracic Surgeons, The Society of Cardiovascular Anesthesiologists, and The American Society of ExtraCorporeal Technology: Clinical Practice Guidelines – Anticoagulation during Cardiopulmonary Bypass. Anesth Analg. 2018.

7. Miles LF, Coulson TG, Galhardo C et al. Pump priming practices and anticoagulation in cardiac curgery: Results from the Global Cardiopulmonary Bypass Survey. Anesth Analg. December, 2017; 125(6):1871–1877.

8. Lemmer JH Jr., Despotis GJ. Antithrombin III concentrate to treat heparin resistance in patients undergoing cardiac surgery. J Thorac Cardiovasc Surg. 2002;123(2):213–217.

9. Chabata CV, Frederiksen JW, Sullenger BA et al. Emerging applications of aptamers for anticoagulation and hemostasis. Curr Opin Hematol. 2018;25 (5):382–388.

Conduct of Cardiopulmonary Bypass

Christiana Burt, Timothy A Dickinson, Narain Moorjani and Caitlin Blau

The safe conduct of cardiopulmonary bypass (CPB) requires excellent teamwork, clear communication and collaboration between surgical, anesthetic, perfusion and nursing teams. A comprehensive understanding of both the mechanics and physiology of CPB is essential to achieve optimum benefit and reduce the risks.

The goals of CPB are to provide a still and bloodless field for the surgeon to operate while not damaging the heart muscle. This chapter reviews the conduct of CPB starting with cannulation (arterial and venous), general management of both the mechanical and physiological aspects of CPB and finishes with a section regarding important aspects of CPB relating to minimally invasive cardiac surgery (MICS). It is important that each institution has detailed protocols and procedures for CPB, and many of the points discussed in this chapter will be performed within the construct of these protocols.

Arterial Cannulation

The arterial cannula is usually the narrowest part of the CPB circuit. The resultant high resistance and pressure gradients produce high velocity jets and turbulence. The effect of the jets on the interior wall of the aorta can lead to arterial dissection, embolization and flow disturbances in the head and neck vessels.

The hemodynamic properties of an arterial cannula can be assessed by their "performance index," which is defined as the ratio of pressure gradient to cannula outer diameter at any given flow rate. Ideally for every case the cannulae are chosen to minimize this value. To optimize hemodynamic performance the narrowest portion of the catheter that enters the aorta should be as short as safely possible and the diameter should then gradually increase in size to minimize the gradient. Pressure gradients greater than 100 mmHg can cause excessive hemolysis and

should be avoided. Cannula selection can be guided using pressure to flow charts, which are provided by the manufacturers. It should be noted that these chart values are usually derived with water as the test fluid. Many different types of cannulae are available and are discussed further in Chapter 2.

"Straight" arterial cannulae are the most commonly used type, with some having a flange to allow secure fixation to the aorta with minimal tip within the vessel. The straight design allows non-turbulent blood flow through the cannula, but results in a single jet of blood, which can cause damage to the aortic wall. The straight nature of the cannula means that the flow direction is reliant on the surgical placement (see Figure 7.1).

Right-angled cannulae have been designed to allow the jet to be directed around the aortic arch, assuming correct placement. Right-angled "diffusion" cannulae, with side holes and a sealed end, may attenuate the damaging jet effect by changing the flow characteristics inside the aorta. However, concern has been expressed regarding an increased risk of hemolysis due to the more turbulent flow through the cannula. These cannulae are not suitable for placement at any site other than the ascending aorta. In certain situations cannulation of the ascending aorta or aortic arch can be performed with a guidewire using a Seldinger technique, either to minimize trauma to the aorta, or in the presence of acute aortic dissection, to ensure placement of the cannula into the true lumen in conjunction with transesophageal echocardiographic guidance.

In addition to direct placement of the arterial cannula in the aorta, arterial return can also be achieved by peripheral arterial cannulation, such as via the femoral, axillary or innominate artery, cannulation of the side arm of a prosthetic graft or in rare circumstances via the left ventricular apex, and they are discussed in the following section.

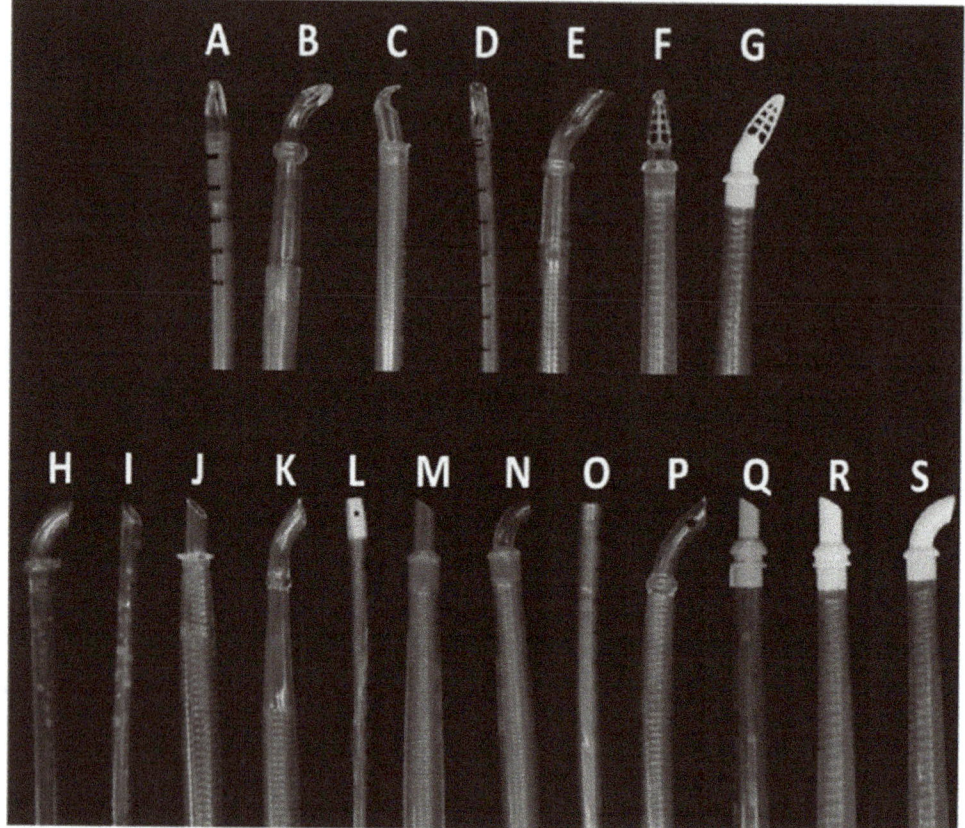

Figure 7.1 Aortic cannula options. Dispersion cannulae on top row (A–G). Non-dispersion cannulae on the bottom row (H–S). (Reproduced from: McDonald et al. "Hydrodynamic evaluation of aortic cardiopulmonary bypass cannulae using particle image velocimetry." *Perfusion* 2016; 31(1): 78–86.)

Connecting the Patient

The usual cannulation site is the ascending aorta, which offers the following advantages:

- ease
- safety
- single incision
- ability to deliver antegrade flow
- size not usually limited by mismatch between vessel and cannula outer diameter (typical sizes range from 18 Fr to 24 Fr)
- no risk of limb ischemia.

Although the site for cannulation in the ascending aorta is traditionally determined by intraoperative digital palpation for calcific atherosclerotic plaques, newer techniques such as epiaortic ultrasound scanning have been shown to be more sensitive at determining plaque-free areas for cannulation (see Figure 7.2). If the extent of the atherosclerosis is significant enough to make aortic cannulation and cross-clamping unsafe because of the risk of stroke due to dislodgement and embolization of atherosclerotic material, alternative cannulation sites should be considered. Retrograde perfusion via femoral arterial cannulation is not without risk of embolization of atheroma either and subclavian or innominate arterial cannulation may be preferable. In the event of a totally calcified "porcelain aorta," alternative strategies that minimize aortic handling, such as off pump coronary artery bypass grafting (OPCAB), the use of deep hypothermic circulatory arrest (DHCA) or alternative catheter based techniques may be appropriate. If the ascending aorta has ruptured in a patient with acute aortic syndrome, the arterial cannula can be placed directly in the true lumen following transection of the ascending aorta.

After ensuring that the patient is sufficiently anticoagulated (see Chapter 6) prior to insertion of the aortic cannula, the chosen site is prepared with placement of opposing purse-string sutures and clearance

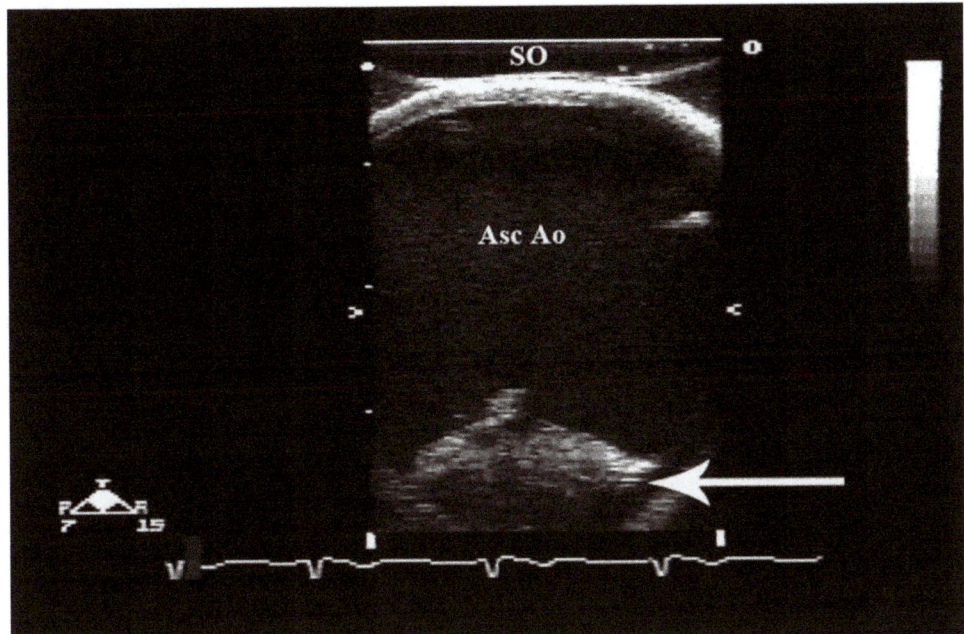

Figure 7.2 Epiaortic ultrasonographic short-axis image of mid ascending (*Asc*) aorta (*Ao*) with significant atheroma (*arrow*) obtained with linear-array transducer. *SO*, Saline standoff to enhance acoustic transmission. (Reproduced from Glas KE, Swaminathan M, Reeves ST et al.; Council for Intraoperative Echocardiography of the American Society of Echocardiography; Society of Cardiovascular Anesthesiologists; Society of Thoracic Surgeons. Guidelines for the performance of a comprehensive intraoperative epiaortic ultrasonographic examination: Recommendations of the American Society of Echocardiography and the Society of Cardiovascular Anesthesiologists; endorsed by the Society of Thoracic Surgeons. Anesth Analg. 2008 May;106(5):1376–1384.)

of the adventitial tissue within the boundaries of these sutures. With the mean arterial pressure between 60 and 70 mmHg to avoid excessive bleeding or trauma, a full-thickness incision is made in the aortic wall through which the aortic cannula is passed. Only 1–2 cm of the cannula tip is advanced and directed toward the arch to avoid inadvertent cannulation of the head and neck vessels or trauma to the posterior wall. The aortic cannula is immediately de-aired by allowing blood to fill the tubing, which is then clamped and secured with the purse-string sutures. Once securely in place, the aortic cannula is connected to the arterial inflow tubing of the bypass circuit, also ensuring that no air is present at the connection site. Once connected, the perfusionist will inform the surgeon of the presence of pulsatility and corresponding mean arterial line pressure within the system to confirm correct intraluminal placement of the cannula – seen as a "good swing" on analog manometers.

Complications of Aortic Root Cannulation

If air is introduced into the arterial limb of the CPB circuit during cannulation, it must be disconnected from the aortic cannula and the air removed from i)

the circuit by pumping fluid into the field and ii) from the cannula by bleeding back prior to reconnection. If gross air embolism is noted in the aortic line during established CPB, it may be possible for the perfusionist to remove the air via recirculation lines within the circuit with only a brief interruption to pump flow. If gross systemic air embolism occurs, de-airing of the cerebral circulation has priority. The first step is to terminate CPB, followed by removal of the arterial cannula leaving the purse-string sutures loose. Simultaneously, the anesthesiologist places the patient in Trendelenburg position and performs bilateral carotid compression. The source of air should be identified and remedied followed by de-airing of the CPB circuit. The arterial line cannula is then inserted into the superior vena cava (SVC) or, if present in bicaval cannulation, is connected to an existing SVC cannula. Retrograde cerebral perfusion (RCP) via the SVC using low flow rates of 1–2 liters per minute, at a blood temperature of 20°C, will enable de-airing of the cerebral circulation back to the aorta. This should be performed for 2–3 minutes or until no more air can be seen coming out of the aortotomy site. The aorta can be re-cannulated upon completion of RCP,

Table 7.1. Complications of ascending aortic cannulation

Inability to introduce the cannula
- Adventitia occluding the incision site
- Inadequate incision size
- Atheromatous plaque within the aortic wall

Intramural placement

Embolization of atheromatous plaque

Air embolization on connection to the circuit

Persistent bleeding around cannula or peri-aortic hematoma

Malposition of tip toward the aortic valve or into the arch vessels

Dissection of the aorta

Inadequate size leading to high pressure and low flow generation

Aneurysm formation at the site of cannulation at a later stage

Table 7.2. Complications of peripheral cannulation

Trauma to the vessel

Retrograde arterial dissection with retroperitoneal hemorrhage or extension of dissection to the aortic root

Thrombosis or embolism

Hemorrhage

Limb ischemia (which can be reduced by using an end to side polytetrafluoroethane (PTFE) or Dacron™ graft sutured to the vessel)

Malperfusion of cerebral and systemic circulation as a result of cannulation of the false lumen of an aortic dissection

Lymph fistula or lymphocele

Infection

Damage to neighboring neurovascular structures, such as femoral vein or brachial plexus

Late vascular stenosis

and upon recommencing CPB should be run in hypothermia for 30–45 minutes. The use of relative hypothermia increases the solubility of gaseous emboli and may reduce the extent of cerebral injury. Once surgery is completed and the patient has been stabilized, CPB should be discontinued at a core temperature of 35°C.

Further potential complications of aortic root cannulation are summarized in Table 7.1.

Peripheral Arterial Cannulation

Peripheral arterial cannulation, most commonly via the femoral or axillary route, is used in the following instances:

1. Establishment of CPB prior to sternotomy or anesthetic induction due to hemodynamic instability
2. Selected redo-sternotomy procedures to allow for controlled conditions during sternotomy and exposure of the heart
3. Aortic aneurysm surgery
4. Aorta not suitable for cannulation due to calcification, such as a "porcelain aorta"
5. Thoracic surgery
6. Minimally invasive cardiac surgery (MICS)
7. Extracorporeal membrane oxygenation (ECMO)

Femoral cannulation necessitates the of use smaller 15–21 Fr. cannulae due to the size of the femoral vessels, with consequent higher pressure gradients, jet effects and possibly lower flow rates. This may be improved by cannulation of iliac arteries. The femoral arterial cannula is inserted over a guidewire, either percutaneously or via a cut-down, and advanced into the aorta. Transesophageal echocardiography (TEE) is used to visualize the guidewire and arterial cannula in order to achieve optimal placement and minimize vascular injury.

The axillary artery is less likely than the femoral artery to have atherosclerotic disease or dissection and also has good collateral flow, with less risk of limb ischemia. In addition to these benefits, it provides antegrade flow, with reduced risk of cerebral embolization. Direct arterial cannulation is uncommon. End to side placement of a polytetrafluoroethane (PTFE) or Dacron™ graft is preferable to direct cannulation, as it allows for improved limb perfusion distal to the cannulation site. In lieu of using an arterial cannula, a 3/8 inch tubing connector is tied onto the end of the graft and attached to the arterial line of the CPB circuit.

The potential complications of peripheral cannulation are summarized in Table 7.2.

Venous Cannulation

Venous drainage is vitally important as it not only influences perfusion pressure in vital organs but also because it is essential for providing the blood source necessary for pump flow. Blood flow into the CPB circuit is usually achieved by gravity drainage, using the "siphon" effect. Gravity siphoning as the means of obtaining adequate drainage relies on:

1. no air being present in the tubing between the patient and the pump, otherwise an "air lock" can develop and stop drainage,
2. the venous reservoir being kept below the level of the patient's thorax and
3. the absence of venous line obstructions (e.g. kinks or clamps).

The degree of venous drainage is determined by

- the patient's central venous pressure (CVP)
- the difference in height between the patient and the top of the blood level in the venous reservoir
- the resistance exerted by the circuit (cannulae, lines and connectors).

The creation of excessive negative pressure in the venous line may cause the veins to collapse around the cannula with intermittent reduction in venous drainage (e.g. venous line chatter) and the potential for generation of gaseous microemboli (GME) in the circuit, a phenomenon referred to as "cavitation." GME are a known risk of CPB and a specific concern for postoperative neurocognitive dysfunction. Efforts to ameliorate cavitation include partial occluding of the venous line, reducing vacuum assist venous drainage (VAVD) pressure and decreasing venous cannula size.

The various available types and sizes of venous cannulae are discussed in Chapter 2. The cannula tip is the narrowest component in the venous circuit and therefore the limiting factor for venous drainage. The appropriate size is selected based on the flow characteristics of the cannula (detailed in the manufacturer's guidelines) and the required cardiac index for the patient. One-third of total flow is derived from superior vena cava (SVC) drainage and two-thirds from inferior vena cava (IVC) drainage.

Connection to the Patient

This is usually achieved via right atrial (RA) cannulation. The two most common approaches include cavo-atrial and bicaval. In urgent situations, a single cannula can be placed through the RA appendage.

- **Cavo-atrial** – This uses a "two-stage" cannula, which has a wider proximal portion with side holes that lie in the RA, and a narrow extension, with end and side holes, that extends into the IVC. This cannula is typically inserted through the right atrial appendage and cannot be used if the right heart is to be opened as it will invariably entrain air.
- **Bicaval** – Purse-string sutures are placed on the posterior-inferior RA wall and the RA appendage to enable direct cannulation of the IVC and SVC respectively. Tapes or snares are passed around the venae cavae, with the cannulae in place to ensure that the patient's entire venous return flows into the CPB circuit and to prevent air from entering the venous lines when opening the RA, or blood leaking past the cannulae into the RA. This is referred to as caval occlusion or total CPB and is the technique of choice if the right heart is to be opened.

Most coronary (CABG) and aortic valve (AVR) surgery is performed with venous drainage via cavo-atrial cannulation, while mitral and tricuspid valve procedures require bicaval cannulation. While this approach usually provides adequate drainage, it is essential to constantly monitor right heart decompression and for the perfusionist to communicate any interruptions in venous return as cannula adjustments can be necessary during the operation to accommodate changes in heart position or cannula migration. Rarely, the right heart may need to be vented via the pulmonary artery to prevent right ventricular (RV) distension due to return of blood into the RA via the coronary sinus. Occasionally, high SVC or even innominate vein cannulation may be required to facilitate resection of an RA tumor or during an operation requiring access to the SVC, such as some heart transplant or heart-lung transplant procedures (Domino heart).

Air entry into the venous side of the circuit may lead to an "air lock," causing obstruction of venous drainage, or to systemic GME. The most common reason for air entry is failure to seal the site around the cannulae adequately or excessive negative venous line pressure. Care must be taken to ensure that purse-string sutures are airtight, and negative venous line pressure is not causing cavitation. If cavitation

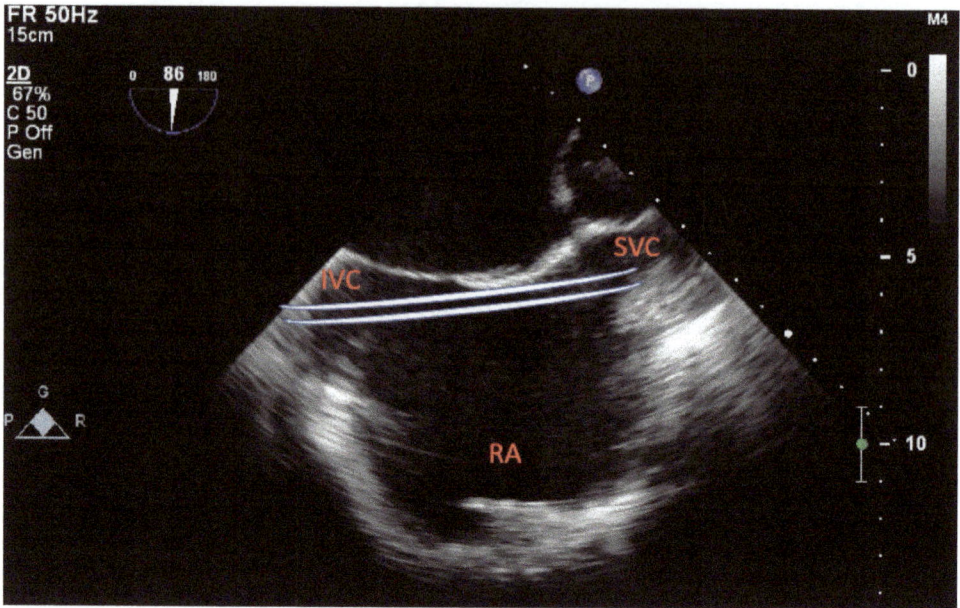

Figure 7.3 Schematic of multistage cannula position across inferior vena cava (IVC), right atrium (RA) and superior vena cava (SVC).

persists, the surgeon should check that the cannulation purse-strings are secure and the perfusionist can either reduce VAVD or partially occlude the venous line. The perfusionist should notify the surgeon anytime venous air entrainment is visualized.

In semi-emergency situations, a single stage cannula – often referred to as a Ross Atrial Basket – can be introduced into the RA and, with the arterial cannula in place, CPB can be rapidly initiated.

Peripheral Venous Cannulation

This is usually performed via the femoral or iliac veins. Indications for peripheral venous cannulation are the same as for peripheral arterial cannulation, with the exception of a calcified aorta.

Drainage through peripheral cannulation is achieved by using an appropriately sized cannula and passing it so the tip is located in the caval/RA junction often using TEE guidance. A multistage cannula can be placed via the femoral vein with drainage holes in the IVC, RA and SVC (see Figure 7.3). Selecting femoral venous cannulae that have numerous side holes permits greater venous drainage and subsequent better arterial blood flow.

An additional cannula can be placed in the SVC via the right internal jugular vein to optimize venous drainage. Typically, a 15–18 Fr peripheral cannula is

utilized in this approach. The SVC cannula is generally placed percutaneously and under TEE guidance.

Venous drainage and subsequent systemic blood flow can be dramatically augmented utilizing VAVD. There are potential hazards associated with VAVD, including cavitation and air embolism. Using an approved vacuum regulator that restricts maximum vacuum to −80 mmHg and positive and negative pressure relief valves on the venous reservoir help mitigate against these complications.

Further possible complications associated with venous cannulation are listed in Table 7.3.

General Sequence of Events for the Conduct of CPB

Before commencing CPB the perfusionists must have completed a series of "checks" as detailed in Chapter 4.

Connecting the Patient to the CPB Circuit

- The surgeon will ask for permission to divide the CPB lines
- The pump flow is slowly reduced, and the venous line clamped, followed by the arterial line and all recirculation lines
- The ACT is confirmed to be adequate for bypass

Table 7.3. Complications of venous cannulation

Low cardiac output due to compression of the heart during IVC purse-string placement

Damage to SVC/IVC/right pulmonary artery while passing tapes around cavae

Reduction in cardiac output prior to commencement of CPB when cannulae are in place

Atrial dysrhythmia

Malpositioning of the cannula tip	SVC cannula into the azygos vein IVC cannula into the hepatic vein RA cannula into LA in the presence of an atrial secundum defect

RA trauma and bleeding from cannulation sites

SVC or IVC laceration on manipulation of cannulated RA

Narrowing of cavae after decannulation and closure of purse-string sutures

- The surgeon will cannulate the aorta or peripheral arterial vessel
- As required, the arterial pump is turned to assist in an air free connection
- When the line is free of air the surgeon will connect the arterial line
- The clamp is removed from the arterial line
- The perfusionist confirms that the arterial line is reading correctly and is consistent with patient pressures. If using a manometer this is confirmed by an appropriate pulse pressure ("good swing")
- The patency of the arterial cannula should be tested by administering a test dose of pump prime to the patient while watching for a spike in the arterial line pressure. The perfusionist states if the test was successful
- If the perfusionist has any doubts about the cannulation, they must inform the surgeon immediately and continue to voice their misgivings until they are confident that the cannula is satisfactorily placed
- The surgeon will cannulate the venous circulation as required
- The pump suckers are ready for salvaging any blood loss and the shed blood can be retransfused through the arterial line ("give what you are getting")

Initiating CPB

- If the gases have not yet been switched on, they are now correctly set according to the patient's anticipated full flow
- The perfusionist clearly informs the rest of the team that the patient is "going onto bypass"
- The clamp, or electronic occluder, on the arterial line is opened and the pump is turned on slowly, gradually increasing the rpm
- When going onto bypass with a centrifugal pump, forward pressure must be generated before the line clamp is removed. The drive motor is therefore turned on while the aortic line is still clamped, in order to generate sufficient forward pressure, to exceed the patient's arterial pressure; above 1500–2000 rpm is usual
- The perfusionist must monitor the line pressure during this stage, looking for any sign of obstruction, at the same time as monitoring the venous and arterial pressures and the blood level in the venous reservoir, as the pump speed is increased
- Having raised the pressure on the venous side, the venous clamp, or the electronic venous occluder, is slowly opened, and the perfusionist should control the venous pressure by adjusting venous clamping until they have achieved full flow for the patient. In situations where air is left in the venous line prior to initiation of bypass, the venous clamps may need to be opened more rapidly to avoid air locks, until this air has been removed
- The team is informed when full flow has been achieved, the anesthesiologist may discontinue ventilation at this point
- Any difficulty in achieving a full venous return is reported immediately to the surgeons, so that they can make any adjustment to the venous cannulation that may be necessary; persistent venous air should also be reported to the surgeons
- Once a steady state of perfusion (e.g. target arterial blood flow and blood pressure) has been attained, the aorta has been clamped, and cardioplegia has been administered, laboratory tests should be sent (see also Chapter 10)

The Rewarming Phase

The majority of cases done on CPB are conducted at temperatures in the range of 30–34°C with the patient allowed to passively drift to target temperature,

63

Table 7.4. Temperature management

Arterial Blood Temp	13–37°C
Core Temp	16–37°C
Target Core Temp for separation from CPB	≥35°C
Warming Gradients (Arterial to Venous)	• Core temp below 30°C: ≤10°C • Core temp above 30°C: ≤4°C
Rewarming Rate (Core Temp)	≤0.5°C/min

Table 7.5. Adequacy of perfusion

Parameter	Target
Mean Arterial Pressure	60–80 mmHg
Cardiac Index	>2.4 L/min/m²
DO_2 Index	>280 mLO$_2$/min/m²
Hemoglobin	70–80 g/L
SvO_2	>65%
Cerebral Oximetry	>50% and/or <20% drop from baseline

although some surgeons prefer to stay normothermic. More complex operations are often conducted at moderate or deep hypothermia (between 28° and 18°C).

Rewarming begins after consultation with the surgeon. Once commenced, appropriate adjustments to gas flows and to blood flows must be made as a rapid drop in S_VO_2 may be experienced. An arterial blood gas sample should be taken during the mid-warming phase, in order to give sufficient time for any corrective action to be taken before coming off bypass. Final blood samples may be taken once a core temperature of >35°C has been attained.

- The arterial blood temperature and patient core temperature are used to guide rate and extent of rewarming
- A gradient of 10°C between arterial outlet and venous inflow on the oxygenator should not be exceeded
- The target arterial outlet blood temperature should not exceed 37.0°C
- The duration of rewarming has to allow time for distribution of heat between core and peripheral tissues, using vasodilators, if needed, to enhance peripheral blood flow and thus heat distribution
- It is reasonable to limit the rate of rewarming, when the arterial blood temperature is greater than 30°C, to ≤0.5°C per minute
- Post-CPB an "after drop" in core temperature occurs as heat is redistributed from core to peripheral tissues; this after drop can be lessened if adequate time is allowed for thorough rewarming

The general principles of temperature management are summarized in Table 7.4 and this is discussed in more detail in Chapter 9.

Monitoring during CPB

Following commencement of CPB and after the patient is on full flow with adequate decompression of the heart, ventilation can be switched off or adjusted, based on the lung protection strategy. Various patient parameters should be continuously monitored to ensure adequate perfusion. Table 7.5 outlines these parameters and their respective targets, which should be adjusted for each patient's need (see Chapter 3 for detailed review of monitoring).

Pressure Management

Mean arterial blood pressure (MAP) – is determined by flow rate and arteriolar resistance. An acceptable MAP on CPB is one which provides adequate tissue perfusion. Adequate tissue perfusion is not only influenced by the MAP, but also by pump flow, core body temperature, and patient comorbidities. In general, it is recommended to maintain higher pressures in the presence of known cerebrovascular disease, in particular carotid stenosis, renal dysfunction or left ventricular hypertrophy.

There mostly is a transient drop in systemic pressure on commencement of CPB. This is the result of:

1. vasodilatation associated with the sudden decrease in blood viscosity resulting from hemodilution through the CPB prime and
2. the systemic inflammatory response associated with CPB.

As CPB continues, vascular resistance gradually increases as a result of equilibration of fluid between the vascular and tissue "compartments," hemoconcentration from diuresis, the increase in blood viscosity seen with hypothermia and the progressive increase in circulating levels of catecholamines and renin as part of the stress response to CPB. However, intermittent boluses of vasopressor are commonly required to maintain an acceptable MAP during CPB.

It is important to emphasize that manipulation of MAP alone is not sufficient to guarantee adequate organ perfusion. Neither a low MAP with a high flow nor a high MAP with a low flow are sufficient in themselves. We advise that whole body oxygen delivery (DO_2) be optimized, and vascular resistance adjusted with vasopressors or dilators to bring the MAP into the autoregulatory range for critical organ beds.

Pulmonary artery (PA) and left atrial (LA) pressure – the PA and LA pressures should be close to zero on CPB. LA pressure monitoring can be useful during CPB to assess left ventricular distension, in particular in cases where an increase in blood flow back to the left heart is expected (cyanotic heart disease, large bronchial flow in chronic lung disease or aortic regurgitation). It is therefore most commonly used during bypass in complex pediatric and adult congenital surgery. LA pressure is usually measured using a transduced catheter or needle directly placed into the left atrium or placed into the left atrium via the right superior pulmonary vein. In cases where a pulmonary artery catheter has been inserted, the pressure reading at the tip of the catheter can be taken as a surrogate of LA pressure but may not always be accurate, particularly if pulmonary vascular pathology is present. Care must be taken with PA catheters to ensure that the catheter tip does not migrate proximally, leading to "wedging" and subsequent PA rupture or lung infarction. Interrogation of the PA catheter position with TEE and frequent observation of the PA waveform are best practice to avoid this complication.

Central venous pressure (CVP) – on CPB, the CVP is expected to be close to zero and no more than in single digits. If a potential issue with the central venous catheter has been excluded, an increase in CVP generally indicates impaired venous drainage. A high CVP during bypass reduces effective perfusion of critical organs. A bulging right heart and/or engorgement of the patient's head and eyes should prompt immediate corrective action. Common causes are inadequate cannula size, obstruction to the cannula tip and insufficient height difference between the patient and the reservoir to enable gravity drainage.

Adding VAVD should be considered if correcting the above does not improve the situation.

Electrocardiogram (ECG) – the ECG must be observed throughout CPB to ensure that it remains isoelectric during cardioplegic arrest. Persistent ST segment changes following removal of the aortic clamp and resumption of myocardial activity may indicate ischemia from inadequate re-vascularization, coronary ostial obstruction, such as by an incorrectly seated aortic valve prosthesis, or air/particulate embolization into the coronary arteries.

Temperature – the principal reason for hypothermic CPB is to protect the heart and other organs by reducing metabolic rate and thus oxygen requirements. Temperature can be measured in the following locations: nasopharynx, tympanic membrane, pulmonary artery, bladder or rectum, arterial inflow, water entering heat exchanger and venous return. Nasopharyngeal temperature probes underestimate, but approximate to brain temperature, while the mixed venous temperature on the CPB circuit is an approximation of average body temperature.

For more detail see Chapters 9 and 11.

Urine output – urine output on CPB is monitored as an indicator of renal perfusion. Indications for diuretic use during CPB include hyperkalemia, hemoglobinuria and hemodilution. Mannitol is an osmotic diuretic which is commonly added to the priming fluid of the bypass circuit in order to stimulate urine production during bypass. The aim is to help reduce hypervolemia and may enable hemoglobinuria to be more effectively cleared, however there is little clear evidence for or against its routine use. Urine output would be expected to be >1 ml/kg/hr (and is often much higher that this) but it is important to note that acute kidney injury can occur via many different mechanisms and may still develop despite adequate urine production.

Laboratory investigations – are discussed in detail in Chapter 10. At a minimum, monitoring during CPB requires measurement of PO_2, PCO_2, base excess (BE), hemoglobin, HCT, pH, potassium, glucose, lactate, and coagulation status using ACT or heparin concentration.

Transesophageal echocardiography (TEE) – TEE is applied increasingly as a routine part of cardiac surgery. It is a useful tool to assess adequacy of de-airing of the heart, intracardiac structures (valves, sub-valvular apparatus, prostheses, septal walls, left and right ventricular outflow tracts) and global and regional wall motion. The opportunity to obtain routine images of cardiac and valvular function usually ends once the patient is transitioned onto cardiopulmonary bypass, due to the fact that blood is diverted away from the heart, and the chambers will no longer be full. There are a few circumstances however in which TEE can still be of use:

- Sudden loss of venous drainage is often the result of a two-stage or IVC cannula tip migrating into a hepatic vein. This can often be visualized on TEE prior to the surgeon withdrawing the cannula by the appropriate amount.

- In circumstances where the LV cannot be adequately assessed visually (e.g. during minimally invasive surgery or due to extensive scar tissue in redo surgery), TEE can be used to see whether aortic regurgitation is resulting in filling and dilation of the LV during administration of aortic root cardioplegia. It is extremely important to avoid LV dilation as the increase in wall tension leads to a reduction in subendocardial perfusion and possible ischemic complications. If the LV is seen to be dilating on TEE, cardioplegia must be stopped and the LV vent started to empty out the chamber before restarting cardioplegia. The degree and speed of LV dilation and the ability to achieve asystole on the ECG will determine whether this cardioplegia strategy is persisted with.

- Positioning of coronary sinus cannula: Correct position inside the coronary sinus can usually be visualized (see Figure 7.4). It is important to monitor the pressure in the cannula during administration of retrograde cardioplegia to avoid over-pressurizing as pressures greater than 30mmHg may risk rupturing the vein which can be extremely difficult to repair and can be a catastrophic complication. Sometimes the cannula can slip back into the right atrium despite correct initial positioning and will most commonly be picked up via the lack of rise in pressure on administration of cardioplegia.

- The descending aorta can still be adequately visualized on bypass and this can aid with the positioning of an intra-aortic balloon pump. TEE examination can confirm the presence of the wire in the aorta and can guide placing the balloon tip just distal to the left subclavian artery origin or distal to the arch if the origin of the left subclavian

artery is not visible. The tip is seen as being a mobile echogenic structure which moves around inside the blood vessel when the balloon pump is switched on (see Figure 7.5). Visualization of the descending aorta or arch can also be used to interrogate for the presence of an aortic dissection in circumstances where there is a rise in pressure in the arterial limb of the bypass circuit or there are difficulties achieving adequate perfusion.

Maintaining a Bloodless Surgical Field

The main aim of CPB is to create a motionless and bloodless surgical field. Several different techniques are used to work in concert to achieve that:

Cardiotomy Suction

After systemic heparinization and confirmation of an adequate ACT, designated cardiotomy suckers are used to collect shed blood in the reservoir for recirculation within the CPB circuit. Cardiotomy suction is most commonly generated by use of a roller pump. If the pump rate is too high the negative pressure at the sucker tip may lead to hemolysis and occlusion of the sucker. Regular adjusting of the pump rate by the perfusionist and of the sucker position by the surgeon helps avoid that problem.

It is essential that the direction of the cardiotomy suckers is confirmed prior to use. The perfusionist and the surgical team need to ensure that they are indeed sucking and not blowing air toward the patient. They are generally tested by submerging the tips in clear fluid and observing that the fluid is being sucked away from the field and air is not exiting the sucker creating bubbles. Assessments such as this must be included in pre-bypass checklists.

In extreme cases of hemorrhage, such as injury of the right ventricle during chest entry in a redo operation, after heparinization and with the arterial cannula in situ, the patient can be placed on "sucker bypass," where the shed blood in the operative field provides venous return to the CPB circuit until formal venous cannulation can be secured.

Adverse Effects of Cardiotomy Suction

Blood suctioned from the surgical field is highly "activated." Hemolysis, coagulation products,

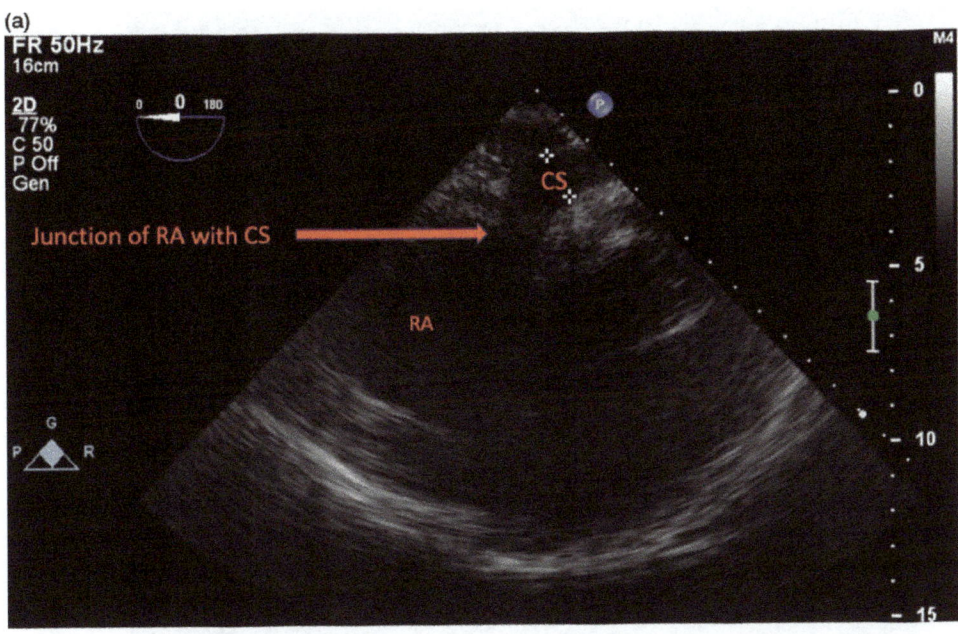

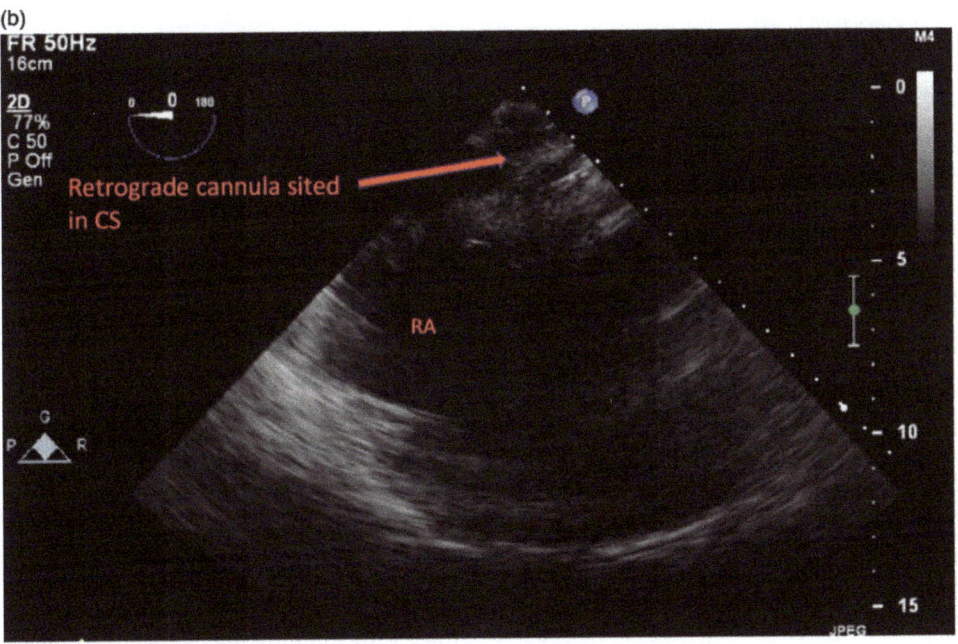

Figure 7.4 Right atrium (RA) with coronary sinus (CS) shown before (a) and after (b) insertion of retrograde cannula into coronary sinus.

microparticles, fat, cellular debris and aggregates cause a surge in inflammatory mediators (tumor necrosis factor alpha (TNF-α), interleukin-6 (IL-6), C3a) and endotoxins. Another potential determinant of injury caused by cardiotomy suction is the amount of room air co-aspirated with blood.

Commonly used strategies to reduce the side effects of cardiotomy suction are shown in Table 7.6.

67

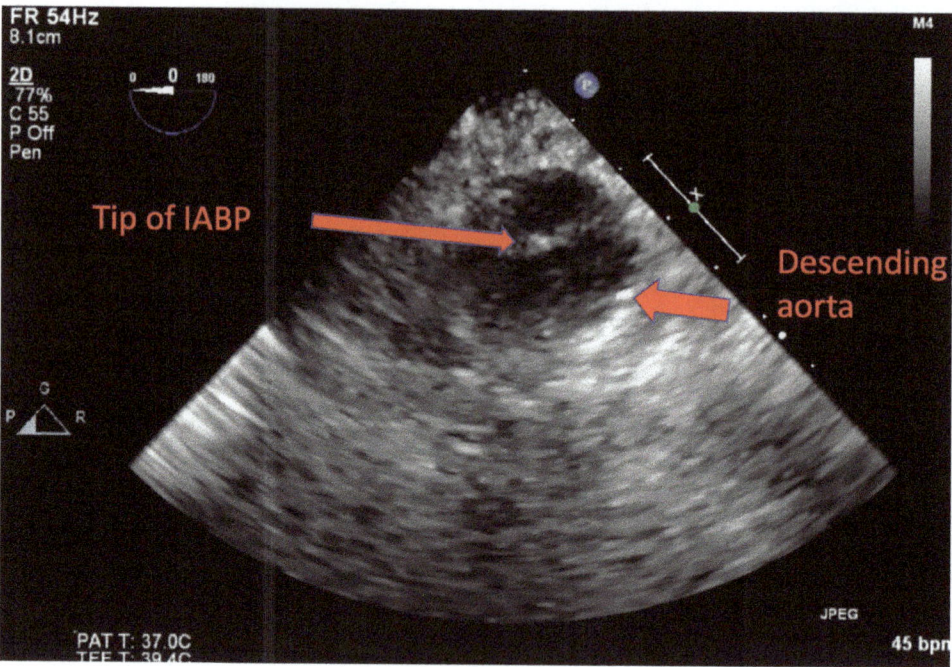

Figure 7.5 TEE image of IAPB tip placed in the proximal descending aorta.

Table 7.6. Strategies to reduce the side effects of cardiotomy suction

Hemostasis throughout operation to minimize shed blood	
Minimize aspiration of air through the cardiotomy suction by	Avoidance of high negative pressures
	Slow rates of suction
	Not sucking the surgical field dry
	Keeping the suction tip under level of blood
Filtration of cardiotomy suction blood (leukocyte depletion)	
Cell salvage blood instead of cardiotomy suction	
MiECC	

Keeping the Heart Relaxed

While on CPB, the left side of the heart receives blood from bronchial arteries and Thebesian veins and the right heart receives blood from the coronary sinus and "leakage" around the venous cannulae. As the ventricles are unable to eject during the period of arrest, they may be vented to protect the heart from distension. Ventricular distension is undesirable because excessive myocardial stretching increases myocardial oxygen demand, impairs subendocardial perfusion and may result in myofibrillar disruption.

On occasions, blood can return from abnormal sources. These include:

● left-sided SVC
● patent ductus arteriosus (PDA)
● atrial septal defect/ventricular septal defect
● anomalous venous drainage
● aortic regurgitation
● systemic to pulmonary shunt.

Detection of LV Distension

The left ventricle needs to be vented if it is filling from any source but not ejecting. It will fill primarily because of aortic insufficiency, or during cardioplegia administration. Surgical inspection and palpation of the LV to monitor the degree of distension is crucial on commencing CPB, during aortic cross-clamping and during initial administration of cardioplegia. Although LA and PA pressure monitoring can help detect moderate LV distension, TEE is probably best placed to assess this. If the heart is well decompressed and empty, it will not be possible to obtain recognizable images. However if there is blood present in the heart then TEE views will be obtainable and can be used to assess for active chamber enlargement.

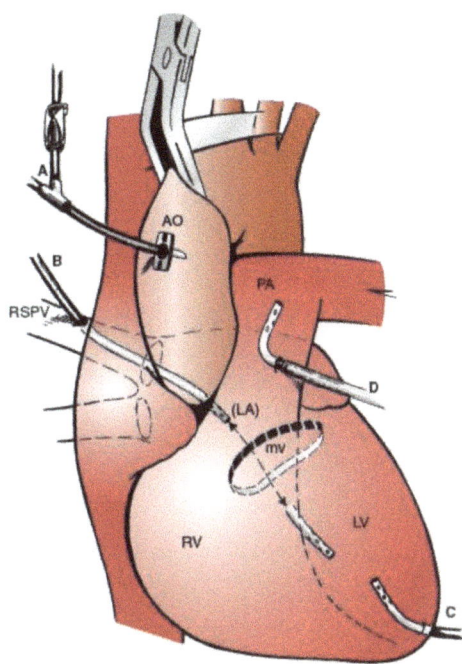

Figure 7.6 Sites to use to vent the heart during cardiopulmonary bypass A) aortic root, B) right superior pulmonary vein, C) left ventricular apex, and D) pulmonary artery. LA = left atrium; MV = mitral valve; RV = right ventricle; AO = aorta; PA = pulmonary artery; LV = left ventricle. (Reprinted from: Hessel EA II. Circuitry and cannulation techniques. In Gravlee GP et al. *Cardiopulmonary bypass*. Philadelphia, PA: Lippincott Williams & Wilkins; 2008:90.)

Venting the Heart

Vent suction is most commonly achieved using a roller pump. The principle is similar to that governing cardiotomy suction and therefore the direction of the pump must also be confirmed via a "sucker (fluid) test." The potential for fatal air embolism exists if a sucker attached to an aortic root vent was to pump air into the patient instead of removing blood. A one-way valve must also be included to further reduce the risk of air being inadvertently introduced via the vent site.

The venous cannula effectively vents the right side of the heart, keeping it empty of blood except for any "leakage" past the cannula, which can be minimized by using bicaval cannulation and caval snares. When antegrade cardioplegia is administered, releasing the caval snares will permit venting of cardioplegia solution returning via the coronary sinus to the right heart.

Placement of a pulmonary arterial vent will keep the right ventricle empty of fluid. The presence of a persistent left SVC requires additional drainage of the coronary sinus or RA in most cases.

The most common vent sites, as illustrated in Figure 7.6, are:

- ascending aorta via aortic root cardioplegia cannula with vent line – this method does not allow venting during cardioplegia administration
- right superior pulmonary vein – a vent is passed into the left atrium and through the mitral valve into the LV
- aortic root, using a cardiotomy sucker placed through the aortic valve into the LV (in patients undergoing an aortic valve replacement)
- left ventricular apex
- pulmonary artery – this may not be effective at venting the LV when there is aortic regurgitation with a competent mitral valve.

It must be remembered that venting the heart is not without complications. These can be immediate or delayed:

- "Steal" of systemic perfusion may occur if the heart is vented excessively in the presence of aortic regurgitation
- If the vents are not removed with great care, the process can be the source of systemic air embolism. Pressures and filling state should be modified during vent placement and removal to mitigate this risk
- Bleeding can occur from the vent site, particularly if an LV apical vent is used
- Later complications include stenosis of the pulmonary vein or pulmonary artery, or aneurysm of the LV apex, depending on the vent site used.

Suggested Further Reading

1. Cheung AT, Stafford-Smith M, Heath M (2019). Cardiopulmonary bypass: Management. In NA Nussmeier (Ed.), UpToDate. Retrieved September 18, 2019, from www.uptodate.com/contents/cardiopulmonary-bypass-management#H3676286842

2. Wahba A, Milojevic M, Boer C et al. EACTS/EACTA/EBCP Committee Reviewers. 2019 EACTS/EACTA/EBCP Guidelines on cardiopulmonary bypass in adult cardiac surgery. *Eur J Cardiothorac Surg.* October 2, 2019

3. Hessel EA 2nd. What's new in cardiopulmonary bypass. *J Cardiothorac Vasc Anesth.* August, 2019;33(8):2296–2326.

4. Ramchandani M, Al Jabbari O, Abu Saleh WK et al. Cannulation strategies and pitfalls in minimally invasive cardiac surgery. *Methodist Debakey Cardiovasc J.* January–March, 2016;12(1):10–3.

Minimal Invasive Extracorporeal Circulation

Kyriakos Anastasiadis, Polychronis Antonitsis, Helena Argiriadou and Apostolos Deliopoulos

Minimal invasive extracorporeal circulation (MiECC) is a recent development in perfusion science. MiECC's unique characteristics include advances such as closed circuits with elimination of blood-air interaction, reduced hemodilution, biocompatible surfaces, and lack of scavenging and reinfusion of unprocessed shed blood. Contemporary hybrid (modular) systems allow perfusionists to safely employ MiECC in the full spectrum of cardiac surgery. MiECC provides the base for developing a multidisciplinary intraoperative strategy which encompasses a surgeon's particular technique and goal-directed perfusion, as well as modified heparin/protamine management. Proponents of MiECC are convinced that it will ultimately replace conventional CPB and become standard practice in cardiac surgery once the potential clinical benefits have been widely accepted. As with traditional extracorporeal circulaton (ECC) techniques, MiECC requires close collaboration of surgical, anesthesiology and perfusion colleagues for optimal outcome.

The Evolution of Minimal Invasive Extracorporeal Circulation

MiECC has its roots in Extracorporeal Life Support (ECLS), where a single circuit with low systemic inflammation, low hemodilution, and enhanced biocompatibility to reduce anticoagulation is required. The successful use of such systems opened a new era in short-term mechanical circulatory support. Subsequently, during the mid-90s multidisciplinary teams developed minimally invasive CPB systems for coronary surgery. These first systems comprised of short arterio-venous lines without cardiotomy reservoir in order to reduce hemodilution and transfusion requirements. Kinetic venous drainage with integration of a centrifugal pump allowed for a compact closed circuit that could be installed close to the patient's chest. In order to improve biocompatibility,

to reduce injury to blood cells and to minimize expression of inflammatory mediators, all lines and oxygenator were coated with heparin, while priming volume was reduced to a minimum. Shed blood from the surgical field was collected, washed and transfused with a cell salvage device, avoiding the adverse effects of recirculating unprocessed shed blood from the operating field into the CPB circuit.

The last two decades have witnessed numerous additional advancements in MiECC technology along with encouraging clinical results. This evolution led to the foundation of the multidisciplinary Minimal Invasive Extracorporeal Technologies International Society (MiECTiS) in order to promote research, clinical use and standards to further develop minimally invasive perfusion. MiECTiS advocates a multidisciplinary strategy involving surgery, anesthesiology and perfusion to promote maximum benefit from this technology.

The term MiECC has replaced all other descriptive terminology previously used for minimal extracorporeal circulation circuits, such as: miniaturized extracorporeal circulation (MECC), mini extracorporeal circulation (mECC), minimized extracorporeal circulation or mini cardiopulmonary bypass (mCPB, mini-CPB).

Table 8.1 summarizes the mandatory and additional components of a contemporary MiECC circuit.

Classification of MiECC systems

MiECTiS has adopted a classification of MiECC systems that reflects how they have evolved over the last decade. Figure 8.1 illustrates a Type III / IV circuit, which is the type most commonly used today.

- Type I systems are derived from ECLS circuits with the addition of a line to administer cardioplegia. These systems are suitable for performing closed-heart surgeries. Soon after

Table 8.1. Components of MiECC

Mandatory Components	Closed CPB circuit
	Biocompatible surfaces
	Reduced priming volume
	Centrifugal pump
	Membrane oxygenator
	Heat exchanger
	Cardioplegia system
	Venous bubble trap/venous air removing device
	Shed blood management system
Additional Components	Vents
	• Aortic root
	• Pulmonary artery / vein
	Reservoir
	• Soft bag / soft-shell
	• Hard-shell (modular systems)
	Regulated smart suction
	Arterial line filter

their introduction significant safety concerns emerged: there was a risk of air entrainment and air lock, requiring stopping the pump and manually de-airing the circuit.

- Type II circuits addressed the air entrainment issue seen with Type I systems by integrating a venous bubble trap or air removal system.
- Type III systems were driven by the desire to use MiECC technology for open-chamber heart surgery, such as valve replacement. The addition of a soft-bag or soft-shell reservoir allows for the management of the circulatory volume during CPB, which is particularly important in patients with preoperative volume overload, such as in aortic or mitral insufficiency.
- Type IV are modular, hybrid systems which integrate a heparinized venous reservoir as a standby component, readily available for conversion to an open, conventional CPB system. This configuration allows the use of MiECC in the full spectrum of cardiac surgery including

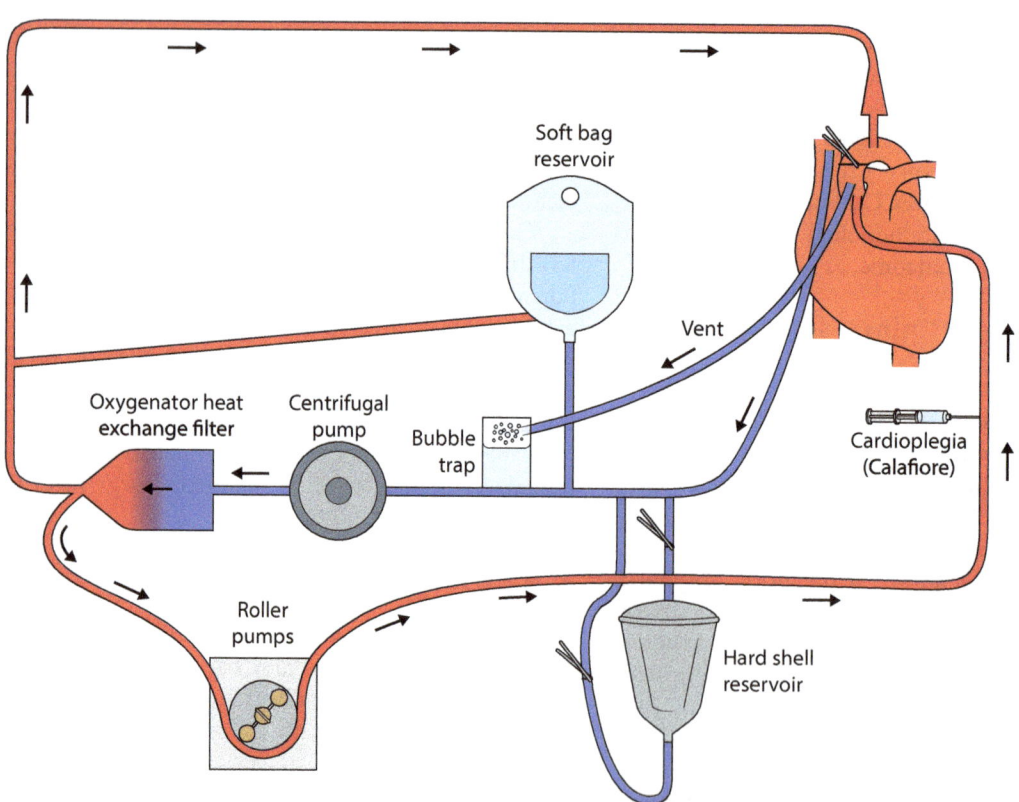

Figure 8.1 Typical Type III circuit, which can easily be converted into Type IV by removing the clamps from the afferent and efferent tubing from the hardshell reservoir. Any cell salvage, if used, needs to be reinfused into the hardshell reservoir.

complex patients and procedures, as any unexpected perfusion scenarios, such as massive air entry to the venous side of the circuit or accidental excessive blood loss to the mediastinum, can be managed by an easy switch to standard CPB.

The Team Approach to MiECC

It is of utmost importance that all members of the team not only comprehend perfusion technology, but that they understand the unique characteristics of MiECC, particularly what it can and what it cannot deliver. Continuous excellent communication with the perfusionist is of utmost importance, particularly during critical moments, such as during retrograde priming of the circuit with patient blood via the aortic cannula (retrograde autologous prime [RAP]), when securing the vent for the cardioplegia line or when removing a vent, in order to avoid accidental air entrainment into the system.

Surgeon's perspective

Firstly, the surgeon must appreciate that when operating on MiECC shed blood does not recirculate into the bypass circuit and is not available for the circulating volume. Meticulous operative technique is mandatory and special attention must be paid to avoiding blood loss, not dissimilar to requirements of beating-heart surgery.

Secondly, all cannulation sites must be secured in a way that provides an airtight seal. The venous cannula is commonly secured with two purse-string sutures and two silk ties; some surgeons arm the purse strings with Teflon pledgets, particularly when the right atrial appendage is of poor quality tissue. Some advocate double-snaring the inferior and superior vena cava cannulae during mitral valve surgery to mitigate against air entrainment. Any manipulations of the heart must be done very carefully in order not to displace the venous cannula(e). Lines are connected with due diligence to avoid introducing air. Accurate positioning of the venous cannula is essential to achieve optimum drainage, which can be assisted by placing a pulmonary artery vent.

Anesthesiologist's perspective

MiECC systems are closed and, without the option of easily adding fluids as necessary, they effectively make the patient's venous compartment the reservoir. This means that fluids have to be used judiciously, i.e. filling up the venous compartment sufficiently without losing the benefit of minimal hemodilution with low prime volume. Appropriate use of vasoconstrictor or inotropic support before initiating CPB can help maintain hemodynamic goals.

Standard perioperative hemodynamic monitoring with invasive, continuous mean arterial pressure (MAP), central venous pressure (CVP) and transesophageal echocardiography (TEE) is often expanded by using pulmonary artery catheters (PAC) and continuous cardiac output (CCO). Some centers opt to use near infrared spectroscopy (NIRS) monitoring of cerebral oxygenation as an index of global perfusion.

Some advocates of MiECC use its unique characteristics – minimal hemodilution, biocompatible surfaces, elimination of blood-air interaction and elimination of unprocessed shed blood reinfusion – to use less anticoagulation, aiming for an ACT value >300 seconds for coronary surgery and >400 seconds for valve and more complex procedures.

Perfusionist's perspective

MiECC integrates all advancements in perfusion technology in a single circuit, but also provides a challenge for the perfusionist.

Centrifugal pump flow is largely dependent on a balance between the filling status of the patient and the systemic vascular resistance and therefore needs regular adjusting. All commercially available centrifugal pumps are fitted with bubble detectors, which cause the pump to stop when air reaches the sensor. In that case the perfusionist has to immediately de-air the bubble trap by applying suction to it, while at the same time adding volume to the circuit. Devices that can purge air automatically can be integrated into the circuit, removing the need for the perfusionist to intervene.

The perfusionist has to appreciate the principles of a closed circuit, where the patient's venous compartment acts as the reservoir. The patient's volume status is monitored via several surrogate measures: negative venous drainage pressure, arterial pressure, cardioplegia pressure and the amount of blood drained from the aortic root vent. Pump flow is another sensitive parameter, as it decreases with hypovolemia. Moving the operating table into Trendelenburg position and volume replacement and/or administration of vasoconstrictors are measures to increase the preload. On the other hand, hypervolemia can cause difficulties in off-loading the heart and in obtaining a bloodless surgical field. In this case, surplus blood volume can be decanted into the soft-shell reservoir or the table can be moved into the reverse-Trendelenburg position.

Understanding the principles of kinetic-assisted venous drainage produced by the centrifugal pump is of paramount importance as the negative pressure at the venous line provides important information on the filling status of the patient. Exceeding -70 mmHg can result in cavitation with the creation of gaseous microemboli and can lead to high blood velocity thereby increasing shear stress and hemolysis at the level of the entrance holes of the cannula and at the wall of the cannula. Increasing the assisted venous, and thus the negative pressure, is not a solution for correcting improper cannula position or hypovolemia.

Major determinants of negative pressure are the type, the size and the position of the venous cannula. When increasing the negative pressure, drainage initially increases linearly with pressure until any further increase collapses the surrounding venous wall and no further advantage in flow will be seen. The ratio between the diameter of the cannula and the vein should be around 0.6 in order to avoid collapse of the vein around the side holes of the cannula. Repositioning of the venous cannula may be required to provide appropriate flow. In case of bicaval cannulation, the perfusionist should prompt the surgeon to check flow in every cannula separately.

In case of a temporary excess in negative pressure due to venous cannula displacement while lifting the heart, the perfusionist might need to add volume to compensate and ensure adequate flow.

During surgery with MiECC it is imperative to use blood mini-cardioplegia (i.e. Calafiore regime) in order to avoid excessive volume. The cardioplegic solution is delivered with a roller pump in combination with a high-speed syringe driver. Hyperkalemia during cardioplegia delivery can cause transient vasodilation but rarely warrants an intervention.

Since there is no cardiotomy reservoir in the MiECC circuit, shed blood is collected into a cell saver. The collected blood is processed and administered as required after weaning off CPB. In case of excessive bleeding, the collected blood can be given back into the circuit directly. Type IV circuits are best equipped to deal with sudden massive blood loss.

Advantages of a Modular Design

Modular MiECC systems (i.e. Type IV) represent the latest evolution in the field of extracorporeal circulation. They integrate contemporary advancements in perfusion technology and address safety concerns. As previously described, they are Type III circuits with a standby hard-shell reservoir connected in parallel to the venous line to allow immediate conversion into a conventional circuit if required. The circuit configuration of the AHEPA University Hospital Thessaloniki prototype Type IV MiECC circuit is shown in Figure 8.2.

Two recently published series show that modular configuration ensured 100% technical feasibility for performing every type of cardiac surgery including aortic arch replacements. They reported conversion rates to conventional CPB of 0.8 and 6%. Modular configuration is advocated for all cardiac surgical procedures, including isolated coronary artery bypass grafting, in order to promote more widespread adoption of MiECC technology in modern cardiac surgical practice.

Training

A MiECC training program can be divided into five stages (see Figure 8.3). After appropriate proctorship, a dedicated team of surgeon, anesthesiologist and perfusionist can start operating on coronary cases, using at least a Type II MiECC system. Experience shows that tangible results, particularly in reducing transfusion requirements, materialize after about 50 cases.

After having completed 50 cases, it is feasible to progress to uncomplicated open-chamber heart surgery, such as aortic valve replacement. Although these operations are doable with a Type II circuit, the integration of a soft-shell reservoir (Type III circuit) is highly recommended for volume management.

After gaining experience in aortic valve cases, more complex mitral and tricuspid valve procedures can be pursued with a Type III circuit, although a modular design is advocated as a "safety net." With a high level of expertise and confidence in using Type IV circuits, any cardiac procedure, even emergency aortic dissection repair or demanding redo cases, can be performed using MiECC technology.

Type IV circuits can obviously be used even from the first coronary cases, obviating the need for a staged approach, as part of the learning strategy.

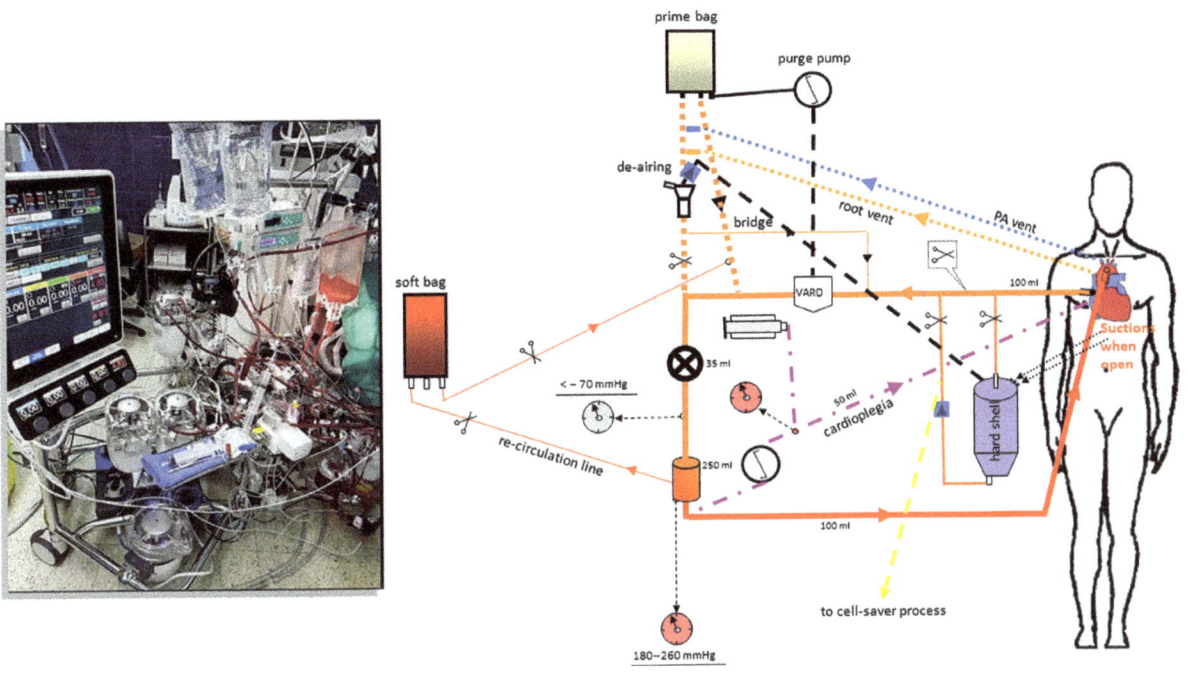

Figure 8.2 The prototype modular type IV AHEPA MiECC circuit (left). Schematic configuration (right). PA: pulmonary artery, VARD: venous air removal device.

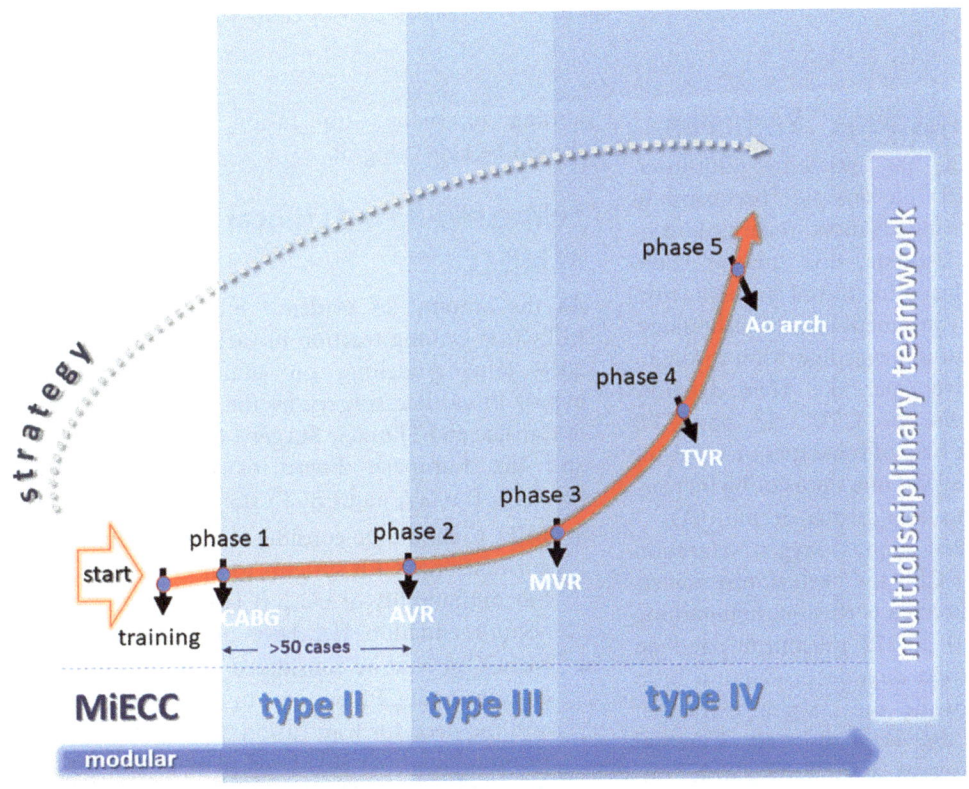

Figure 8.3 Proposed MiECC training pathway. Ao arch: aortic arch, AVR: aortic valve replacement, CABG: coronary artery bypass grafting, MVR: mitral valve replacement, TVR: tricuspid valve replacement.

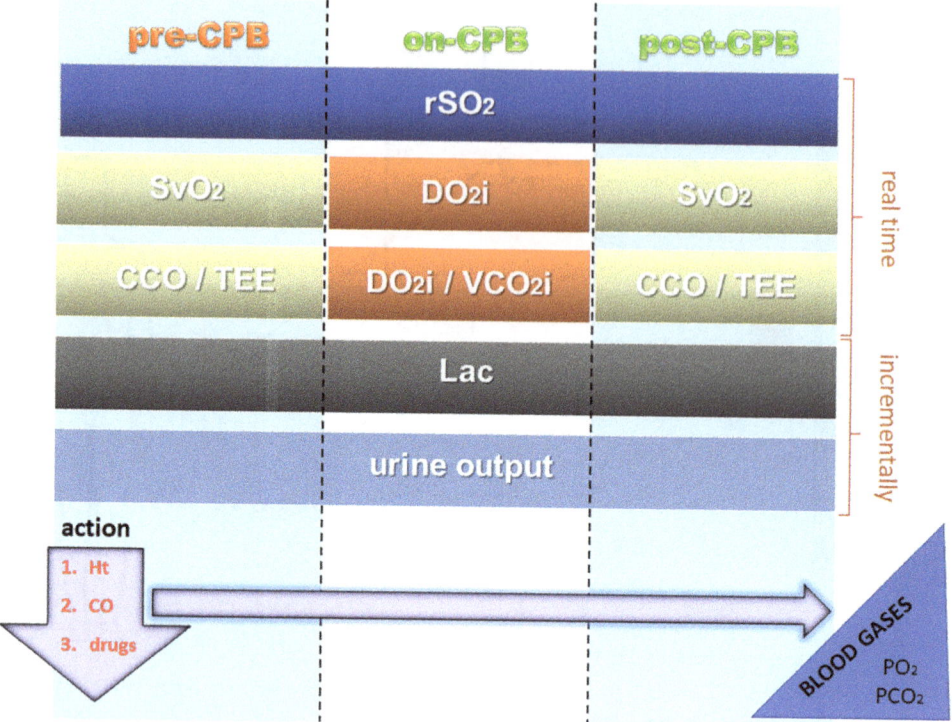

Figure 8.4 Schematic diagram of perioperative strategy to optimize the use of MiECC. CCO: continuous cardiac output; CO: cardiac output/ circulatory flow; CPB: cardiopulmonary bypass; Ht: hematocrit; Lac: lactate levels; POC: point-of-care; rSO_2: cerebral oxygen saturation; TEE: transesophageal echocardiography.

The Quest for "Physiologic" Perfusion

Development of MiECC has initiated a multidisciplinary strategy toward "physiologic" perfusion in cardiac surgery. Despite all advances in surgical techniques and cardiac anesthesia, this concept could never have been introduced in clinical practice without the concomitant advancement in CPB technology. Figure 8.4 proposes a monitoring algorithm throughout the perioperative period. Hemodynamic management during the pre-CPB and post-CPB period – either with the help of inotropes or vasoconstrictors, with optimizing volume status or by increasing pump flow – aims to keep cardiac output (CO) > 2.4 $L/min/m^2$ and mixed venous oxygen saturation (SvO_2) > 70%. During CPB the perfusionist adjusts their strategy to goal-directed perfusion, maintaining oxygen delivery (DO_2i) > 272 $ml/min/m^2$ and an oxygen delivery to carbon dioxide production ratio (DO_2i/VCO_2i) > 5, while the oxygen extraction ratio (O_2ER) should be kept at <30. Cerebral oximetry monitoring serves as a 'level alarm' on- and off-CPB and a drop of >20% from the baseline needs to prompt immediate intervention. While aiming to reduce transfusion, hemoglobin level should be kept >8 g/dl.

Evidenced-Based Clinical Advantages of MiECC

As the amount of evidence increases, the use of MiECC is gaining traction in various guidelines. The 2019 joint guidelines on adult cardiopulmonary bypass in cardiac surgery by the European Societies of Cardiac and Thoracic Surgery, Cardiac Anaesthesia and the European Board of Cardiac Perfusion (EACTS, EACTA and EBCP) state that:

- MiECC should be considered over standard conventional CPB systems to increase the biocompatibility of ECC. (Class of recommendation: IIA, Level of evidence: B.)
- MiECC should be considered over standard conventional CPB systems to reduce blood loss and the need for transfusion. (Class of recommendation: IIA, Level of evidence: B.)
- A combination of MiECC features – such as coating, the centrifugal pump, the separation of

Table 8.2. MiECC Practice Recommendations

	Level of Evidence
Class I	
MiECC systems reduce hemodilution and better preserve hematocrit as well as reduce postoperative bleeding and the need for RBC transfusion.	A
MiECC systems reduce the incidence of postoperative atrial fibrillation.	A
MiECC systems preserve renal function.	A
MiECC is associated with improved myocardial protection.	A
Class IIA	
Inflammatory response assessed by specific inflammatory markers is attenuated with use of MiECC.	B
MiECC systems can reduce cerebral gaseous microembolism and preserve neurocognitive function.	B
MiECC exerts a subclinical protective effect on end-organ function (lung, liver, intestine) which is related to enhanced recovery of microvascular organ perfusion.	B
Class IIB	
Within a MiECC strategy, less thrombin generation may permit reduced heparin dose targeted to shorter ACT times. When such a strategy is followed, individual heparin dose should be determined using heparin dose-response monitoring systems.	B
MiECC appears to offer survival benefit in terms of lower 30-day mortality after CABG procedures.	B
Use of short-acting opioids in combination with propofol or volatile anesthetics, and hypnotic effect monitoring by processed EEG, is recommended for induction and maintenance of anesthesia for MiECC-based surgery. TEE findings pertinent to institutional management of MiECC should be communicated during the preoperative surgical safety time out.	C

ACT: Activated Clotting Time; CABG: Coronary Artery Bypass Grafting; EEG: Electroencephalogram; MiECC: Minimal Invasive Extracorporeal Circulation; RBC: Red Blood Cells

cardiotomy suction blood and the use of closed systems – should be considered to improve conventional CPB. (Class of recommendation: IIA, Level of evidence: C.)

The 2017 EACTS/EACTA guidelines on patient blood management for adult cardiac surgery recommend considering MiECC to reduce perioperative blood transfusion. A position paper produced by MiECTiS in 2016 provides a detailed overview of practice recommendations, which are summarized in Table 8.2

A meta-analysis including 2,700 patients from 24 randomized controlled trials showed that MiECC is associated with reduced postoperative morbidity and lower mortality (0.5% versus 1.7%; p = 0.02) in coronary surgery when compared to conventional CPB. A large network analysis including 22,778 patients showed that MiECC and OPCABG reduce the odds of 30-day all-cause-mortality, and particularly stroke, new onset atrial fibrillation and renal dysfunction, over CABG done on conventional CPB.

There was no difference in the odds for developing a postoperative myocardial infarction. The authors conclude that MiECC may represent an attractive compromise between OPCAB and conventional CPB.

Incorporating the Lessons Learned from MiECC into Practice

Cardiac surgery is by definition a "non-physiologic" intervention. MiECC attempts to apply physiology to perfusion. On a cellular level it shows less impairment of microcirculation and a faster recovery of physiologic flow compared with conventional flow. At least in low-risk coronary surgery, this seems to translate into improved organ protection and clinical outcomes appear to be better than those of patients operated on using conventional CPB (see Figure 8.5).

Some teams have introduced the term "optimized ECC" (opECC), representing a shift from conventional

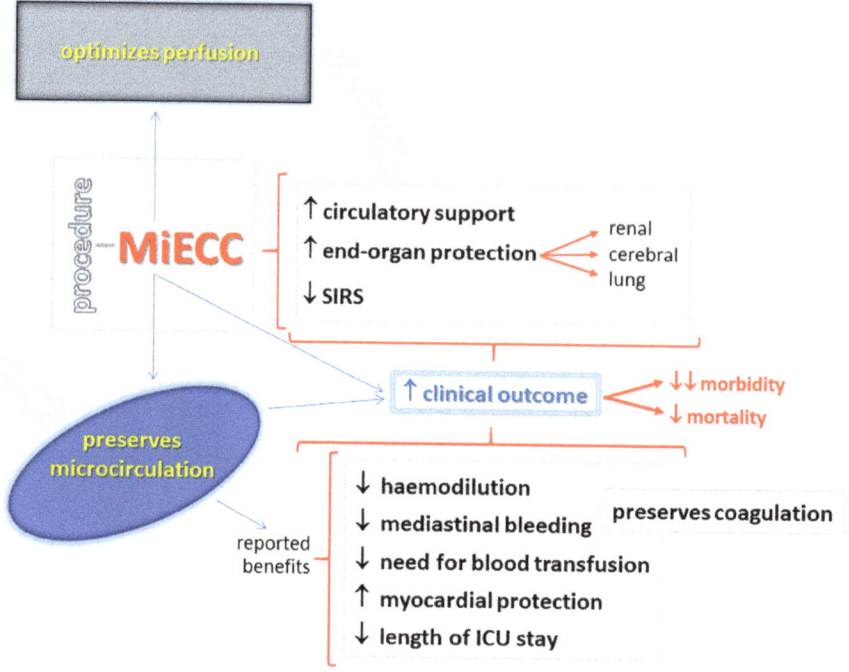

Figure 8.5 Schematic representation of the pathophysiologic pathway that leads from preserved microcirculation to improved clinical outcome with MiECC use.

CPB to advanced perfusion circuits. This trend highlights the change in mindset that MiECC has offered to perfusion, leading perfusionists to improve CPB technology. An opECC circuit often follows a custom-made design, incorporating relatively easy-to-make changes, such as using short tubing with biocompatible surfaces, centrifugal pumps, low prime oxygenators and assisted venous drainage. They might not reach the efficacy of a MiECC system but are a step toward more physiological perfusion becoming global practice.

The success of MiECC depends on the engagement of all three stakeholders of the cardiac surgical team in order to obtain the maximum benefit. Combining a multidisciplinary strategy with technological advances has the potential to make MiECC a "therapy" for cardiac surgery. The evidence is not strong enough at present, but it could at some point in the future replace conventional CPB and become standard practice in cardiac surgery.

Suggested Further Reading

1. D' Agostino RS, Jacobs JP, Badhwar V et al. The Society of Thoracic Surgeons adult cardiac surgery database: 2019 update on outcomes and quality. *Ann Thorac Surg* 2019;107:24–32.

2. Benedetto U, Puskas J, Kappetein AP et al. Off-Pump versus on-pump bypass surgery for left main coronary artery disease. *J Am Coll Cardiol* 2019;74:729–740.

3. Anastasiadis K, Murkin J, Antonitsis P et al. Use of minimal invasive extracorporeal circulation in cardiac surgery: principles, definitions and potential benefits. A position paper from the Minimal Invasive Extra-Corporeal Technologies International Society (MiECTiS). *Interact Cardiovasc Thorac Surg* 2016;22:647–662.

4. Anastasiadis K, Antonitsis P, Argiriadou H et al. Modular

minimally invasive extracorporeal circulation systems; can they become the standard practice for performing cardiac surgery? *Perfusion* 2015;30:195–200.

5. Anastasiadis K, Antonitsis P, Asteriou C et al. Quantification of operational learning in minimal invasive extracorporeal circulation. *Artif Organs* 2017;41:628–636.

6. Alexander Wahba, Milan Milojevic, Christa Boer et al.

EACTS/EACTA/EBCP Committee Reviewers, 2019 EACTS/EACTA/EBCP guidelines on cardiopulmonary bypass in adult cardiac surgery, *European Journal of Cardio-Thoracic Surgery*, 2020;57(2): 210–251.

7. Anastasiadis K, Antonitsis P, Haidich AB et al. Use of minimal extracorporeal circulation improves outcome after heart surgery; a systematic review and meta-analysis of randomized controlled trials. *Int J Cardiol* 2013;164:158–169.

8. Benedetto U, Angeloni E, Refice S et al. Is minimized extracorporeal circulation effective to reduce the need for red blood cell transfusion in coronary artery bypass grafting? Meta-analysis of randomized controlled trials. *J Thorac Cardiovasc Surg* 2009;38:1450–1453.

9. Kowalewski M, Pawliszak W, Raffa GM et al. Safety and efficacy of miniaturized extracorporeal circulation when compared with off-pump and conventional coronary artery bypass grafting: evidence synthesis from a comprehensive Bayesian-framework network meta-analysis of 134 randomized controlled trials involving 22 778 patients. *Eur J Cardiothorac Surg* 2016;49:1428–1440.

10. Donndorf P, Kuhn F, Vollmar B et al. Comparing microvascular alterations during minimal extracorporeal circulation and conventional cardiopulmonary bypass in coronary artery bypass graft surgery: a prospective, randomized study. *J Thorac Cardiovasc Surg* 2012;144:677–683.

Considerations for Operations Involving Deep Hypothermic Circulatory Arrest

Pingping Song and Joseph E Arrowsmith

The technique of core cooling (<28°C) and complete cessation of blood flow is termed "deep hypothermic circulatory arrest" (DHCA). This concept arose from two overlapping eras in the evolution of modern cardiac surgery: a brief period in the early 1950s when "cold immersion" hypothermia, introduced by William Bigelow, was used as the sole method for organ protection, and the current epoch of CPB heralded by John Gibbon and colleagues in 1953. Although CPB-induced hypothermia and DHCA for the management of aortic arch pathology was described in the 1960s, it was not until the mid-1970s that DHCA became established as a safe and relatively simple technique for aortic arch surgery. Nowadays DHCA, either alone or in combination with other perfusion strategies, has become the mainstay of vital organ protection for a variety of pathologies and surgical procedures that necessitate the complete cessation of blood flow.

DHCA provides a near bloodless operating field, albeit of limited duration, while ameliorating the major adverse consequences of vital organ ischemia. Cooling of the brain – the organ at greatest ischemic risk – reduces cerebral metabolic rate, extending the period of "safe" ischemia from 3 to 4 minutes at normothermia to >20 minutes.

Indications

In addition to being used to facilitate cardiac and thoracic aortic surgery, DHCA is used in a number of pulmonary vascular, urological and neurologic procedures (see Table 9.1).

Pathophysiology

In homeotherms, body temperature is maintained within a tight range as a result of the dynamic balance between heat production and heat loss. Stimulation of peripheral cold receptors and temperature sensitive hypothalamic neurons activates sympathetic autonomic, endocrine, extrapyramidal and adaptive behavioral mechanisms to maintain core body temperature. Hypothermia – defined as a core temperature <35°C – occurs when heat losses overwhelm thermoregulatory mechanisms (e.g. cold immersion) or when thermoregulation is impaired by disease or drugs. Thanks to experiences gained in the management of accidents, the physiological effects of hypothermia are well understood (see Table 9.2).

Preoperative Considerations

Preoperative Assessment

DHCA is often used in the context of emergency surgery (e.g. acute type A aortic dissection) and it may not be possible to undertake the usual battery of "routine" preoperative investigations. Significant comorbidities, such as coronary artery and cerebrovascular disease, diabetes mellitus and renal insufficiency, should be anticipated on the basis of the clinical history, if available. With aortopathy (aortic dissection or aneurysm), special attention needs to be paid to the presence of aortic valve pathology, mediastinal mass effect, cardiac tamponade and signs of end-organ malperfusion.

Monitoring Considerations

Standard arterial, central venous and peripheral venous access is required in all cases. The choice of site(s) for arterial pressure monitoring should be tailored to both the pathology and the surgical cannulation strategy. Catheterization of the right radial artery and either a femoral artery or the left radial artery permits arterial pressure monitoring proximal and distal to the aortic arch.

The right radial arterial catheter permits monitoring of cerebral perfusion pressure if antegrade cerebral perfusion (ACP) via the right axillary or innominate artery cannulation is used. In this case

Table 9.1. Clinical applications of deep hypothermic circulatory arrest

Cardiothoracic surgery	Aortic arch surgery
	Descending thoracic aortic aneurysm (DTAA) and thoracoabdominal aortic aneurysm (TAAA) repair
	Pulmonary thromboendarterectomy (PTE)
	Complex congenital cardiac reconstructions
	Re-entry sternotomy with high risk of cardiovascular injury
Neurosurgery	Cerebral tumor resection
	Basilar artery aneurysm surgery
	Intracranial arteriovenous malformation resection
Other	Resection of mass or tumor with atriocaval extension (e.g. renal cell carcinoma)
	Head and neck vessel surgery

additional left radial or femoral arterial monitoring is required because the arterial pressure is interrupted during axillary artery cannulation. Also, the pressure measured from the right radial artery is likely to overestimate systemic perfusion pressure in this setting. Peripheral venous access should be sited in the right arm if division of the left innominate vein (to improve surgical access to aortic arch and epiaortic vessels) is anticipated.

Temperature monitoring at two or more sites is recommended. In most cases, nasopharyngeal or tympanic membrane monitoring provides an indication of brain temperature while bladder or rectal monitoring provides an indication of core temperature.

Surgical Considerations

Arterial Cannulation

In the context of CPB with DHCA, the three most common sites for arterial cannulation are: ascending aorta, right axillary artery and femoral artery. The optimal cannulation site is dictated by both the disease and the goals of surgical reconstruction. In cases of aortic dissection where cannulation of the ascending aorta or a femoral artery is used, perfusion of the true lumen must be confirmed with epiaortic ultrasound or transesophageal echocardiography

(TEE). In situations where sternotomy or ascending aortic cannulation pose a high risk of injury to the major vessels or cardiac chambers (such as type A aortic dissection or re-entry sternotomy), femoral or right axillary arterial cannulation may initially be necessary in combination with femoral venous cannulation. Femoro-femoral or axillo-femoral CPB permits systemic cooling prior to sternotomy and affords a degree of organ protection should chest opening be accompanied by exsanguination secondary to inadvertent injury to the aorta or the heart. After completion of the distal aortic repair, placement of the arterial cannula directly into the prosthetic graft or into a sidearm permits restoration of anterograde flow (Figure 9.1). Femoral arterial cannulation should be avoided in patients with significant thoracic aortic disease to reduce the risk of atheroembolism associated with retrograde blood flow.

If ACP is planned, cerebral perfusion can be initiated easily by inserting balloon catheters into the brachiocephalic and left common carotid arteries (Figure 9.2).

Venous Cannulation

The choice of venous drainage site and cannula type is largely dictated by surgical preference and the degree of access required. Venous cannulae can be placed in the right atrium (RA), a femoral vein or both venae cavae. In situations where sternotomy carries high risk of injury to the major vessels or heart, femoral venous cannulation is preferable. Bicaval cannulation is chosen if retrograde cerebral perfusion (RCP) is to be used with reversal of blood flow in the superior vena cava (SVC). If selective anterograde cerebral perfusion (SACP) is to be used with cannulation of the carotid arteries, adequate cerebral venous drainage must be ensured. Again, bicaval cannulation is preferred to optimize cerebral perfusion pressure and prevent cerebral edema. Removal of a renal or adrenal tumor extending to the inferior vena cava (IVC) and RA requires the use of a Ross atrial basket in preference to bicaval or standard two-stage cannulation to permit full visualization of the cava and to prevent tumor embolization into the lungs.

Descending Thoracic Aortic Surgery

With the development of percutaneously delivered endovascular stent-grafts, open operations on the descending thoracic aorta have become rare. When

81

Table 9.2. Physiological effects of hypothermia

	Mild (33–35°C)	Severe (<28°C)
Neurologic	Confusion Amnesia Apathy – delayed anesthetic recovery Impaired cognitive function	Depressed consciousness Pupillary dilatation Coma Loss of autoregulation
Neuromuscular	Shivering Ataxia Dysarthria	Muscle & joint stiffening Muscle rigor
Cardiovascular	Tachycardia Vasoconstriction Increased BP, CO	Severe bradycardia Increased SVR, reduced CO ECG changes: J (Osborn) waves, widening of QRS complex, prolongation of QT interval, ST changes, T wave inversion, A-V block. VF → Asystole
Respiratory	Tachypnea Left shift Hb-O_2 dissociation curve	Bradypnea Bronchospasm Further left shift HbO_2 curve
Renal **Metabolic**	ADH resistance Cold-induced diuresis Reduced drug metabolism	Reduced GFR Reduced H^+ & glucose reabsorption Metabolic (lactic) acidosis
Gastrointestinal		Ileus Gastric ulcers Hepatic dysfunction
Hematology **Immunological**	Increased blood viscosity & hemoconcentration (2% increase in hematocrit per Celsius drop in temperature) Increased infection risk	Coagulopathy – inhibition of intrinsic/extrinsic pathway enzymes, platelet activation, thrombocytopenia (splenic sequestration) Leukocyte depletion, impaired neutrophil function & bacterial phagocytosis

necessary, though, they can be challenging for the entire team. During surgery for descending thoracic aortic aneurysm (DTAA) and thoracoabdominal aortic aneurysm (TAAA), when the aneurysmal anatomy precludes safe cross clamping of the proximal aorta, DHCA with CPB is necessary for surgical repair and organ protection. The standard surgical approach is via left thoracotomy, although this limits access to the heart and great vessels. CPB is usually established via femoral arterial cannula and a long, fenestrated femoral venous cannula advanced into the RA during TEE guidance. The proximal aortic anastomosis is carried out during DHCA with the aorta open.

When the proximal aorta can be safely clamped, disruption of distal organ perfusion (spinal cord and abdominal viscera) during the proximal aortic anastomosis contributes significantly to the development of ischemic complications. Partial left heart bypass (LHB) provides distal aortic perfusion and unloads the left ventricle during aortic occlusion. Evidence suggests that LHB reduces mortality, neurologic injury and the need for postoperative renal replacement therapy. LHB is achieved by establishing bypass from left atrium or left inferior pulmonary vein to a femoral artery or the descending aorta distal to the aortic cross clamp via an in-line centrifugal pump (see Chapter 13 for more detail).

Perfusion Considerations

Extracorporeal Circulation

DHCA may require modifications to the standard CPB setup:

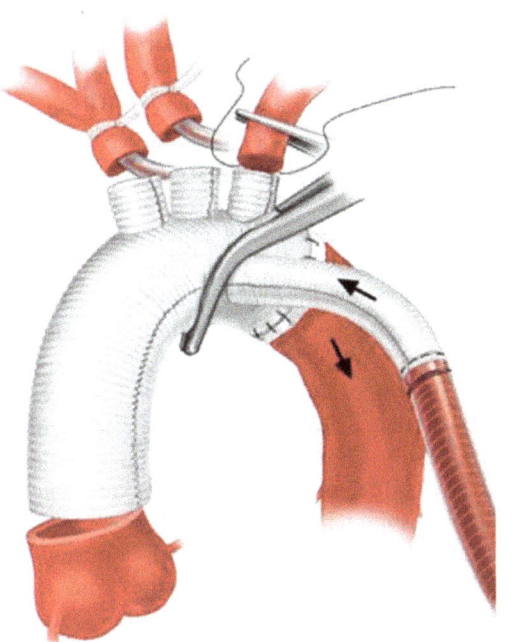

Figure 9.1 Branched arch graft for total arch replacement. After completion of the distal aortic repair, placement of the arterial cannula into a sidearm of the graft permits restoration of anterograde flow. See also the cannulated and snared head and neck vessels for antegrade cerebral perfusion. (From Brown CR, Bavaria JE, Desai ND. Ascending and Arch Aortic Aneurysms. In Cohn LH, Adams DH (Eds.) *Cardiac Surgery in the Adult* (5th ed.) 2016. New York: McGraw-Hill. Reproduced with kind permission from McGraw-Hill.)

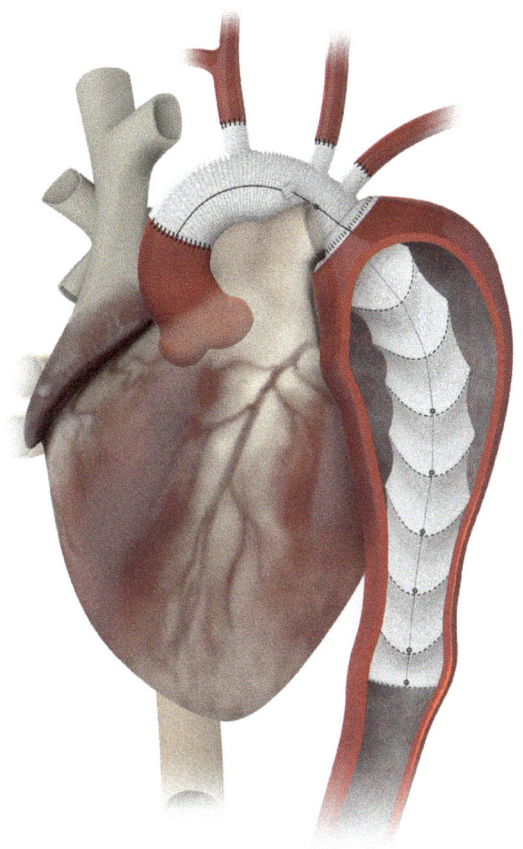

Figure 9.2 Fully implanted "Frozen Elephant Trunk" aortic arch graft. Note the cut and oversewn sidearm used for central aortic perfusion. (Reproduced with kind permission from Terumo.)

- Incorporation of a hemofilter to permit hemoconcentration or ultrafiltration during rewarming.
- Arteriovenous bypass and accessory arterial lines to permit adjunct cerebral or cardiac perfusion strategies (see below).
- Standard blood collection bags (citrate phosphate dextrose adenine, CPDA-1) to facilitate normovolemic hemodilution (see below).
- Selection of a cardiotomy reservoir of sufficient capacity to accommodate the circulating volume during exsanguination immediately before DHCA. A second reservoir may be required for patients with large circulating blood volume.
- Some centers:
  ○ advocate the use of a centrifugal pump – in preference to a roller pump – to reduce damage to blood cells and reduce hemolysis.
  ○ incorporate leukocyte depleting arterial line filters to reduce the inflammatory response to CPB, reperfusion injury and postoperative infective complications.

Hemodilution

Vasoconstriction, increased plasma viscosity and reduced erythrocyte plasticity secondary to hypothermia lead to impairment of the microcirculation and to tissue ischemia. Acute normovolemic hemodilution (ANH) theoretically mitigates against these adverse effects while ensuring adequate tissue oxygen delivery during hypothermia. Hypothermia reduces oxygen consumption, permitting perfusion with a hematocrit (Hct) of 0.18–0.22 at 26–28°C. As yet, there is insufficient evidence to support an "optimal" Hct during hypothermic CPB and DHCA.

The patient is placed "head down" while 1–4 "units" of venous blood are drained into standard CPDA-1 blood collection bags. Not infrequently, a vasoconstrictor is required to maintain systemic blood pressure during this period. The timing of

Table 9.3. Summary of STS/SCA/AmSECT temperature management guidelines

Oxygenator arterial outlet blood temperature is recommended as a surrogate for cerebral temperature

It should be assumed that the oxygenator arterial outlet blood temperature underestimates cerebral perfusate temperature during rewarming

Arterial outlet blood temperature should be limited to <37°C to avoid cerebral hyperthermia

The temperature gradient between arterial outlet and venous inflow on the oxygenator during CPB *cooling* should not exceed 10°C to avoid generation of gaseous emboli

The temperature gradient between arterial outlet and venous inflow on the oxygenator during CPB *rewarming* should not exceed 10°C to avoid outgassing when blood is returned to the patient

Pulmonary artery or nasopharyngeal temperature monitoring may be used during weaning from CPB and in the early postoperative period

It is reasonable to maintain an outflow-inflow gradient ≤4°C and a rewarming rate ≤0.5°C/min when the oxygenator arterial outlet temperature is ≥30°C during rewarming

It is reasonable to maintain an outflow-inflow gradient ≤10°C when the oxygenator arterial outlet temperature is ≤30°C during rewarming

There is insufficient evidence to determine the optimal temperature for weaning from CPB

ANH varies from center to center: in some, blood is removed after induction of anesthesia and before heparinization, whereas in others, heparinized blood is removed immediately before the onset of CPB.

Temperature Management

The most recent guidelines on temperature management during CPB were developed jointly by the Society of Thoracic Surgeons (STS), the Society of Cardiovascular Anesthesiologists (SCA) and the American Society of Extracorporeal Technology (AmSECT). They are summarized in Table 9.3.

Cooling: CPB is typically instituted with a constant flow rate of 2.2–2.4 l/min/m^2 and active cooling immediately commenced. The application of external ice packs or a cooling cap to the head may augment cerebral cooling and help avoid a rise in intracranial temperature during the period of DHCA. Vasoactive drugs are used as required to maintain a mean arterial pressure (MAP) of 50–60 mmHg. The onset of hypothermia-induced ventricular fibrillation (VF) signals the need for either application of an aortic cross clamp (AXC) and administration of cardioplegia, or more commonly, insertion of a vent to prevent left ventricular distension. As much of the planned surgical procedure as possible (e.g. surgical dissection and preparation of any prosthetic grafts) should be carried out during cooling to minimize the duration of DHCA.

The neurophysiologic endpoint of cerebral cooling is electrocortical silence on the electroencephalogram (EEG). Other generally accepted endpoints that ensure sufficient cerebral metabolic protection include a nasopharyngeal temperature of 18–25°C, equilibration of brain and core temperatures at the target temperature for 10–15 minutes and jugular venous oxygen saturation (S$_{JV}$O$_2$) >95%. Cutaneous Near Infrared Spectroscopy (NIRS) sensors applied to the patient's forehead are used to measure oxygen saturation in the frontal lobes. Although NIRS penetration depth is limited and the area measured is necessarily small, it provides a guide to cerebral oxygen delivery. Most centers aim to maintain NIRS within 20% of baseline after induction of anesthesia or ≥50%. Sustained low cerebral oxygen saturation should prompt swift intervention, such as antegrade or retrograde cerebral perfusion. It is important to note that relying solely on any one of these individual measures may not be sufficient to ensure adequate cerebral metabolic suppression. In one published report it was noted that electrocortical silence at a nasopharyngeal temperature of 18°C was not achieved in around half of the patients studied. This emphasizes the need to evaluate all available monitoring parameters, including core and brain temperatures, EEG, evoked potentials, NIRS and S$_{JV}$O$_2$ before initiating DHCA. (See Chapter 18 for more detail.)

Circulatory arrest: The operating table is placed in a slightly head-down position, CPB is stopped and the patient is exsanguinated into the venous reservoir. Once isolated from the patient, blood within the extracorporeal circuit is recirculated via a shunt between the arterial and venous lines in order to prevent stagnation and clotting. The surgical repair proceeds with heed to the duration of circulatory arrest. As the intravenous administration of drugs during DHCA is at best pointless and at worst potentially dangerous, all infusions should be discontinued when the CPB pump is switched off.

Removal of the aortic cross clamp and opening the aorta to the atmosphere exposes both the coronary and cerebral arteries to the risk of air embolism. At the end of DHCA therefore, adequate de-airing and measures such as head-down tilt or flooding the surgical field with crystalloid at 4°C should be undertaken.

Rewarming: This is a critical phase of CPB, during which cerebral injury may be caused or exacerbated. Infusions of anesthetic drugs should be restarted as soon as the circulation is restored to avoid inadvertent awareness during rewarming. Following the reinstitution of CPB, rewarming is typically delayed for approximately 10 minutes. This practice, known as "cold reperfusion," has been shown to reduce reperfusion injury in both animal and human studies. The rewarming process is then initiated while maintaining the temperature gradient between the venous inlet and arterial outlet ≤10°C. Above 30°C, this gradient should be ≤4°C. Rewarming should proceed slowly, with the rate of temperature rise limited to no more than 0.5°C/min to avoid exacerbating any adverse neurological outcome. Excessively rapid rewarming tends to produce a large core-peripheral temperature gradient, which risks significant "after-drop" following separation from CPB. The arterial outflow temperature should not exceed 37°C at any time to avoid cerebral hyperthermia.

Sites typically used for temperature monitoring include the bladder, nasopharynx, tympanic membrane (ear canal) and blood (via the thermistor in the PA catheter), as well as the arterial outlet and venous inlet. Cranial temperature monitoring, using a jugular bulb catheter, should be considered a research modality not used in routine clinical care. Although accurate at "steady-state," studies have demonstrated that temperature monitoring at extracranial sites tends to lag behind and underestimate jugular bulb blood temperature during rewarming. Urinary bladder or rectal temperature is considered to be "core" temperature and used to monitor the equilibrium between the blood and peripheral tissue temperature. Although there is no agreement on the optimal temperature for separation from CPB, the typical core body (bladder or rectal) temperature range is 35.5–36.5°C; the gradient between core and peripheral temperatures should be <5°C at that point.

During the period of rewarming attention should be given to the correction of metabolic abnormalities, particularly the metabolic (lactic) acidosis that inevitably accompanies reperfusion following circulatory arrest. Blood lactate concentration increases gradually after the onset of reperfusion and peaks approximately six hours after DHCA. A higher hematocrit is desirable during rewarming due to the increased oxygen carrying capacity and free radical scavenging effect. Autologous blood, removed prior to CPB, is gradually returned to the cardiotomy reservoir during rewarming to meet the demands of the rising metabolic rate.

Acid–Base Management

There are two strategies to manage blood gases during DHCA – pH-stat and α-stat. The concept is explained in detail in Chapter 10. In neonates undergoing DHCA for repair of congenital heart defects, pH-stat management prior to DHCA appears to be associated with fewer complications than α-stat management and better developmental outcome. Most institutions use α-stat during DHCA in adult patients. On theoretical grounds, using pH-stat during cooling and α-stat during rewarming (the so-called crossover management) has some appeal and is used in some centers.

Glucose Management

Insulin resistance and hyperglycemia are common during hypothermic CPB and DHCA. The STS recommends that the blood glucose concentration should be maintained at <10 mmol/l (180 mg/dl) to reduce mortality and infectious complications. Tight glycemic control during cardiac surgery with or without DHCA has yet to be proven to offer any neuroprotective effect. Where an infusion of insulin is used, the blood glucose concentration should not be allowed to fall below 4.5–6.0 mmol/l (80–110 mg/dl).

Blood Conservation

Prolonged CPB and hypothermia produce a coagulopathy secondary to inhibition of intrinsic and extrinsic pathway enzymes, platelet activation and splenic platelet sequestration. Blood conservation is facilitated by meticulous surgery, the use of autologous blood and the administration of allogenic blood components guided by the results of point-of-care and laboratory tests of coagulation. In the 2011 update to the STS and SCA Blood Conservation Clinical Practice Guidelines, antifibrinolytic agents (e.g., tranexamic acid and ε-aminocaproic acid) are strongly recommended (Class IA evidence) for blood conservation during cardiac surgery.

Following publication of the BART study in 2008, the routine use of aprotinin in cardiac surgery effectively ceased. In recent years – in territories outside North America – there has been a resurgence of interest in the use of aprotinin in cardiac surgery. Results following the reintroduction of the drug are eagerly awaited.

Neuroprotection during DHCA

Hypothermia is the principle neuroprotectant during circulatory arrest. Surgical maneuvers, such as intermittent cerebral perfusion, selective ACP and RCP, may also be used to protect the brain and extend the operating time available to the surgeon.

Hypothermia Alone

Cerebral metabolism decreases by 6–7% for every 1°C fall in temperature below 37°C, with consciousness and autoregulation being lost at 30°C and 25°C respectively. At 18°C, the cerebral metabolic rate for oxygen ($CMRO_2$) is about 17–30% of that at normothermia and the ischemic tolerance is around 10 times that at normothermia (see Table 9.4). Hypothermia alone provides the simplest form of neuroprotection. The main concern is the duration

of the circulatory arrest period that is considered to be safe. Clinical studies in adults undergoing DHCA suggest that a safe period of arrest is roughly 20 minutes at 20°C and 45 minutes at 10°C. Neurologic complications increase when the duration of DHCA alone without any adjunct cerebral perfusion exceeds 40 minutes. Combining the findings of several studies of neurologic deficit after DHCA, an arrest time of 20 minutes should be considered the maximum tolerable period of brain ischemia if using DHCA alone (i.e., bladder temperature 18°C or nasopharyngeal temperature 15°C). Certain patient risk factors (e.g., advanced age, history of stroke, severe atherosclerotic disease) confer a lower margin of safety. The application of external ice packs or a cooling cap to the head delays brain rewarming during DHCA.

Pharmacological Neuroprotection

At present no drug is specifically licensed for neuroprotection during cardiac surgery. Over the last four decades a wide variety of compounds, many with very promising pre-clinical pharmacological profiles, have been evaluated for cardiac surgery. These include anesthetic agents (barbiturates, propofol, volatile agents), calcium channel blockers, immunomulators (corticosteroids, cyclosporin), amino acid receptor antagonists (magnesium, remacemide), glutamate-release inhibitors (lidocaine, fosphenytoin), antiproteases (aprotinin, nafamostat) and free radical scavengers (mannitol, desferrioxamine, allopurinol). Unfortunately none of these agents has demonstrated clinical efficacy (see Chapter 18 for more detail). The observation that thiopental reduces $CMRO_2$ was long used as the rationale for its administration during cardiac surgery or immediately before the onset of DHCA. Although a handful of small studies have suggested reduced operative mortality, any beneficial impact on neurologic outcome has not been demonstrated. Thiopental is no longer available in the USA as production ceased in 2011.

Cerebral Perfusion Strategies

Intermittent Cerebral Perfusion

Intermittent systemic perfusion punctuated by periods of DHCA lasting 20 minutes has been used as an alternative strategy to prolong the total cumulative duration of DHCA. A common application of this technique is during pulmonary thromboendarterectomy

Table 9.4. Calculated maximum duration of hypothermic circulatory arrest

Temperature (°C)	Cerebral Metabolic Rate (% of baseline)	Maximum Duration of HCA (minutes)
37	100	5
30	56 (52–60)	9 (8–10)
25	37 (33–42)	14 (12–15)
20	24 (21–29)	21 (17–24)
15	16 (13–20)	31 (25–38)
10	11 (8–14)	45 (36–62)

(PTE). It is suggested that 10 minute periods of intermittent reperfusion preserve neurologic function by replenishing cerebral high-energy phosphates and removing accumulated waste products. NIRS can be used to guide the durations of DHCA and reperfusion (see neurologic monitoring below).

Selective Antegrade Cerebral Perfusion (SACP)

This technique involves direct cannulation of the innominate, axillary or carotid arteries. SACP can be carried out in either a bilateral or unilateral approach. Bilateral SACP involves direct cannulation of both common carotid arteries or insertion of perfusion cannulae into the ostia of the innominate and left carotid arteries via the open arch at time of DHCA (see Figure 9.1). Unilateral SACP is achieved using right axillary artery cannulation and occlusion of the innominate and left carotid arteries and relies on an intact circle of Willis. Oxygenated blood is pumped via a separate arterial line at 8–12 ml/kg/min to maintain a perfusion pressure of 50–70 mmHg – measured in the ipsilateral radial artery or in a pressure transducer at the end of the cannula. Although SACP permits surgery to be conducted at lesser degrees of systemic hypothermia (e.g., 22–25°C), it often requires greater mobilization of the epiaortic vessels and division of the innominate vein. In addition to increasing complexity and crowding the surgical field with cannulae, SACP is accompanied by the risk of cerebral embolization from manipulation of the epiaortic vessels.

Retrograde Cerebral Perfusion (RCP)

This technique relies on the fact that cerebral veins have no valves and involves the continuous administration of cold (10–15°C) oxygenated blood via an SVC cannula (see Figure 9.3). Blood flow to the brain is most likely to occur via the azygos veins because the internal jugular veins possess valves. The azygos vein has connections to the vertebral venous system and the venous plexus of the foramen magnum and intracranial sinuses. Massive shunting via the superficial and deep venous systems, including the internal and external jugular veins, may result in only a small fraction of the blood entering the SVC actually reaching the cerebral arteries. For these reasons the exact levels of CBF and metabolic

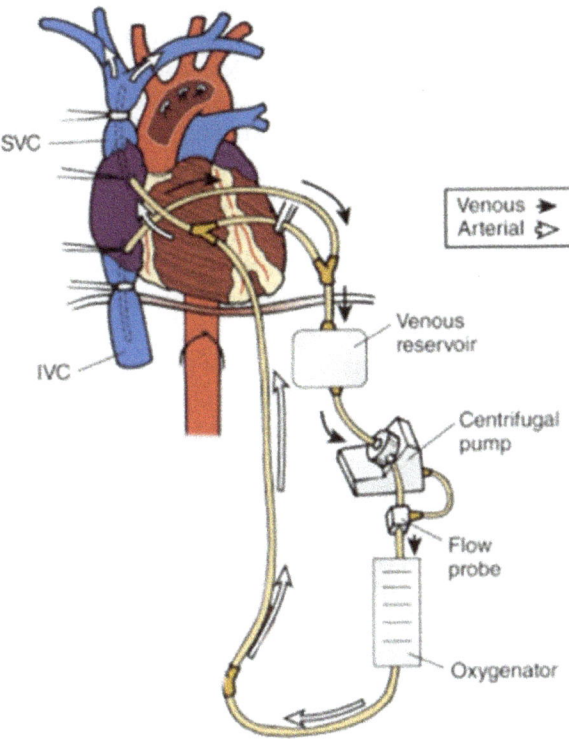

Figure 9.3 Retrograde cerebral perfusion (RCP) established via cannula in the superior vena cava (SVC) which is looped into the CPB circuit via a Y-connector. IVC, inferior vena cava

substrate delivery provided by RCP are poorly defined but are unlikely to fulfill the metabolic demands of the brain even under deep hypothermia. Suggested blood flow rates for RCP are 200–300 ml/min with SVC pressure <25 mmHg to prevent cerebral edema. SVC pressure is typically monitored via the side-port of the introducer sheath in the internal jugular vein.

Theoretical advantages of RCP include:

- more homogenous brain cooling
- washout of embolic material (gaseous and particulate) and metabolic waste products
- prevention of cerebral blood cell microaggregates
- fewer thromboembolic events by avoidance of epiaortic vessel manipulation.

The prolongation of safe DHCA that can be achieved with RCP is less than that with SACP. RCP for >60 minutes is a significant predictor of permanent neurologic dysfunction.

There is currently no expert consensus on which cerebral protection strategy (DHCA alone, DHCA

87

with SACP, DHCA with RCP) is superior. There have been few prospective, randomized trials and the majority of published studies comparing these approaches have been retrospective. The conclusions from the available literature are that:

- an adjunct form of cerebral protection (SACP or RCP) is superior to DHCA alone
- the method of cerebral perfusion – SACP vs RCP – has no impact on the incidence of postoperative stroke or permanent neurologic dysfunction
- SACP reduces the incidence of temporary neurologic dysfunction (delirium, confusion, prolonged obtundation without focal deficits or radiographic signs of structural brain abnormalities) compared to RCP.

A randomized study of DHCA alone versus DHCA with SACP in patients undergoing PTE found no difference in postoperative cognitive dysfunction.

Neurologic Monitoring

Neurologic monitoring can be considered in three categories: routine clinical observation, monitors of cerebral substrate delivery and monitors of cerebral activity (see Table 9.5). For a monitor to be useful it must prompt a corrective intervention before the onset of irreversible neurologic injury. Due to their

Table 9.5. Neurologic monitoring

Clinical	Arterial pressure
	Central venous pressure
	CPB pump flow rate
	Arterial oxygen saturation
	Hemoglobin concentration
	Arterial PCO$_2$
	Temperature
	Pupil size
Substrate delivery	Transcranial Doppler sonography
	Near infrared spectroscopy
	Jugular venous oxygen saturation
Cerebral activity	Electroencephalography
	Somatosensory evoked potentials
	Auditory evoked potentials
	Motor evoked potentials

significant cost and lack of level 1A evidence of efficacy, neurologic monitoring has yet to be universally adopted as "standard of care."

Near infrared spectroscopy (NIRS) allows non-invasive measurement of regional cerebral oxygen saturation (rSO$_2$). An abrupt bilateral decrease in rSO$_2$ (>20% below the baseline value) may indicate global cerebral ischemia; a significant unilateral decrease of rSO$_2$ may suggest regional compromise of cerebral perfusion or an embolic event. Both situations must be communicated to the surgeon and perfusionist immediately, prompting interventions to improve cerebral oxygen delivery. A decrease of rSO$_2$ >20% from baseline or an absolute rSO$_2$ <50% have been reported to be clinically significant. Simplicity and relatively low cost mean that cerebral NIRS is the most widely used adjunct to routine clinical monitoring.

Measuring venous oxygen saturation at the jugular bulb (S$_{JV}$O$_2$) using a fiberoptic catheter provides a continuous measure of the global balance between cerebral oxygen supply and demand. Catheters need placing under fluoroscopy and only very few centers use this modality routinely. Low S$_{JV}$O$_2$ prior to the onset of DHCA is associated with adverse neurologic outcome. S$_{JV}$O$_2$ monitoring may also be used to monitor the adequacy of SACP.

Transcranial Doppler (TCD) sonography of the middle cerebral arteries is largely an investigational technique used to measure CBF velocity (a surrogate measure of CBF) and as a means for detecting and quantifying cerebral microemboli (gaseous and particulate). Finding acoustic windows in the temporal region of the skull and maintaining probe position are notoriously difficult. TCD is of limited use during DHCA, although it has been used to assess CBF during SACP and RCP.

Chapter 18 provides more in depth discussion of neurologic monitoring.

Spinal Cord Protection

Surgery involving the descending thoracic aorta may interrupt blood flow to the spinal cord via the anterior spinal artery (of Adamkiewicz) and cause paraplegia – a devastating complication that occurs in as many as one in six cases. Risk factors include the extent and severity of aortic atheroma, longer duration of AXC application, emergency surgery, previous surgery to the distal aorta, perioperative hypotension, advanced age and diabetes mellitus. Besides hypothermia, the interventions thought to reduce the risk of spinal cord injury include sequential clamping of the aorta with re-implantation of intercostal and lumbar segmental vessels, LHB to provide distal perfusion, cerebrospinal fluid (CSF) drainage and neurophysiologic monitoring.

Cerebrospinal Fluid Drainage

The production of cerebrospinal fluid (CSF) increases during ischemia, leading to increased intrathecal pressure soon after the aortic cross clamp is applied. Spinal cord perfusion pressure (SCPP) is the difference between MAP and intrathecal pressure (ITP). Typically, during thoracoabdominal aortic surgery the SCPP is maintained at ≥70 mmHg (i.e., MAP >80 mmHg and ITP <10 mmHg). Maintaining MAP at a level higher than is usual during conventional cardiac surgery may require a vasopressor infusion, and intermittent CSF drainage may be required to maintain ITP <10 mmHg.

Both randomized trials and meta-analyses have demonstrated that CSF drainage reduces the incidence of paraplegia after open thoracic aortic surgery. It is recommended in all patients at high risk for spinal cord ischemia (Class IIa recommendation, level B evidence). In many centers a drainage catheter is inserted into the intrathecal space at either the $L_{3/4}$ or $L_{4/5}$ interspace. The catheter is connected to a closed collection system which enables both ITP monitoring and removal of CSF when clinically indicated (Figure 9.4). The risk of direct spinal cord or nerve root damage at this level is small. The timing of catheter insertion is largely driven by institutional practice and concerns about bleeding during insertion (which could progress to epidural hematoma with heparinization during the surgery) sufficient to warrant postponement or cancellation of surgery. Practice ranges from insertion on the day before surgery to insertion immediately before induction of anesthesia. In some centers, however, a CSF catheter is placed *after* induction of general anesthesia but before placement of all invasive lines, which in most cases still allows for a safety margin of at least one hour before systemic heparinization. A CSF drainage catheter may also be inserted after surgery in lower risk patients who develop signs of spinal cord ischemia.

The management of CSF drains varies between institutions. The following general principles apply:

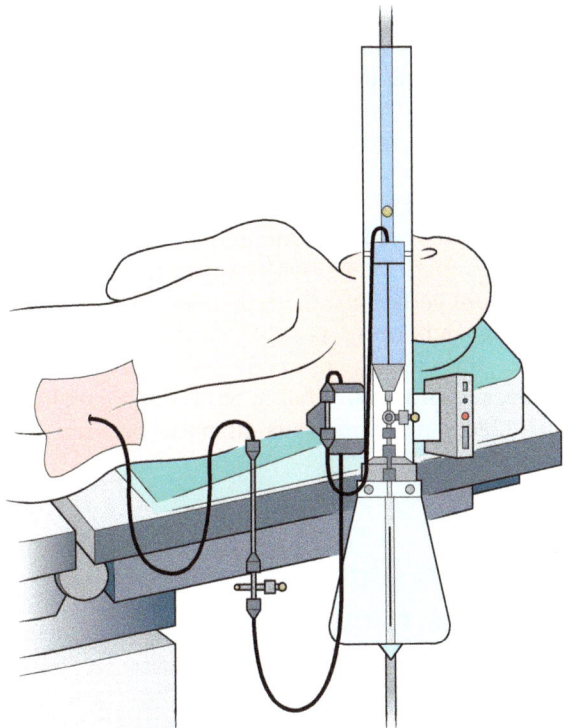

Figure 9.4 Lumbar cerebrospinal fluid drainage system with CSF collection bag. Pressure can either be transduced onto the anesthetic monitoring system or can be read on an analog scale. The pressure transducer is zeroed at the level of the foramen magnum.

The collection system should be mounted on a dedicated IV pole and the CSF drainage stopcock should be closed to the patient at all times except for the time of actively draining the CSF. The transducer should be "zeroed" at the level of foramen magnum or the catheter insertion site. During and immediately after surgery, CSF is allowed to drain passively from the catheter to maintain an ITP of 8–10 mmHg. Once the patient is awake and neurologic signs of ischemia can be monitored, the ITP can be allowed to rise to 15–20 mmHg. CSF drainage should be limited to 20 ml/hr. Rapid drainage of a large volume of CSF should be avoided as an abrupt fall in intracranial pressure may cause tearing of the subdural vessels and subarachnoid hemorrhage.

Neurophysiologic Monitoring

Motor evoked potential (MEP) monitoring is increasingly used to assess descending anterior spinal pathways, thus providing a measure of the adequacy of spinal cord perfusion and guiding the need for selective re-implantation of key intercostal arteries. Profound neuromuscular blockade should be avoided when attempting to use MEP monitoring.

Somatosensory evoked potential (SSEP) monitoring provides a means of assessing the integrity and function of ascending posterior sensory pathways. A fall in SSEP amplitude >50% from baseline should prompt re-implantation of intercostal arteries into the graft, along with measures to improve spinal cord perfusion, mainly increasing mean arterial pressure and, where possible, SCPP. It should be borne in mind, however, that hypothermia produces a progressive fall in SSEP signal amplitude such that some components disappear between 24°C and 17°C.

Pulmonary (Thrombo) endarterectomy (PTE)

The incidence of chronic thromboembolic pulmonary hypertension (CTEPH) in patients surviving acute pulmonary embolism is up to 4%. Medical therapy for CTEPH is limited and ultimately only palliative. When the disease lies proximal enough to allow surgical excision, PTE offers both symptomatic and prognostic benefit as well as the potential to restore normal life expectancy. PTE has been shown to offer superior outcomes to lung transplantation in the CTEPH population (95% one-year survival versus 85% in lung transplant). As the morbidity and mortality (~4%) associated with PTE have fallen, the indications for the procedure have widened to include the elderly and younger patients with mild yet symptomatic pulmonary hypertension.

The surgical setup involves bicaval and ascending aortic cannulation, and the use of a continuous flow "cold jacket" placed behind the heart to augment myocardial protection. To achieve maximal hemodynamic improvement and optimal outcome, a complete endarterectomy to the distal tail ends of each pulmonary arterial branch is essential. Due to the large amount of bronchial circulation usually present in these patients, circulatory arrest is necessary to ensure a bloodless field to perform a thorough endarterectomy. In experienced centers, bilateral endarterectomy on each side can be performed using

two 20-minute periods of DHCA. Cerebral perfusion adjuncts are not usually needed. RCP is not helpful in PTE because it precludes a bloodless surgical field. In most cases, DHCA with intermittent systemic reperfusion is used in preference to SACP, with NIRS to guide the duration of circulatory arrest. A rSO_2 of <40% is widely used as the acceptable minimum.

Complications of PTE include pulmonary artery rupture, reperfusion injury (reperfusion pulmonary edema) and right ventricular failure. The discovery of frank blood in the endotracheal tube following separation from CPB typically indicates pulmonary artery rupture. CPB should be reinstituted immediately to reduce pulmonary blood flow. Further attempts to wean from CPB tend to be futile whereas the institution of central veno-arterial extracorporeal membrane oxygenation (ECMO) is associated with >50% survival to hospital discharge. By contrast, refractory hypoxia secondary to severe reperfusion injury is managed with veno-venous ECMO.

DHCA is an established and widely employed technique for providing optimal operating conditions while preserving organ function. Most patients will tolerate 20 minutes of circulatory arrest at 20°C without significant neurologic impairment. While hypothermia is the main method of cerebral protection, other neuroprotective strategies include pharmacological methods, tight glycemic control, hemodilution, acid–base management, CSF drainage and neurologic monitoring.

Surgical techniques such as SACP and intermittent reperfusion may be used to prolong the safe duration of DHCA. The development of novel branched vascular grafts allows surgeons to undertake repair of the aortic arch in stages, providing the means to restore antegrade blood flow to the distal aorta and cerebral circulation earlier in the surgical procedure, and the opportunity to shorten the duration of CPB with safe, early rewarming. Nevertheless, DHCA inevitably exposes patients to significantly prolonged CPB with all its associated risks and adverse effects. Fastidious attention to temperature management during both cooling and rewarming is essential.

Suggested Further Reading

1. Arrowsmith JE, Ganugapenta MSSR. Intraoperative brain monitoring in cardiac surgery. In Bonser R, Pagano D, Haverich A (Eds.). *Brain Protection in Cardiac Surgery*. London: Springer-Verlag. 2011. pp.83–111.

2. Chan MJ, Chung T, Glassford NJ et al. Near-Infrared spectroscopy in adult cardiac surgery patients: a systematic review and meta-analysis. *J Cardiothorac Vasc Anesth.* 2017; 31(4): 1155–1165.

3. Ghadimi K, Gutsche JT, Setegne SL et al. Severity and duration of metabolic acidosis after deep hypothermic circulatory arrest for thoracic aortic surgery. *J Cardiothorac Vasc Anesth* 2015; 29 (6): 1432–1440.

4. James ML, Anderson MD, Swaminathan M et al. Predictors of electrocerebral inactivity with deep hypothermia. *J Thorac Cardiovasc Surg* 2014; 147(3): 1002–1007.

5. Krüger T, Hoffmann I, Blettner M et al. Intraoperative neuroprotective drugs without beneficial effects? Results of the German Registry for Acute Aortic Dissection Type A (GERAADA). *Eur J Cardiothorac Surg* 2013; 44 (5): 939–946.

6. Misfeld M, Leontyev S, Borger MA et al. What is the best strategy for brain protection in patients undergoing aortic arch surgery? A single center experience of 636 patients. *Ann Thorac Surg* 2012; 93(5): 1502–1508.

7. Scheeren TWL, Kuizenga MH, Maurer H et al. Electroencephalography and brain oxygenation monitoring in the perioperative period. *Anesth Analg* 2019; 128(2): 265–277.

8. Steppan J, Hogue CW Jr. Cerebral and tissue oximetry. *Best Pract Res Clin Anaesthesiol* 2014; 28(4): 429–439.

9. Vuylsteke A, Sharples L, Charman G et al. Circulatory arrest versus cerebral perfusion during pulmonary endarterectomy surgery (PEACOG): a randomized controlled trial. *Lancet* 2011; 378 (9800): 1379–1387.

10. Etz CD, Weigang E, Hartert M et al.Contemporary spinal cord protection during thoracic and thoracoabdominal aortic surgery and endovascular aortic repair: a position paper of the vascular domain of the European Association for Cardio-Thoracic Surgery, *European Journal of Cardio-Thoracic Surgery*, 2015, 47 (6): 943–957.

Metabolic Management during Cardiopulmonary Bypass

Jonathan Brand and Edward M Darling

The metabolic management of patients on cardiopulmonary bypass (CPB) is a complex process, involving several key biochemical and physiological parameters essential to maintaining homeostasis and reducing morbidity and mortality associated with CPB and cardiac surgery. There is movement toward goal-directed perfusion (GDP), using indexed parameters such as carbon dioxide production, oxygen delivery and oxygen consumption to individualize perfusion strategies. This chapter provides an overview over the fundamental principles surrounding the metabolic management of the patient on CPB.

Cardiopulmonary Bypass and the Challenges of Metabolic Management

The primary challenge for safe and effective extracorporeal circulation is to maintain optimal metabolic conditions for physiological homeostasis. CPB management must maintain systemic perfusion and physiological metabolic processes and must adapt to the particular demands of each patient. CPB-induced challenges that must be accounted for to ensure optimal metabolic management and prevention of end-organ dysfunction include:

- Non pulsatile flow and its distribution
- Hemodilution
- Altered hemodynamics and vascular tone
- Electrolyte shifts
- Temperature changes and blood gas strategies

Any attempt at successful metabolic management during CPB must address these challenges.

Effective Bypass and Circuit Design

Optimizing metabolic management during CPB begins with the ability to achieve technically "good bypass." Good bypass is predicated upon the ability to decompress the venous system and empty the heart

(venous drainage) while at the same time providing adequate arterial pump blood flow with good oxygenator function. The perfusionist should be able to achieve the necessary pump flow without constantly having to add fluid to the circuit or empty the venous reservoir. Sufficient venous drainage (assessed hemodynamically by low central venous or pulmonary pressure with a non pulsatile arterial pressure trace and visually by the heart being relaxed and collapsed) is the essential starting point to optimizing metabolic management.

Metabolic Markers during CPB

Classic markers of adequate perfusion include achieving the calculated flow, target arterial pressure, satisfactory blood gases and a normal mixed venous oxygen saturation (S_vO_2) as shown in Table 10.1.

CPB Blood Flow

The desired pump flow rate during CPB is traditionally determined according to body surface area (BSA) and temperature. At normothermia, an indexed flow rate of 2.2–2.8 l/min/m^2 is targeted by most clinical teams. For the obese patient (BMI > 30 kg/m^2), the traditional target flow calculations may overestimate flow requirements and can be modified to more closely represent the metabolic need based on lean body mass. By setting a BMI of 28 kg/m^2 and using the patient height (m) to calculate mass (kg), a new BSA can be derived, and a "lean" target flow calculated (see sample calculation in Figure 10.1).

Measuring oxygen delivery (DO_2) as part of a GDP strategy, in addition to standard metabolic and oxygenation parameters, has been suggested as the most accurate means of assessing the adequacy of pump flow.

The majority of CPB is undertaken using a continuous flow. It is possible to use pulsatile flow by using specifically designed pumps or modifying standard pumps. A heterogeneity of literature exists around this topic with some papers indicating that pulsatile perfusion may reduce renal complications in high-risk patients. More recent publications have either shown there to be no difference between continuous and pulsatile flow or the latter to be causing hemolysis. Pulsatile flow is not a widely accepted practice.

Table 10.1. Standard adult CPB metabolic management parameters

	Target	Monitoring
Blood Flow Rate C.I. (l/min/m²)	2.2–2.8	Centrifugal pump: ultrasonic flow probe distal to any shunts Roller pump: calculated from RPM/ultrasonic flow probe distal to any shunts
Mean Arterial Pressure (mmHg)	60–80	Arterial pressure transducer
Arterial and Venous Blood Gases	"normal" *	Intermittent sampling from circuit ports and/or real time in-line sensors
Hematocrit/ Hemoglobin	>24% >8.0 g/dl	Optical cell in venous line of CPB circuit
SvO₂ (%)	>75%	Optical cell in venous line of CPB circuit
Urine Output	>4 ml/ kg/ hour	Catheter bag
Blood Lactate	<2.0 mmol/l	Intermittent sampling

* See Table 10.2.

Mean Arterial Pressure (MAP) during CPB

In analogy to the physiological circulation the primary determinants of MAP during CPB are:

- pump flow and
- systemic vascular resistance.

Ensuring an acceptable MAP during CPB is an important determinant in maintaining appropriate perfusion of vital end-organs, particularly the brain and kidneys, both of which rely on MAP across a range of 35–100 mmHg during physiological flow to maintain intrinsic autoregulation. Despite published standards and prevailing clinical practice having established a MAP between 50 and 80 mmHg during CPB as an acceptable range, the optimal MAP for each individual patient is still subject to debate. It has been suggested that MAP during CPB should be determined by the individual patient's cerebral autoregulation range (based on the preoperative MAP) rather than universally set ranges. More recent studies suggest a reduced incidence of stroke with higher (>70 mmHg) when compared to lower MAPs.

There are many reasons why blood pressure will vary during CPB. Higher MAPs may result from inadequate anesthesia/analgesia, systemic vasoconstriction or catecholamine release and may require deepening of anesthesia or the addition of vasodilators to correct. Conversely, and more commonly,

Traditional Calculation	Lean Flow Calculation
Height = 173 cm	Height = 173 cm
Weight = 125 kg	Adjusted Weight = 28 kg/m² x (1.73m)² = 83.8 Kg
BMI = 41.8	Adjusted BMI = 28
BSA = 2.45	Adjusted BSA = 2.01
Target Flow (2.4 C.I) = 5.9 L/min	Target "Lean" Flow (2.4 C.I) = 4.8 L/min

BMI = weight/height²

$$BSA = \sqrt{\frac{weight \; x \; height}{3600}}$$

Figure 10.1 Obese patient lean flow sample calculation.

Table 10.2. Typical blood gas parameters during CPB

	Circuit Arterial Blood Gas	Circuit Venous Blood Gas
pH	7.35–7.45	7.33–7.44
$PaCO_2$	4.6–6.0 kPa 35–45 mmHg	5.0–6.4 kPa 37.5–48 mmHg
PaO_2	13–33 kPa 100–250 mmHg	>5.2 kPa >39 mmHg
Oxygen saturations (SaO_2)	>95%	>75%
Bicarbonate (HCO_3^-)	22–26 mEq/L (mmol/l)	22–26 mEq/L (mmol/l)
Base excess	−2 to +2	−2 to +2

MAP may reduce during CPB. Common causes include increased anesthetic depth with hypothermia, hemodilution, inflammatory response, ongoing sepsis (e.g. endocarditis), perioperative antihypertensive medication (particularly ACE inhibitors) and vasoplegic syndrome. Current literature supports the use of alpha agonists, such as phenylephrine, as primary vasopressors when treating low MAP on bypass (in addition to addressing potential underlying causes).

Blood Gas Parameters

Blood gas management during CPB typically aims for the ranges shown in Table 10.2. The air/oxygen blender allows titration of both the inspiratory oxygen concentration (FiO_2) and gas flow (sweep) through the oxygenator gas phase, providing excellent control of arterial O_2 and CO_2. Sampling arterial blood gases from the circuit every 30 minutes and continuous S_vO_2 in-line monitoring are recommended standards.

Continuous In-line Blood Gas Monitoring

Sensors placed in the arterial and venous lines of the CPB circuit can provide near real time changes in a variety of key parameters including arterial oxygen saturation (SaO_2), pH, pCO_2, pO_2, hematocrit, bicarbonate, base excess and potassium. When combined with pump flow rate, these monitors provide continuous measures of DO_2 and oxygen consumption (VO_2). Continuous monitoring allows necessary changes to be made immediately while also being able

to see the success of an intervention in a timely manner, which is a clear advantage of over intermittent sampling.

Acid-Base Balance

Acid-base balance during bypass is integral to the maintenance of physiological homeostasis. Metabolic derangement, particularly acidosis, often results from DO_2/VO_2 mismatch which can be corrected by methods described later in this chapter. The bicarbonate (HCO_3^-) buffer system plays a vital role in maintaining physiological pH. At times of significant metabolic acidosis during CPB, it becomes necessary to add HCO_3^- to correct a persistently low pH (< 7.2) or a base excess lower than -5. The following simple formula can be used to guide HCO_3^- administration during CPB: [body weight (kg) $\times$ 0.15] $\times$ base deficient $=$ mmol $NaHCO_3^-$. Care must be taken to avoid the inherent consequences of the high sodium load that comes with buffering. The use of hemofiltration may also correct an ongoing acidosis. It is important to consider the potential causes of ongoing metabolic acidosis rather than just correcting its sequela.

Hematocrit on CPB

Hematocrit (Hct) is an important determinant of DO_2. Hemodilution (and hence reduced Hct) is not uncommon during CPB, particularly when using asanguinous circuit prime. Importantly, Hct values below the accepted range of 22–24% have been associated with poor outcomes and increased morbidity and mortality; conversely, excessive increases in the Hct with blood transfusion are also associated with increased morbidity and mortality. It is prudent to consider strategies such as retrograde autologous prime, ultrafiltration and minimizing prime volume to optimize Hct to reduce the use of bank blood.

Mixed Venous Oxygen Saturation (S_vO_2)

Historically, an $S_vO_2 > 75\%$ during CPB has been considered the primary indicator for an even balance between DO_2 and VO_2. The S_vO_2 should be considered in the context of patient temperature. While organ metabolic demand decreases with hypothermia, the solubility and hemoglobin affinity of oxygen increases at the same time. The S_vO_2 should therefore increase with decreasing temperature provided perfusion is adequate. Venous saturations of 65–75% at

35–37°C, 76–85% at 32–34°C and 85–100% at 20–32°C are typical.

It is a standard of perfusion practice to monitor S_VO_2 continuously with an in-line optical sensor. A declining S_VO_2 suggests an imbalance of DO_2 relative to VO_2 and the perfusionist will respond by increasing pump flow and ensuring optimal Hct or hemoglobin. Although a low SVO_2 indicates a problem with systemic DO_2 and is associated with poor postoperative outcomes, a normal S_VO_2, does not necessarily guarantee that CPB pump flow is meeting regional and/or organ specific VO_2.

Urine Output

Acute kidney injury (AKI) is common following cardiac surgery. The kidneys are particularly sensitive to hypoperfusion, and urine output (UO) is traditionally used as an organic marker of adequate perfusion. UO <2 ml/kg/h can be associated with higher rates of AKI. Limitations of this parameter are that UO changes can be a late indicator of renal injury, and that it is affected by multiple other factors unrelated to the adequacy of metabolic support. Chapter 19 discusses the impact of CPB on renal function and AKI in more detail.

Blood Lactate

Lactate is the predominant metabolic component of glucose metabolism and under normal conditions feeds into the aerobic pathway of glucose utilization. Despite lactate disturbances commonly occurring during periods of low flow or hypothermic CPB, it is recognized that increased lactate levels may be indicative of inadequate perfusion, in particular of a mismatch between DO_2 and VO_2, leading to increased anaerobic metabolism. Numerous studies have demonstrated that hyperlactatemia (>2.0 mmol/l) is associated with significantly worse outcomes. Recently there has been a shift toward attention to lactate as a dynamic parameter with an increase of lactate by more than 200% from baseline (and irrespective of the baseline level) being associated with significantly higher mortality. Increased lactate levels are not always the result of inadequate perfusion and alternative reasons must be borne in mind: hypothermia, inadequate hepatic metabolism (resulting from reduced function or perfusion), oral hypoglycemic agents, altered glycolytic flux or inhibition of pyruvate dehydrogenase. Treatment strategies generally aim to correct the presumed cause and include increasing the pump flow, rewarming to normothermia, and checking that the venous pipe does not impede venous drainage from the liver. Although generally done with every blood gas analysis, the intermittent sampling of blood lactate has the risk of delaying timely intervention.

Goal-Directed Perfusion Parameters in Metabolic Monitoring during CPB

Goal-directed perfusion is a strategy that algorithmically monitors both oxygen delivery and carbon dioxide production during CPB. It uses this information, combined with the classic metabolic and hemodynamic parameters (of stroke volume, end diastolic volume index, MAP and cardiac index), to provide tailored and optimal perfusion for each individual patient by avoiding a mismatch between oxygen delivery and consumption. Various studies have demonstrated a reduction in postoperative morbidity associated with the use of GDP. Important constituents of this approach are described below and illustrated in Table 10.3. GDP parameters tend to be indexed to the patient's BSA.

Oxygen Delivery

Oxygen delivery is influenced by both pump flow and hematocrit and is one of the most significant determinants of "optimal" perfusion. Cardiac surgery is associated with a 22–40% incidence of AKI and inadequate DO_2 is a likely contributor. It has been demonstrated that maintaining an indexed DO_2 (DO_2i) > 270–300 $mlO_2/min/m^2$ may reduce the incidence of AKI. Monitoring and maintaining DO_2i levels by adjusting pump flow and/or Hct is an important aspect of optimizing metabolic management. In addition to maintaining DO_2, monitoring the indexed VO_2 (VO_2i) can be informative. In an anesthetized patient on CPB, VO_2i will normally be in the range of 40–50 $mlO_2/min/m^2$.

CO_2-derived Parameters

Monitoring CO_2 production (VCO_2i) may allow early real time detection of inadequate perfusion. Increases in VCO_2i are often the result of carbon dioxide production under anaerobic conditions. They can be indicative of buffering of hyperlactatemia by the bicarbonate system. Therefore, in the presence of

95

Table 10.3. Goal-Directed perfusion parameters and ratios

All targets are based upon normothermic temperatures during CPB.

Parameter	Measurement Calculation	Targets	Considerations & Management
Oxygen Delivery Indexed (DO_2i)	$DO_2i = CI \times C_aO_2 \times 10$	Maintain > 270 mL/min/m^2	If below target, increasing pump flow rate and/or increasing the Hb should be considered
Oxygen Consumption Indexed (VO_2i)	$VO_2i = CI \times (C_aO_2 - C_vO_2)$	Normally 40-50 ml O_2/min/m^2 under anesthesia	Higher than expected VO_2i → consider the depth of anesthesia and temperature
Carbon Dioxide Production Indexed (VCO_2i)	$VCO_2i = (V_E \times ePCO_2{}^* \times 1.315)$ /BSA	<60 mL/min/m^2	>60 mL/min/m^2, rule out CO_2 field flooding
GDP ratio	DO_2i/VCO_2i	Target ratio > 5.0	Increase DO_2i if outside target
Oxygen Extraction Ratio (O_2ER)	VO_2i/DO_2i	<40	>40 may suggest trigger for RBC transfusion
Respiratory Quotient	VCO_2/VO_2i	Normal $= 0.8-1.0$	>1 corresponds to increase in lactate production

$ePCO_2$ = exhaled CO_2

inadequate DO_2i, VCO_2i is considered to be a rapid, indirect marker of lactate generation. The CO_2 production is measured at the gas outlet site of the oxygenator.

O_2 and CO_2 Ratios in Metabolic Monitoring during CPB

- *GDP Ratio* – Pairing DO_2i and VCO_2i in a ratio is a key component in the GDP concept. A study by deSomer et al. found that a DO_2i/VCO_2i less than 5.3 was a predictor of postoperative AKI. This cutoff value has not yet reliably been reproduced in other studies, the goal of the GDP ratio is rapid detection and prevention of anaerobic metabolism by maintaining a DO_2i above 270 mL/min/m^2, $VCO_2i < 60$ mL/min/m^2 and the $DO_2i/VCO_2i > 5$.
- *O_2 Extraction Ratio* – The oxygen extraction ratio (O_2ER) is the ratio of VO_2 to DO_2. There is some evidence that O_2ER is better than a hemoglobin value for guiding transfusion decisions on CPB. Some studies have demonstrated using O_2ER as a measure of tissue hypoxia and aiming for a value of over 40 was associated with a reduction in single organ failure and length of hospital stay.

- *Respiratory Quotient* – The respiratory quotient (RQ) is the ratio of CO_2 produced (VCO_2) to O_2 consumed (VO_2). During CPB, anaerobic metabolism and lactate production have been shown to positively correlate with RQ > 0.9.

These three quotients provide the foundation of emerging GDP practice and metabolic management. Although it might be tempting, practitioners should not fall into the trap of seeing them in isolation but need to evaluate them in the context of other parameters such as blood chemistry and temperature.

Electrolytes

Electrolytes play fundamental roles in metabolism and cellular energy production alongside generation of resting membrane potentials in both nerve and muscle cells. It is essential to prevent electrolyte disturbances during CPB. The effects of any imbalances can be cumulative when more than one deficiency exists.

Potassium

Potassium is the predominant intracellular cation and abnormalities during bypass are common.

Hyperkalemia often results from cardioplegia administration and is mostly self-limiting, rarely needing active treatment. Potassium has many cellular re-uptake pathways, promoting the restoration of electrochemical balance, particularly in response to fluid shifts and urine production. The tolerance for hyperkalemia varies between patients and some with chronic kidney disease tolerate high levels of 6mmol/l or above. The presence of ECG abnormalities and plasma levels above 6.5 mmol/l are often triggers for instituting treatment. Commonly used treatments include IV bolus doses of calcium, dextrose-insulin infusion or forced diuresis with a loop diuretic. Zero-balance ultrafiltration with a potassium free solution (usually sodium chloride) is another option to lower high potassium levels when removal of excess plasma water is required at the same time, although care must be taken to avoid hypernatremia or hyperchloremia. When hyperkalemia exists in the presence of an acidosis, the use of sodium bicarbonate may help to promote the intracellular movement of potassium. The clinical team should keep in mind that there might be other reasons than cardioplegia for hyperkalemia. They include red cell transfusion, hyperglycemia, renal failure, ongoing ischemia from reduced bypass flow or malignant hyperthermia and rhabdomyolysis.

Hypokalemia is a common preoperative finding, often resulting from hemodilution, concomitant diuretic use or secondary hyperaldosteronism in congestive cardiac failure. Untreated hypokalemia can precipitate significant arrhythmias and poor ventricular function, which can pose serious problems when weaning from bypass. Initial treatment of hypokalemia is usually by replacement of potassium at a dose of 10–20 mmol, which can be given straight into the reservoir.

Magnesium

Magnesium is another intracellular cation involved in energy production and utilization. It also plays an important role in the stabilization of electrically excitable cells and in the regulation of vascular tone. Depletion of magnesium during cardiac surgery is common, often resulting from the concomitant use of preoperative loop diuretics, hemodilution by the pump prime, low magnesium in cardioplegic solutions, or ultrafiltration. In both adult and pediatric populations, hypomagnesemia (defined as a plasma level of <0.7 mmol/l) is associated with the presence of arrhythmias (in particular atrial fibrillation but also supra- and ventricular arrhythmias), seizures and worsening of clinical outcomes.

Intravenous magnesium supplementation with up to 2g is common during cardiac surgery as there is suggestion that this can help prevent arrhythmias. Magnesium may also be given in an analgesic dose (50 mg/kg) as part of enhanced recovery protocols after cardiac surgery. Ideally any magnesium supplementation should be titrated against plasma levels to avoid hypermagnesemia.

Calcium

Hypocalcemia (defined as a plasma level <2.1 mmol/l) is another common electrolyte abnormality, often resulting from hemodilution, hemofiltration and chelation with citrate in processed blood. Correction of hypocalcemia is required due to the ubiquitous role of calcium in cardiovascular and coagulation physiology. This is typically achieved by the administration of either calcium chloride or calcium gluconate as a bolus dose. Hypocalcemia should only be corrected after a period of normothermic myocardial reperfusion, following cross clamp removal, because of the role it plays in the cellular signaling of apoptosis and the possibility of worsening reperfusion injury if given too early.

Phosphate

Phosphate plays a role in many intracellular enzymatic and energy producing pathways and in maintaining cellular resting membrane potential. Despite many patients having postoperative hypophosphatemia, presumably as a result of intracellular shifting resulting from alterations in acid-base status, intraoperative supplementation is not a routine practice in the majority of institutions. Failure to correct phosphate levels can lead to undesirable clinical effects such as respiratory failure, muscle weakness, or impaired cardiac function with reduced cardiac output. Correcting phosphate levels should be part of the postoperative treatment.

Chloride

Chloride is a key component of both normal saline and unbalanced colloid solutions. Excessive use of normal saline or unbalanced fluid solutions as either infusion fluid, priming volume or as part of intraoperative cell salvage can lead to a hyperchloremia, in turn leading to a metabolic acidosis. Despite an absence of literature detailing the effects on outcome, normal physiological levels should be targeted, and consideration given to the role of chloride in contributing to any metabolic acidosis.

Glucose

Hyperglycemia is common during CPB and often requires an insulin infusion to control blood sugar levels. The main causes are:

i. the physiological stress response evoked by surgical insult leading to decreased insulin sensitivity,

ii. many cardiac surgical patients are diabetic, and quality of sugar control varies widely,

iii. sicker hearts are unable to utilize glucose as an energy substrate, predisposing these patients to hyperglycemia,

iv. the use of some inotropic agents, namely epinephrine, induce a rise in plasma glucose,

v. addition of steroids to the circuit prime,

vi. glucose containing cardioplegia solutions.

Hyperglycemia leads to poor outcomes. Morbid conditions associated with poor perioperative blood sugar control include neurological dysfunction, mediastinitis and increased risk of infection and sepsis. Tight intraoperative blood glucose control using a titrated insulin infusion has been associated with improved patient outcomes and reduced mortality in a number of studies. However, there is some debate about the actual blood sugar target required. Tight control to normal glucose levels (4.0–5.5 mmol/l; 70–100 mg/dl) is difficult to achieve, can lead to rebound hypoglycemia and is not recommended. This has led to a more recent "liberal" approach being favored, particularly in diabetic patients. This approach allows blood glucose to rise to 10 mmol/l (180 mg/dl) in diabetics, with non diabetic patients only being treated at levels above 7.8 mmol/l (140 mg/dl). The goal in glucose management is to maintain near to normal blood glucose levels for every patient while not forgetting the dangers of too tight glycemic control.

Drug Metabolism

CPB will often cause significant changes in both the pharmacokinetic and dynamic properties of drugs.

Table 10.4 summarizes the effects on the most important anesthetic drugs. There are four principal mechanisms that are responsible for altered drug behavior during CPB:

- The dilutional effects of priming volume changes drug and plasma protein concentrations. Altered plasma protein concentrations may alter the ratio of bound versus free drug leading to differing pharmacological activity depending on whether a drug is active in its free or bound state.

- The materials, which various components of the bypass circuit are made of, may affect drug binding while some drugs like vancomycin are sequestered by certain oxygenators.

- Drug metabolism and clearance behave proportional to decrease in microcirculatory flow and hypothermia, both of which lead to reduced elimination and the potential for prolonged pharmacological activity. The effect of some neuromuscular blocking agents is increased by decreasing systemic temperature.

- Pulmonary drug sequestration, resulting from lung isolation during aortic cross clamping, may lead to increased plasma levels of drugs such as fentanyl on full reperfusion at the time of separation from bypass.

Volatile anesthetic agents are widely used in cardiac anesthesia and can be given throughout the operation, i.e. both on and off bypass, to maintain general anesthesia. The blood:gas partition coefficient of an agent determines the rate of physiological response, with higher coefficients representing slower response rates and vice versa. This coefficient is altered as soon as a patient is put on CPB – hemodilution reduces it, increasing the response rate; hypothermia increases it, slowing the response down. Perfusionists must be mindful of the effect that both temperature and hemodilution have on the activity and concentrations of volatile anesthetic agents. It is recommended that anesthetic agent monitoring is attached to the exhaust line of the oxygenator. Anesthetic agents (intravenous and volatile) may contribute to systemic vasodilation, potentially reducing MAP.

Nitrous oxide should not be used before or after bypass due to its insolubility in blood. It can enlarge systemic air bubbles, thereby worsening the consequences of any residual systemic air. In addition, it can depress myocardial function.

Table 10.4. Summary of the effects of CPB on key anesthetic drugs

Drug	Effects of bypass
Volatile anesthetics	• Uptake and elimination are inversely proportional to blood:gas solubility coefficient – the higher the coefficient, the more soluble the agent and the slower the onset of action. • Increases in sweep gas flow increases uptake, changes in pump flow do not. • Hemodilution reduces protein binding, increasing the response rate. • Hypothermia increases the blood:gas solubility coefficient, reducing the speed of onset of volatile anesthetics. • Rewarming reduces the volatile anesthetic blood:gas solubility coefficient and can increase depth of anesthesia. • Volatile anesthetic agent transfer across the oxygenator membrane can differ between models, making agent monitoring essential.
Propofol	• Free drug concentration increases with hemodilution and reduced plasma protein concentration, leading to increased efficacy of propofol on CPB.
Opioids	• Free drug concentration increases with hemodilution and reduced plasma protein concentration. • Hypothermic CPB increases the elimination half-life due to reduced hepatic clearance. • Remifentanil elimination is temperature-dependent, a reduction of infusion rates should be considered during hypothermic CPB.
Muscle relaxants	• Free drug concentration decreases with hemodilution. • Requirements fall during CPB.
Benzodiazepines	• Free drug concentration decreases with hemodilution • Plasma levels can be increased after CPB due to prolonged elimination.

Temperature Management

Temperature is an important determinant in the metabolic management on CPB. Traditional perfusion strategies have involved the use of controlled hypothermia as a protective strategy to reduce systemic metabolic demand and to protect organ function. Cerebral oxygen consumption ($CMRO_2$) decreases by 7% for every degree Celsius reduction in temperature. Together with the subsequent reduction in CO_2 production, hypothermia is protective against cerebral, and by inference, systemic ischemic injury. This is supported by work using the temperature coefficient Q_{10}, described as the $CMRO_2$ at a temperature T divided by the $CMRO_2$ at 10°C lower. The higher the Q_{10}, the more cerebral (and other vital organ) metabolic activity is suppressed. The less desirable physiological consequence of hypothermia is the leftward shift of the oxygen dissociation curve, increasing the affinity of hemoglobin for oxygen, thus reducing tissue oxygen delivery.

CPB is mostly conducted in mild (32–35°C) hypothermia, although normothermia (36–37°C) is becoming increasingly popular. Moderate (28–32°C), severe (27–25°C) or deep (<25°C) hypothermia can be used depending on the complexity and duration of a surgical procedure, the degree of organ preservation required and often surgical preference. Deep hypothermic circulatory arrest (DHCA) is a technique that can be used to protect brain and organ function in both adult and pediatric surgical procedures where aortic cross clamp placement is not possible or total absence of blood flow is required. The specific considerations for DHCA are discussed in depth in Chapter 9. Hypothermic bypass has numerous benefits including inhibition of catabolic and destructive enzyme and neurotransmitter activity, suppression of free radical production and reduction of the metabolic requirements in peripheral tissues. Additionally, systemic oxygen delivery can be titrated to oxygen consumption by reducing pump flow or allowing for further reductions in hematocrit.

Hypothermia can be achieved passively by letting the patient cool down or actively using the heater/cooler unit on CPB. Current recommendations

Table 10.5. Summary of the adverse effects of hypothermic bypass

System	Consequences
Cardiovascular	• Vasoconstriction and reduced microcirculatory flow • Hypokalemia and arrhythmias • Reduced delivery of oxygen (leftward shift of oxygen dissociation curve)
Hematological	• Increased plasma viscosity • Impairment of coagulation • Impairment of platelet function
Cerebral	• Reduction in cerebral blood flow • Ischemic injury during rewarming phase
Metabolism	• Metabolic acidosis • Hyperglycemia due to impairment of glucose metabolism • Altered drug metabolism and excretion • Altered ABG management
Renal	• Reduced GFR • Impairment of renal blood flow and increased AKI risk
Infection	• Increased infection risk • Altered antibiotic handling

suggest that the temperature gradient between venous inlet and arterial outlet on the oxygenator should not exceed 10°C to reduce the risk of micro-emboli forming. Much debate exists on the optimal site of systemic temperature measurement as a reflection of cerebral temperature. Commonly used sites include pulmonary artery catheter tip, nasopharynx, esophagus, ear, bladder and rectum. Recently the oxygenator arterial outlet temperature has gained support as the most appropriate surrogate for cerebral temperature. Practically, many centers monitor temperature at more than one site.

Despite the benefits of hypothermic bypass, it has a number of adverse unfavorable consequences, which are summarized in Table 10.5.

Hypothermic Bypass ABG Management: Alpha versus pH Stat

Gas solubility increases as temperature decreases. As a result, during hypothermia temperature corrected

blood gas values have reduced PaO_2 and $PaCO_2$ values and increased pH values, although content remains largely unchanged. There are two strategies to manage this in clinical practice:

• Alpha stat management - does not correct for hypothermia, measuring samples at 37°C and allowing alkalosis to occur without intervention during cooling. It is based on the fact that the dissociation constant (pK) of the imidazole group of histidine changes with temperature, providing consistency of its ionization state (alpha) in order to maintain a constant intracellular pH. The aim is to allow continued cellular, protein and enzyme activity in a normal environment. Clinical studies demonstrate better preservation of cerebral autoregulation, flow and neurovascular coupling, although this comes at the expense of less homogenous brain cooling and limited reduction in oxygen consumption of the brain. The disadvantages of this method include increasing the "steal" phenomenon from cerebral to pulmonary circulation in congenital cardiac surgery.

• pH stat management – blood gas analysis is corrected to the actual core body temperature and the pH is maintained at 7.4 throughout the period of hypothermia with the addition of CO_2 to the oxygenator gas flow. The higher CO_2 content leads to the loss of cerebral autoregulation and to cerebral vasodilation, increased cerebral oxygen delivery and more homogenous cooling of deeper brain structures, albeit with the increased risk of cerebral edema and a potentially higher micro-embolic load. In pediatric practice, where intraoperative brain injury is the likely result of global ischemia, this approach has been shown to reduce shunt flow and it potentially improves neurobehavioral development.

Both management strategies work well, however, evidence would suggest alpha stat is preferable in adults, while pH stat is preferable in pediatric practice, particularly with DHCA.

Rewarming from Hypothermic Bypass

Cautious rewarming following hypothermia is recommended to avoid the risk of cerebral hyperthermia, which is associated with cerebral injury, poor postoperative neurological outcomes, increased infection risk and renal injury. The $CMRO_2$ is uncoupled from cerebral blood flow in the hyperthermic brain, with subsequent supply and demand mismatch and the potential for cellular and neuronal injury. Current recommendations suggest that the temperature gradient between oxygenator venous inflow and arterial outlet does not exceed 10°C and ideally remains less than 4°C. The rate of rewarming should be slow and guided by a temperature gradient of less than 5°C between patient core and periphery. The oxygenator arterial outlet temperature should be limited to less than 37°C to avoid the risk of underestimating true cerebral temperature and causing inadvertent cerebral hyperthermia. Rewarming from therapeutic hypothermia is discussed in more detail in Chapter 9.

Suggested Further Reading

1. Murphy GS. Hessel EA 2nd, Groom RC. Optimal perfusion during CPB: an evidence-based approach. *Anesth Analg* 2009; 108:1394.

2. Baker RA, Nikolic A, Onorati F et al. 2019 EACTS/EACTA/EBCP guidelines on CPB in adult cardiac surgery: a tool to better clinical practice. *Eur J Cardiothorac Surg* 2020; 57: 207– 209.

3. Reves JG. Toward understanding cerebral blood flow during CPB: implications for the central nervous system. *Anesthesiology* 2019; 130: 609–613.

4. American Society of ExtraCorporeal Technology Standards and Guidelines For Perfusion Practice. 2017. Available from www.amsect.org/d/do/1370

5. Svenmarker S, Hannuksela M, Haney M. A retrospective analysis of the mixed venous oxygen saturation as the target for systemic blood flow control during CPB. *Perfusion* 2018; 33: 453–462.

6. Engelman R. Baker RA, Likosky DS et al. The Society of Thoracic Surgeons, the Society of Cardiovascular Anesthesiologists, and the American Society of ExtraCorporeal Technology: Clinical practice guidelines for CPB temperature management during CPB. *J Cardiothorac Vasc Anesth* 2015; 29: 1104–1111

7. Govender P, Tosh W, Burt C et al. Evaluation of increase in intraoperative lactate level as a predictor of outcome in adults after cardiac surgery. *J Cardiothorac Vasc Anesth.* 2020 Apr;34(4): 877–884.

8. Ranucci M, Carboni G, Cotza M et al. Carbon dioxide production during CPB: pathophysiology, measure and clinical relevance. *Perfusion* 2017; 32: 4–12.

9. Society of Thoracic Surgeons Blood Conservation Guideline Task Force. Ferraris VA, Brown JR, Despotis GJ et al. Update to the Society of Thoracic Surgeons and the Society of Cardiovascular Anesthesiologists blood conservation clinical practice guidelines. *Ann Thorac Surg* 2011; 91: 944–982.

10. Kunst G, Milojevic M, Boer C et al. 2019 EACTS/EACTA/EBCP guidelines on CPB in adult cardiac surgery. *BJA* 2019; 123: 713–757.

Myocardial Preservation during Cardiopulmonary Bypass

Gudrun Kunst, Luc Puis and Tom Gilbey

Avoiding unnecessary myocardial damage has been at the forefront of cardiac surgery since its early days. The ability to arrest and immobilize the heart and revive it again without loss of function has facilitated more and more complex surgeries. Effective myocardial protection, particularly for the duration of aortic cross clamping, involves multimodal strategies, consisting of temperature management, cardioplegic solutions delivered by various routes as well as noncardioplegic techniques like ischemic preconditioning through intermittent cross clamping or pharmacological protection.

As in many other aspects of cardiac surgery, myocardial protection depends on good communication and teamwork.

History of Myocardial Protection

The basic principle of myocardial protection consists of minimizing the myocardium's oxygen demand during times of low supply, mainly during the period when the surgeon requires a bloodless and still operating field and the aortic cross clamp is on.

The most important discoveries occurred:

i. at the end of the nineteenth century, when Ringer showed the effect of electrolytes on the regulation of the heartbeat.
ii. in 1935, when Zwikster and Boyd showed that potassium could reversibly arrest the heart.

Systemic and topical hypothermia was advocated early in the use of extracorporeal circulation to provide an extra margin of organ protection as it was feared that the then available technology could not provide sufficiently high blood flows and gas exchange to satisfy oxygen demand. The concept of lowering the metabolism through hypothermia was quickly adopted into the science of myocardial protection.

The term "cardioplegia" was first described by Melrose in 1955. Melrose also induced the first elective cardiac arrest using potassium. Potassium concentrations of 35 to even 50 mmol/l were common. During the 1960s the negative effects of these high dose strategies, namely myocardial necrosis and irreversible, ischemic myocardial contracture (stone heart), became increasingly apparent. This led to the development of solutions with lower concentrations. Today solutions typically have concentrations of 12–25 mmol/l.

Building on this, in the 1970s Buckberg's group led the effort of developing blood cardioplegia and other techniques like warm, substrate-enriched cardioplegia and reperfusion modalities, such as warm hyperkalemic reperfusion immediately prior to removal of the aortic cross clamp (terminal hot shot), not only to protect the heart from ischemia but to aid recovery from damage. The concept of retrograde cardioplegia delivered continuously via the coronary sinus was explored at the same time.

The 1980s saw an increasing interest in combined, intermittent, ante- and retrograde administration of cardioplegia to provide better protection for the right heart.

The concept of ischemic preconditioning – where short episodes of ischemia prior to a prolonged ischemic event are thought to confer protection from myocardial reperfusion injury, even if the ischemia is administered at a remote region of the body – caused much excitement after its first description by Murry in 1986. Subsequent clinical trials were not able to reproduce the initial results and this technique is hardly used today.

Despite much research there is still a lack of agreement on numerous aspects of cardioplegia. The debates on crystalloid versus cold blood cardioplegia or on whole blood microplegia versus diluted blood cardioplegia – to name but two – are still ongoing. Several metanalyses have not been able to demonstrate superiority of any of the currently available techniques.

Ischemia/Reperfusion Injury and Key Intracellular Modulators of Cell Survival

Many cardiac surgical procedures require the myocardium to be immobile and bloodless while the heart-lung machine maintains circulation. The associated insult to the myocardium is twofold:

i. Cross clamping of the aorta leads to myocardial ischemia, despite the cardioplegic arrest.
ii. Reperfusion after release of the aortic cross clamp causes ischemia-reperfusion injury.

Myocardial Ischemia

As tissue hypoxia develops after aortic cross clamping, acidosis ensues and lactate accumulates in minutes as ATP is consumed much faster than it can be produced in the mitochondria. The intracellular proton accumulation activates the Na^+/H^+ ion exchanger and subsequently the Na^+/Ca^{2+} exchanger, resulting in intracellular Ca^{2+} accumulation. Prolonged, untreated ischemia leads to disruption of the cell membrane, resulting in the leakage of intracellular components into the extracellular compartment.

Mitochondria supply ATP to cardiomyocytes, but they have also been identified as activators of cell death pathways, modulating the balance between pro-survival and death. The mitochondrial permeability transition pore (mPTP) is a nonselective channel of the inner mitochondrial membrane. The acidosis during ischemia causes the mPTP to remain closed. This provides a degree of protection as mPTP opening causes depolarization and uncoupling of oxidative phosphorylation, resulting in intracellular ATP depletion and cell death.

Ischemia/Reperfusion

Myocardial reperfusion results in different types of cardiac dysfunction:

i. Stunning – reversible, mechanical dysfunction.
ii. No-reflow phenomenon – the inability to reperfuse an ischemic region.
iii. Reperfusion arrhythmias, which are usually treatable.
iv. Lethal reperfusion injury, mostly driven by the presence of reactive oxygen species (ROS), intracellular calcium overload and inflammation.

Mitochondrial Based Protection

Mitochondrial based protection has been focused on inhibiting the opening of the mPTP and on opening of the mitochondrial ATP-dependent potassium (K_{ATP}) channel. Two protective pathways are activated by myocardial ischemia, via the G-protein-coupled cell surface receptors (reperfusion injury salvage kinase [RISK] – pathway) and via the tumor necrosis factor (TNF)-alpha receptors (survivor activating factor enhancement [SAFE] pathway).

Cardioplegia Techniques

Delivering a cardioplegic solution to the myocardium in order to induce diastolic arrest, topping it up intermittently to keep the heart protected during the arrest, and re-perfusing the myocardium after surgical repair is a well-trodden path, repeated the world over millions of times each year.

The principle behind cardioplegia and hypothermia is to continually match myocardial oxygen supply and demand to limit any damage. This means that the main determinants of myocardial energy consumption – electromechanical activity and left ventricular end-diastolic wall tension (LVEDP) – need to be controlled. Rapid onset of diastolic arrest without distending the left ventricle immediately after aortic cross clamping is important. Protection can be further enhanced by decreasing the metabolic rate and suppressing electrical activity through cooling (see Figure 11.1).

Physiology of Cardioplegia

There is an electrical potential between the intra- and extracellular space. This electrical gradient is maintained by ions on either side of the cell membrane. Cardioplegia solutions are able to rapidly induce cardiac arrest by altering the electrical gradient across the cell membrane of myocytes and by doing so eliminate electrical activity and subsequent mechanical contraction.

A cell's resting membrane potential is determined by the selective permeability of its membrane to ions.

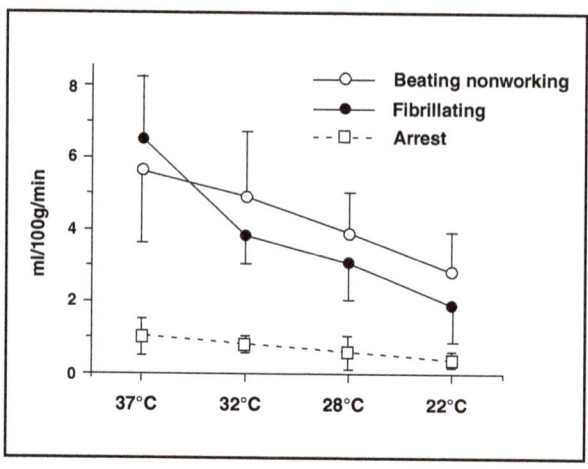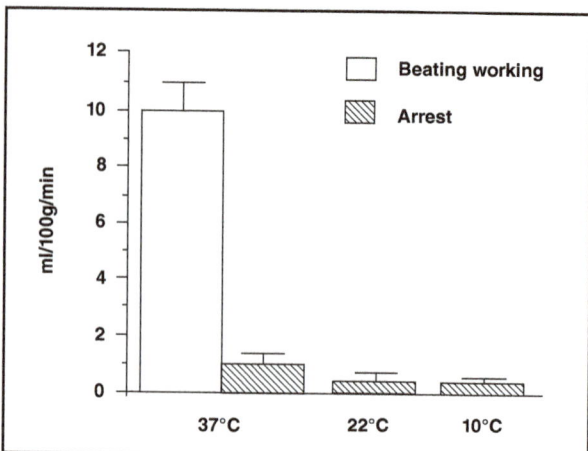

Figure 11.1 Myocardial O_2 demand at various working modes and temperatures.

$$E_{mK} = 61.5 \log_{10}\left(\frac{Co}{Ci}\right)$$

E_{mK} = K⁺ equilibrium potential (mV), Co = extracellular K⁺ concentration, Ci = intracellular K⁺ concentration

Figure 11.2 Simplified Nernst equation for K⁺.

At equilibrium, the ionic flows into and out of the cell are equal in magnitude and there is no net current. The myocyte membrane is most permeable to K⁺ and relatively impermeable to other ions; its resting membrane potential is therefore dominated by the K⁺ equilibrium and is relatively negative at –90 mV. Movement of other ions across the membrane is mainly determined by voltage gated channels, which open or close at specific membrane potentials. The equilibrium potential for any ion may be calculated using the Nernst equation (see Figure 11.2).

The normal value of Co/Ci for K⁺ is 4/140, i.e. the K⁺ equilibrium potential is calculated as –94 mV. If the extracellular K⁺ concentration rises to 20 mmol/L, the value for Co/Ci changes to 20/140, and the equilibrium potential is –52 mV. Using this simple tool helps appreciate how manipulating the extracellular environment changes the equilibrium potential of the cardiac myocyte.

Figure 11.3 shows the normal electrical cycle of a cardiac myocyte. Phase 4 represents the resting membrane potential of the cell and coincides with ventricular diastole. Normally, as an action potential propagates through the heart's conduction system, the myocyte membrane becomes less negative, to approximately –70 mV, and once this threshold

potential is reached, the fast Na⁺ channels open. This allows Na⁺ to rush into the myocyte which very rapidly raises the membrane potential further and depolarizes the cell. Continued Na⁺ entry creates a +20 mV potential (Phase 0). The positive membrane potential closes the voltage controlled Na⁺ channels and opens the voltage gated K⁺ channels, allowing K⁺ to leave the cell, thereby reducing the membrane potential to +5 mV (Phase 1). At this point the voltage gated Ca²⁺ channels open and Ca²⁺ enters the myocyte (Phase 2). Calcium influx into the cell results in contraction and this coincides with ventricular systole. These Ca²⁺ channels only remain open transiently and, as soon as they close, the membrane potential returns to approximately –90 mV, as K⁺ is still able to leave the cell via the voltage gated K⁺ channels, and the cell membrane repolarizes. The intracellular calcium is reduced, and the cell relaxes again.

Displacing blood using extracellular cardioplegia with a high K⁺ concentration makes the cell membrane potential less negative thus allowing it to depolarize more readily. The depolarization causes the voltage gated Ca²⁺ channels to open and the transient calcium influx results in contraction (systole); once the calcium is locked away in the

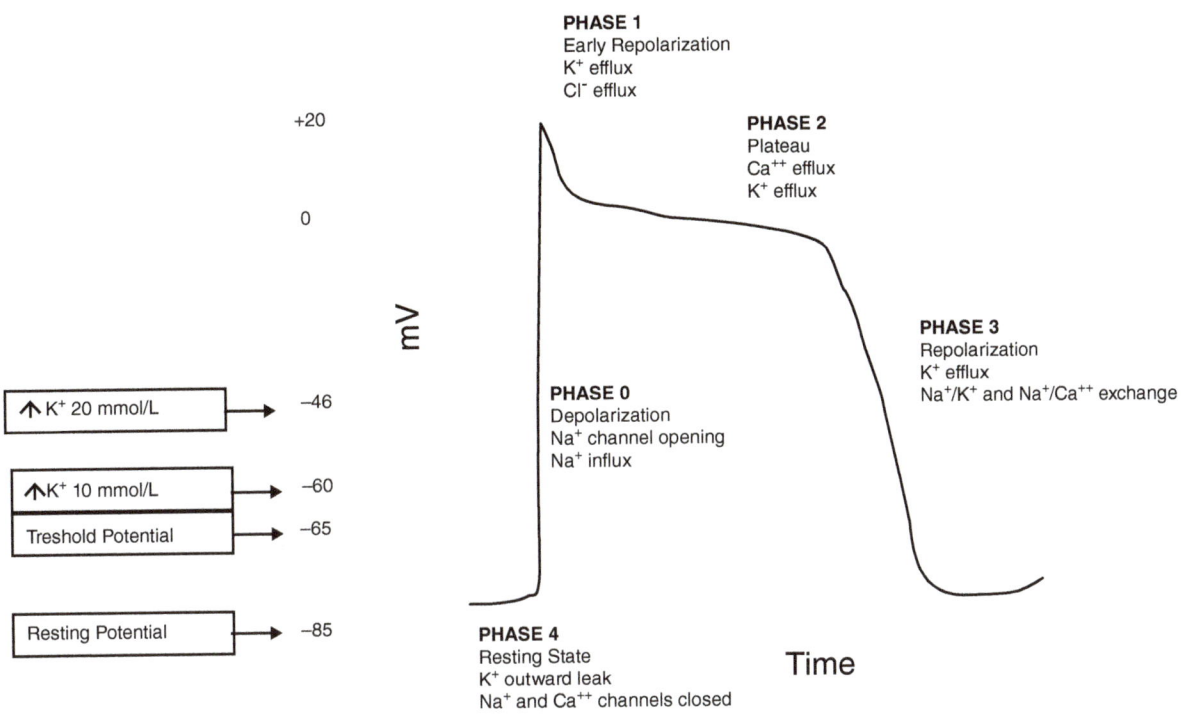

Figure 11.3 Cardiac myocyte action potential. The resting membrane potential is −85 mV and the threshold potential for depolarization is −65 mV. Increasing the extracellular potassium leaves the myocytes above the threshold potential and in an arrested state.

sarcoplasmic reticulum again the cell relaxes (diastole). Rather than this cycle continuing, the high extracellular potassium concentration now prevents repolarization and the cell stays depolarized. When the resting potential approaches −50 mV, Na^+ channels are deactivated resulting in diastolic arrest.

Potassium is not the only ion which could be used to manipulate the myocyte electrical membrane potential. Hyponatremia, hypocalcemia and hypermagnesemia will all ultimately cause diastolic cardiac arrest. Hypercalcemia, if profound enough, may cause systolic cardiac arrest.

Cardioplegia Solutions

Cardioplegia solutions can be divided into crystalloid and blood-based solutions, with crystalloids further subdivided into either intracellular or extracellular solutions. The key features of cardioplegia solutions are summarized in Table 11.1.

- Extracellular-like solutions – The earliest cardioplegia solutions consisted of crystalloids with a very high potassium content. While these were rapidly able to achieve cardiac arrest they were also profoundly depolarizing and caused myocardial damage due to excessive intracellular calcium accumulation. Subsequent work focused on reducing the potassium content. The prototypical extracellular-like crystalloid solutions are referred to as St Thomas' solution.

- Intracellular-like solutions – Bretschneider and coworkers pursued a different strategy in the 1970s. They developed a calcium free, low sodium cardioplegia solution, which works by reducing the trans-membrane Na^+ gradient sufficiently to stop enough Na^+ entering the myocyte during phase 0 to cause depolarization. The membrane remains hyperpolarized and arrested in diastole. This solution is known as histidine-tryptophan-ketoglutarate (HTK), Bretschneider's or Custodiol solution. It is classified as an intracellular cardioplegia solution as its composition is closer to that of the intracellular environment, in contrast to the K^+ based extracellular environment-like solutions. It has a large buffering capacity and is often given as a single shot designed to protect for up to two hours

Table 11.1. Different cardioplegic solutions and their components

Components	Extracellular		Intracellular		Blood	
	St. Thomas Hospital 1 (STH)	St. Thomas Hospital 2 (STH2, Plegisol)	Custodiol (HTK, Bretschneider's)	Del Nido	Microplegia (Miniplegia)	Buckberg
NaCl (mMol)	144	110	15			
KCl (mEq)	20	16	9	26	≈28	≈28
NaHCO₃ (mEq)	* added prior to use	10		13		
MgCl₂ (mmol/L)	16	16	4	6.6	≈2–4	
CaCl₂ (mmol/L)	2.2	1.2	0.015	0.4		
Mannitol (g/L)			30	0.4		
Histidine (mmol/L)			180			
Histidine-HCl (mmol/L)			18			
Tryptophane (mmol/L)			2			
KH2- ketoglutarate (mmol/L)			1			
THAM (mmol/L)						≈50
CPD (mmol/L)						≈20
Other additives	procaine			lidocaine	lidocaine (adenosine)	citrate; glutamate/ aspartate on reperfusion

without interruption. However, hemodilution and hyponatremia can be problematic side effects, particularly in pediatric cases. Mannitol is added to correct the osmolarity of the solution and minimize fluid shifts.

- Blood cardioplegia – Buckberg and colleagues developed the concept of blood cardioplegia, which promised many theoretical advantages including high buffering capacity, oxygen and carbon dioxide transport, free radical scavenging and minimal hemodilution. They also advanced the idea of a myocardial protection strategy with different ingredients and concentrations administered at various stages of the surgical procedure, for

example high potassium for rapid arrest (20 mmol/L) followed by moderate potassium for maintenance (10 mmol/L). These techniques have evolved into cold, tepid, warm and combined strategies, with centers adapting to either a single-shot approach or to recurrent, intermittent doses (every 15–20 minutes). Blood and cardioplegia solution are generally mixed in a 4:1 ratio, but variations are common.

- Perhaps the logical evolution of blood cardioplegia is the so-called miniplegia, where oxygenated blood coming from the CPB is minimally diluted by adding concentrated potassium, magnesium and other additives via a syringe driver rather than mixed from a crystalloid solution. This technique provides maximal control of cardioplegia delivery and least hemodilution.

- Del Nido Cardioplegia – Many clinicians feel that blood is the optimum basis for cardioplegic solutions and Del Nido popularized the use of a single shot mixed blood/crystalloid cardioplegia (1:4) in pediatric cases in the 1990s. This concept is now gaining traction in adult surgery. Del Nido Cardioplegia (DNC) is given as a single shot and consists of 26 mEq of potassium chloride, 13 mL of 1% lidocaine, 3.2 g/L of mannitol, 2 g magnesium sulfate, 13 mEq of sodium bicarbonate, all in 1000 mL of Plasma-Lyte A. The advantages are an uninterrupted procedure with potentially shorter clamp and pump times and less hemodilution. Any clinical outcome advantages, however, have yet to be determined.

Additives

Many constituents have been proposed both as primary arrest-inducing agents and as additives to improve myocardial protection. In the former category high-dose magnesium and the short acting beta-blocker esmolol are promising, whereas in the latter category amino acids, sodium channel blockers, buffers and low-dose magnesium are all added according to institutional and surgeon preference and case-specific factors.

- Magnesium offers additional arresting potential by limiting the calcium influx into cells. It provides a veno-dilating effect, making it useful when administering cardioplegia through vein grafts during CABG procedures.
- Citrate-Phosphate-Dextrose (CPD) has calcium-chelating properties, making it useful as an additive to prevent calcium overload, although the supporting evidence is poor.
- Tris (hydroxymethyl) Aminomethane (THAM) is sometimes used as a buffer to prevent acidosis, but its usefulness is contested when using blood cardioplegia.
- Sodium bicarbonate ($NaHCO_3$) is also used as a buffer but is even more controversial.
- Aspartate and glutamate are amino acids and have been advocated due to a theoretical ability to provide ATP in an anaerobic milieu. The evidence of their use is poor.

- Mannitol is added to augment the osmotic pressure and prevent myocardial edema.

Delivery of Cardioplegia

Cardioplegia needs to be delivered directly to the myocyte membrane to induce and then maintain diastolic arrest. Depending on the patient's pathology, the operation and on surgical preference, delivery can be either antegrade via the coronary arteries and/or retrograde through the coronary sinus into the heart's venous system (see Figure 11.4).

Cardioplegia delivery is mostly controlled by the perfusionist. A system consisting of one or two electronically linked pumps provides the mix of blood and crystalloid cardioplegia, via a separate heat exchanger, to the surgeon, who connects it to the desired delivery site. Adequate de-airing and close temperature and pressure monitoring need to be provided. The heart has to be completely emptied and relaxed before the aorta is occluded and cardioplegia is given.

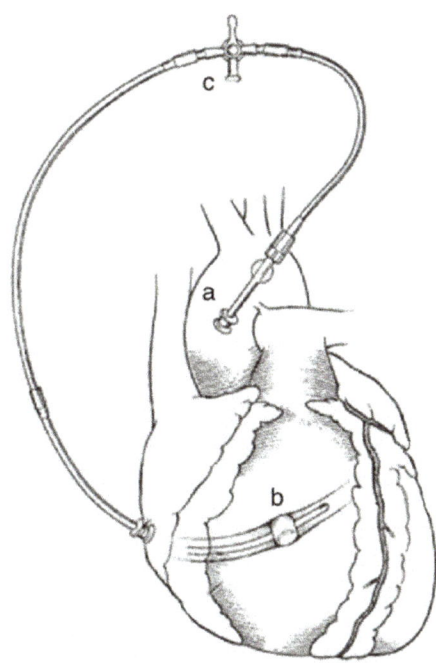

Figure 11.4 Antegrade and retrograde cardioplegia delivery circuit. a = aortic cannula, b = coronary sinus cannula, c = 3-way tap to connect cardioplegia line from HLM and easily switch between delivery mode.

(a)

(b)

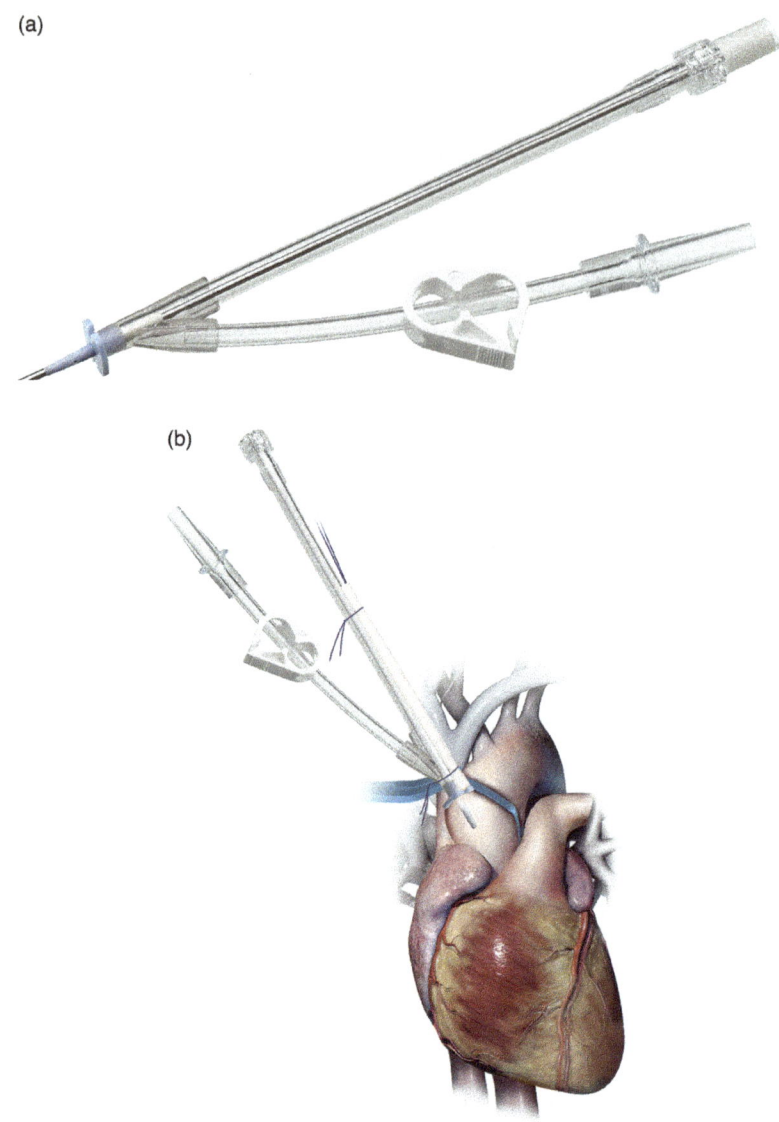

Figure 11.5 (a) DLP™ Double-lumen aortic root cannula, which can be used to deliver cardioplegia and as an aortic root vent. (b) Schematic drawing of antegrade cardioplegia delivery. (Reproduced with ©2020 Medtronic. All rights reserved. Used with the permission of Medtronic.)

Excellent communication between the perfusionist, the surgeon and the anesthesiologist is crucial during cardioplegia delivery.

Antegrade Delivery

Antegrade cardioplegia is most commonly delivered through a cannula placed in the aortic root, proximal to the aortic clamp, utilizing the native coronary circulation (Figure 11.5a and b). Flows of 250–350 ml/min with a pressure of 80–120 mmHg after aortic occlusion forces the aortic valve to close and the cardioplegia solution into the left and right coronary ostia. The perfusionist controls the flow while the pressure is servo regulated to avoid excessive values, which are associated with myocardial edema.

Successful delivery through the aortic root requires a competent aortic valve. Even a small degree of aortic insufficiency can lead to cardioplegia leakage into the left ventricle. Not only does this lead to insufficient perfusion of the myocardium and delayed arrest, but it

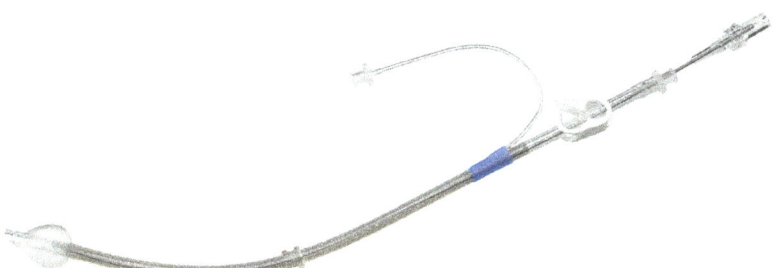

Figure 11.6 DLP™ Retrograde cardioplegia delivery cannula. (Reproduced with ©2020 Medtronic. All rights reserved. Used with the permission of Medtronic.)

can cause left ventricular distension, further impairing delivery of cardioplegia to the sub-endocardial tissues.

There are several options available if the aortic valve is found to be regurgitant:

- Direct ostial cardioplegia – the aorta is opened after cross clamping and the cardioplegia is delivered directly into the coronary ostia using either a basket-tipped or a gel-tipped special cannula. The left coronary artery is generally perfused first as the left ventricle is more susceptible to ischemia. Once cardiac arrest has been achieved the right ostium is perfused before topping up the left side again. Flows and pressures are generally lower with this technique in order not to cause endothelial damage or dissect the coronaries. If an intermittent cardioplegia technique is used, the operation needs to be interrupted every 15–20 minutes.
- Retrograde cardioplegia (see below).

Achieving timely arrest is a concern particularly in patients with severe proximal left main and/or right-sided stenoses. The addition of retrograde delivery is often chosen in these cases to decrease the risk and extent of myocardial injury.

Retrograde Delivery

Retrograde cardioplegia should be considered whenever antegrade delivery is deemed to be technically difficult to achieve or to provide insufficient myocardial protection (e.g. redo CABG with partially patent grafts, severe mainstem stenosis, ongoing myocardial infarction). It can be achieved by placing a cannula in the coronary sinus, which is the final drainage zone of the venous coronary circulation. The cannula is most commonly placed by palpation and transesophageal echocardiography (TEE) offers some guidance. A circumferential, inflatable balloon near the distal end of the catheter provides a seal between catheter and the sinus wall, allowing delivery of cardioplegia

(see Figure 11.6). Retrograde delivery should always be done with continuous sinus pressure monitoring, preferably using a servo regulated pump. The pressure should be kept below 40 mmHg to avoid endothelial damage or even rupture of the coronary sinus.

Proponents of this technique emphasize that it offers continuous delivery without interruption of the procedure, is not dependent on a competent aortic valve and supplies all of the subendocardial tissue, regardless of coronary artery stenoses. Despite these advantages it is regarded as inferior to antegrade methods because:

- Right-sided protection can be impaired, especially if the catheter is placed too deep into the sinus, past the posterior interventricular vein
- Placement of the catheter is sometimes time-consuming, not always accurate and risks damage to the sinus
- Catheters can also slip out of the sinus unnoticed during manipulation of the heart
- Induction of cardiac arrest requires more time than with antegrade delivery.

Both techniques are often combined, commonly giving an induction dose antegrade, followed by retrograde maintenance.

Delivery through Vein Grafts

Cardioplegia can be delivered through vein grafts once the distal anastomosis is completed. When this is done through a pump using a set pressure, this technique can give the surgeon the confidence about graft patency and quality of the anastomosis. Flows of 80–100 ml at a pressure of 100 mmHg are desirable.

Cardioplegia Techniques for Minimal Access Surgery

As minimal access surgery increased in popularity, new methods of achieving myocardial protection were needed.

Longer aortic cannulas and the extended Chitwood cross clamp enable standard antegrade cardioplegia delivery. A different approach is the use of an endoballoon catheter, which is advanced from the femoral artery and placed into the ascending aorta under TEE guidance. Once safely in situ, the balloon is inflated to occlude the aorta and cardioplegia is delivered in standard antegrade manner proximally to the balloon through one lumen of the catheter. The catheter provides two transducers, one to measure the aortic root pressure during cardioplegia delivery and the second one to monitor the balloon inflation pressure. Specific catheters that are inserted through the jugular vein and can be positioned in the coronary sinus have been developed for retrograde delivery. Intracellular cardioplegia solutions, allowing longer clamp times and longer intervals between doses, are often used during minimal access surgery.

Extremely good communication and coordination between perfusionist, surgeon and anesthesiologist are crucial during these operations.

Temperature Management and Cardioplegia

Myocardial oxygen demand decreases with decreasing temperature, as Figure 11.1 illustrates. Before the introduction of myocardial cardioplegia, systemic hypothermia was the mainstay of myocardial protection; it remains an adjunct to cardioplegia today. Crystalloid cardioplegia appears to be most effective when administered cold, with delivery temperatures as cold as 4°C seen commonly. Cold cardioplegia is often supplemented with "bathing" the heart in ice-cold water during the period of delivery. Oxygenated blood cardioplegia is more likely to transfer oxygen to the myocardium if administered warm, as this minimizes the shift of the oxygen dissociation curve to the left. Warm blood cardioplegia (i.e. 37°C) has been shown to maintain myocardial ATP levels more efficiently. This explains why many surgeons opt to induce arrest with cold blood cardioplegia and give top up doses warm.

Non-Cardioplegic Methods of Myocardial Protection

Numerous techniques have been investigated over the years as adjuncts or alternatives to cardioplegia. The second aspect of myocardial protection that has been the focus of academic efforts is the avoidance of ischemia/reperfusion injury. Although many concepts have shown promise in preclinical and small-scale clinical trials, none have so far found their way into mainstream cardiac surgery.

Intermittent Cross Clamping/Fibrillation

The technique of intermittent cross clamping/fibrillation (ICC) is used in several centers, especially in coronary artery bypass graft surgery. It never was accepted widely, as operating on a fibrillating heart is technically more challenging than on a still, flaccid and bloodless field. There is no consensus as to how many consecutive episodes of cross clamp/fibrillation can be considered safe, how long each one should maximally last and how much time is needed to reperfuse between them. There is also an increased risk of embolic complications associated with repeated application of the aortic cross clamp.

During ICC, the patient is on CPB and cooled to 28–32°C. While cross clamped, the heart is completely emptied and a fibrillatory electrode is placed behind it to induce ventricular fibrillation to reduce myocardial oxygen consumption and also ventricular motion. ICC is the archetypical form of ischemic preconditioning.

Despite the skepticism toward it, ICC has been shown to be safe in coronary surgery with clinical results similar to those with cardioplegic arrest. The fibrillator provides a useful rescue technique to immobilize the myocardium and reduce oxygen consumption when cardioplegia administration unexpectedly fails and other means of myocardial perfusion are unavailable.

Off Pump Surgery (OPCABG)

Avoiding CPB, aortic cross clamping and cardioplegia is seen by some as the ultimate form of myocardial protection. For obvious reasons this is only possible for coronary artery surgery. However, recent large analyses have not shown better long-term outcomes associated with this technique.

Ischemic Preconditioning

After commencing CPB, the aorta or the left anterior descending coronary artery is occluded several times followed by short periods of reperfusion before applying the aortic cross clamp and giving cardioplegia. This technique showed initial promising results in small clinical trials, but overall clinical results were inconclusive.

Remote Ischemic Preconditioning

This technique is based on the concept that the ischemic conditioning stimulus can confer protective effects on the heart if applied to distal tissues such as arms or legs. It involves up to four episodes of 5-minute inflation/deflation of a standard blood pressure cuff on the patient's arm after induction of anesthesia. After initially promising results two major multicenter studies did not show improved patient outcome with this technique.

Sodium Hydrogen Exchanger Isoform-1 (NHE-1)

The pharmacological inhibition of the sodium hydrogen exchanger isoform-1 (NHE-1) reduces intracellular calcium overload and resulted in myocardial protection in experimental studies. Whereas subsequent clinical trials in cardiac surgical patients confirmed the beneficial effect on the myocardium by a significant reduction in myocardial infarction, overall mortality was increased in patients treated with sodium hydrogen exchanger inhibitors, due to an increase in cerebrovascular events.

Cyclosporine

Cyclosporine as an additive to cardioplegia solutions may be beneficial in protecting the myocardium from ischemia reperfusion injury, by inhibition of mPTP. This potential protective effect has not been demonstrated convincingly in clinical studies and the immunosuppressive effect of the drug can potentially be harmful.

Volatile Anesthetic Agents

Experimental studies suggested that volatile anesthetics may protect the myocardium from ischemia/reperfusion injury. So far clinical studies have yielded inconclusive results and further trials, particularly involving the delivery of volatile agents through the HLM while the lungs are not ventilated, are ongoing. Their long-term utility is questionable, though, due to the significant environmental impact of volatile anesthetics.

Cardioplegia and hypothermia remain the pillars of myocardial protection during cardiac surgery. Several initially promising new strategies did not show any benefits in clinical trials.

Suggested Further Reading

1. Yellon DM, Hausenloy DJ. Myocardial reperfusion injury. *N Engl J Med.* 2007; 357: 1121–1135

2. Xia Z, Li H, Irwin MG. Myocardial ischaemia reperfusion injury: the challenge of translating ischaemic and anaesthetic protection from animal models to humans. *Br J Anaesth.* 2016; 117: ii44–ii62

3. Davidson SM, Andreadou I, Garcia-Dorado D et al. Shining the spotlight on cardioprotection: beyond the cardiomyocyte. *Cardiovasc Res.* 2019; 115: 1115–1116

4. Kunst G, Klein AA. Peri-operative anaesthetic myocardial preconditioning and protection – cellular mechanisms and clinical relevance in cardiac anaesthesia. *Anaesthesia.* 2015; 70: 467–482

5. Buckberg GD. Update of current techniques of myocardial protection. *Ann Thorac Surg* 1995; 60: 805–814

6. Spellman J. Pro: in favor of more generalized use of del Nido cardioplegia in adult patients undergoing cardiac surgery. *J Cardiothor Vasc Anesth* 2019; 33: 1785–1790

7. Gorgy A, Shore-Lesserson L. Del Nido cardioplegia should be ssed in all adults undergoing cardiac surgery: con. *J Cardiothor Vasc Anesth.* 2019; 33: 1791–1794

8. Salerno TA, Ricci M, eds. *Myocardial Protection.* First edition. Oxford: Blackwell Publishing Ltd. 2004

9. Ali JM, Miles LF, Abu-Omar Y et al. Global cardioplegia practices: results from the Global Cardiopulmonary Bypass Survey. *J Extra Corpor Technol.* 2018; 50: 83–93

10. Murry CE, Jennings RB, Reimer KA. Preconditioning with ischemia: a delay of lethal cell injury in ischemic myocardium. *Circulation.* 1986; 74: 1124–1136

Weaning from Cardiopulmonary Bypass

Joanne F Irons, Kenneth G Shann and Michael Poullis

The transition from cardiopulmonary bypass (CPB) to normal circulation requires numerous mechanical, physiological and pharmacological factors to be coordinated efficiently within a short period of time. Weaning from CPB is often a routine process, however preexisting poor cardiac function or difficulties during the operation may make it complex and challenging. Complications encountered during the weaning phase may contribute to significant additional perioperative morbidity.

Communication and Teamwork

There is a strong correlation between adverse events and poor communication and coordination during this vital time. Communication between team members and in particular the perfusionist, surgeon and anesthesiologist are key to successful weaning from CPB. Important information, including surgical interventions, diagnostic data, such as filling status and transesophageal echocardiography (TEE) findings, and therapeutic decisions surrounding pharmacological support and an accurate assessment of the CPB prior to weaning, need to be conveyed intelligibly and in a timely manner to prevent morbidity. Simulation training of standard separation and crisis management should be considered to improve non-technical skills and team performance in real-life situations.

Weaning Checklist

Separation from CPB requires the heart to resume its inherent pump function. In order to achieve a smooth transition, cardiac function must be optimized prior to weaning. Delays in either recognizing or treating abnormal physiological parameters may lead to poor cardiac performance or failure to separate from CPB necessitating a return to extracorporeal circulatory support.

Several authors have proposed weaning checklists, which follow the general themes outlined in Table 12.1. Mnemonics help practitioners remember important points in the checklists, both in routine and in high stress cases. Two common mnemonics used as a checklist prior to weaning are "CVP" and "TRAVEL" (see Table 12.2) and are discussed below. It should be recognized that a number of these steps occur concurrently.

Temperature

Patients must be rewarmed prior to separation from CPB. There is currently insufficient evidence on the optimal temperature for weaning. It should be based on a balance between avoidance of cerebral hyperthermia with excessive rewarming and minimization of coagulopathy and transfusion with inadequate rewarming.

Rewarming targets of nasopharyngeal (NP) or esophageal temperatures of 36.5°C and bladder or rectal temperatures of 35°C are commonly employed.

Chapters 7 and 9 provide in more depth discussion of temperature management during bypass and on rewarming from hypothermia.

De-airing

Cardiac surgical procedures that require opening of cardiac chambers will inevitably allow introduction of air. Air in the right-sided chambers is usually relatively innocuous if its volume is not substantial enough to prevent forward flow and there are no intracardiac shunts. Air in the left side is dangerous and presents two major risks:

1. cerebral air embolus with postoperative morbidity, ranging from transient confusion to widespread neurological damage; and
2. coronary air embolus, which may cause transient and possibly widespread regional ventricular dysfunction and, in the extreme, irreversible myocardial damage.

Table 12.1. Preparation for weaning from CPB

Warm patient to target temperature

Correct electrolytes and acid-base status

Have blood and blood products available

Ensure sufficient volume in pump reservoir

Achieve target hemoglobin

Restart ventilation

Assess heart rate, rhythm and conduction

Control arrhythmias

Ensure pacing wires work and start pacing if required

Consider mechanical support if difficulties are anticipated

Table 12.2. Checklist mnemonics to aid weaning

"CVP"

C	V	P
Cold	Ventilation	Predictors
Conduction	Vaporizer	Protamine
Calcium	Volume	Pressure
Cardiac Output	Visualization	Potassium
Coagulation	Vasopressors	Pacer

"TRAVEL"

T	Temperature
R	Reperfusion Rate Rhythm
A	Air
V	Ventilation
E	Electrolytes (including Hemoglobin, Acid-base)
L	Level

It is therefore vital that meticulous attention to de-airing is applied. Direct cardiac agitation, syringing of air from left-sided chambers and venting of the aorta or left-sided chambers is started prior to aortic unclamping and continued until the air has disappeared. Hand-bagging the lungs vigorously during the de-airing process displaces air that accumulates in the pulmonary veins. The aortic root vent generally runs at a rate of 500–1000 ml/min and the operating table can be manipulated in a way that it sits at the highest point. TEE can assist with de-airing by identifying air "pockets" and tracking the success of de-airing until the amount of residual intracardiac air is considered acceptable (see Figure 12.1).

Reperfusion

Following removal of the aortic cross clamp and prior to attempting to wean from CPB, adequate reperfusion of the myocardium is important to allow myocytes time to replenish metabolic substrates, specifically high-energy phosphates (ATP), and "wash out" the products of anaerobic metabolism and residual cardioplegia.

Initial reperfusion can often be complicated by tachyarrhythmias or heart block. Some centers prefer to reduce the risk of reperfusion arrhythmias by giving prophylactic anti-arrhythmic agents, such as lidocaine, prior to cross clamp release. There are many parameters that influence myocardial and end-organ recovery and there is significant variation in routine practice across institutions. Clear and practical advice on blood pressure during or the time needed for reperfusion is not available in the literature, although it is generally accepted that an increased reperfusion time is associated with a more complete restoration of myocardial function. Full recovery usually takes at least 20 minutes and during this time there is an increase in myocardial metabolic demand. Surgical sequence may accommodate time for myocardial reperfusion – for example, the aortic anastomoses of coronary grafts may be performed during the reperfusion period.

Rate/Rhythm/Contractility

Cardiac function should be assessed prior to weaning from CPB, focusing primarily on heart rate, rhythm and contractility – visual (right ventricle) and echocardiographic guided (left ventricle). Communication between the surgeon and anesthetist is important as agreement is needed to formulate a weaning plan in cases where contractility is decreased.

Ventricular and supraventricular tachycardia at this time should be treated with electrical cardioversion or defibrillation and anti-arrhythmic therapy should be considered to increase success and reduce recurrence. Adding 150–300 mg amiodarone into the pump as well as keeping the potassium

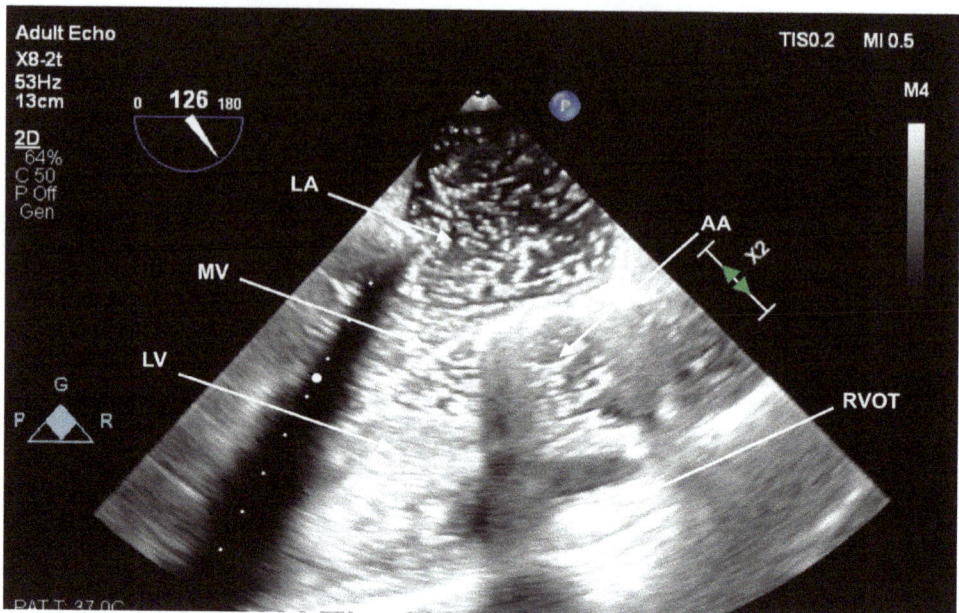

Figure 12.1 Transesophageal echocardiogram (mid-esophageal left ventricular outflow tract view) showing the heart during de-airing following aortic valve surgery. Air is seen as white speckles throughout the left heart with an accumulation in the left ventricular outflow tract (LVOT).

level >5 mmol/l are frequently used when dysrhythmias recur and persist during reperfusion.

Following CPB, the ventricles are generally less compliant and will not have their normal capacity to respond to changes in preload. The heart rate is therefore usually maintained at 80–100 beats per minute to help compensate for this. This "stiff" ventricle phenomenon increases the relative importance of the contribution of synchronous atrial contraction to stroke volume and cardiac output. Thus sinus rhythm is always preferable. Epicardial pacing leads and an external pacemaker, ideally with dual chamber function to allow sequential atrioventricular (AV) pacing if required, have to be immediately available.

Pacing

Evaluating the ECG on the anesthesia monitor for bradycardia or AV block may identify the need for epicardial pacing leads. When possible, atrial pacing is preferable to AV or ventricular pacing. Atrial pacing may be used alone to increase heart rate in patients in sinus rhythm or in a junctional rhythm where AV conduction is intact. Ventricular pacing may be employed in isolation when there is no effective atrial contraction (e.g. chronic atrial

fibrillation). In cases where AV synchronization is likely to be helpful and effective sinus rhythm is not yet established, atrial and ventricular epicardial leads should be placed to facilitate sequential AV pacing.

Prophylactic pacing should be considered in patients with:

1. left ventricular hypertrophy, especially those undergoing aortic surgery, as they require their left atrial "kick" to maintain LV filling,
2. a high risk of conduction defects due to the nature of the surgical procedure – aortic or mitral valve surgery (AVR or MVR), MVR especially via transeptal approaches and atrial or ventricular septum defect (ASD or VSD) repair,
3. atrial fibrillation (AF) and those requiring support with an intra-aortic balloon pump (IABP) as regular heart rate improves IABP efficiency,
4. hypertrophic cardiomyopathy (HCM), especially when undergoing AVR.

Commonly, pacing is set at around 80–100 bpm immediately post-CPB. The pacing rate should be determined by patient requirement and not by protocol. Atrial pacing leads exteriorized on the patient's right side and ventricular leads on the left help to avoid labeling issues and pacing errors.

Inotropes

While the chest is open, direct inspection of the right ventricle (RV) allows assessment of contractility while the left ventricle (LV) can be difficult to see and is better assessed via TEE.

Vasopressors, inotropes and vasodilators must be immediately available. The choice of drugs should be based on the patient's myocardial function, vascular tone and complexity of surgery as well as individual and institutional experience and preference.

Anesthesia

Patients' anesthetic demand increases with rewarming and there is a risk of awareness if this is not managed correctly. Anesthesia, analgesia and neuromuscular blockade must be assessed and supplemented as required. Weaning from CPB may require either a change in anesthetic agent (e.g. intravenous to volatile) or an adjustment to continuing dose delivery. It is vital that anesthesia is maintained continuously on and off CPB and this should be confirmed by team members. The use of processed electroencephalogram (EEG) or bispectral index (BIS) can be helpful.

Alarms

Alarm settings for many parameters displayed on anesthetic monitors and ventilators are adjusted or even disabled during CPB. It is vital that physiological monitoring with appropriate alarm settings is re-enabled prior to weaning from CPB. Similarly, alarms and safety devices of the CPB machine should not be disabled during the weaning process

Ventilation

During CPB the lungs are allowed to deflate fully or remain slightly inflated at low levels of continuous positive airway pressure. Prior to weaning from CPB, full and effective reinflation of the lungs has to be ensured with controlled manual alveolar recruitment. If one or both pleural cavities are open, direct visualization of the lung is possible and the pleural cavities should be drained of any accumulated fluid. Inspection of lung re-expansion should occur if an internal mammary artery is used for coronary bypass grafting as the lung is often "squashed" during vessel harvest. If the pleurae are closed, always exclude a pneumothorax by inspecting for bulging pleura. It may be prudent to apply tracheo-bronchial suction to clear respiratory secretions before ventilation is resumed.

Effective mechanical ventilation of the lungs must be established prior to ventricular ejection when significant pulmonary blood flow is reestablished. The perfusionist must confirm with the anesthesiologist if they are satisfied with ventilation before significantly reducing pump flow or weaning from CPB.

Electrolytes and Acid-Base

Electrolyte abnormalities should be corrected before separation from CPB in order to optimize myocyte function.

- Potassium (4.0–5.5 mmol/l) – increased potassium levels are commonly associated with CPB as a result of giving cardioplegia. In many centers, potassium is maintained at the higher end of the normal range in order to suppress arrhythmias. Hyperkalemia, however, can cause conduction abnormalities and impair contractility. Values above 6.0 mmol/l should serve as an alert and levels above 6.5 mmol/l need to be treated in the majority of patients before weaning. Treatment includes the use of zero-balance ultrafiltration with a low potassium solution, forced diuresis with a loop diuretic such as furosemide, or an insulin/dextrose infusion (e.g. 10 U insulin with 25 g dextrose given over 15 minutes). Hypokalemia can cause arrhythmias and should be treated with 10–20 mmol of K^+ either slow iv or given directly into the reservoir of the CPB circuit if below 4 mmol/l.
- Calcium (1.09–1.30 mmol/l) – the concentration of calcium in plasma may be reduced by hemodilution or transfusion of citrated blood (citrate forms a chelate complex with calcium) leading to impaired contractility, vasodilatation and coagulopathy. Ionized calcium should be maintained above 1.1 mmol/l. Ca^{++} is typically administered as an iv bolus of 1–2 g calcium, either in the form of chloride or gluconate. Practitioners need to be aware of the formulation they are using as a 10% chloride solution contains three times the amount of elemental calcium than 10% gluconate solution does.
- Magnesium (0.80–1.40 mmol/l) – low magnesium is associated with dysrhythmias and should be corrected if below 0.8 mmol/l. Prophylactic magnesium use regardless of the level may also be

indicated to reduce the incidence of supraventricular tachyarrhythmia, AF and ventricular arrhythmias on removal of the cross clamp, although evidence is limited. Treatment consists of 1–2 g of magnesium sulfate either given slowly iv or added to the reservoir of the CPB circuit.

- Glucose (4.0–7.8 mmol/l) – glucose control in the perioperative period has been shown to improve outcome after cardiac surgery. The Society of Thoracic Surgeons (STS) Clinical Practice Guidelines recommend maintaining perioperative glucose levels < 10 mmol/l (180 mg/dL). Hyperglycemia above that level should be treated with intravenous insulin in both diabetic and non-diabetic patients. Tight glycemic control within narrow margins such as 3.5–5 mmol (60–90 mg/dl) has been shown to increase the incidence of hypoglycemic events and the risk outweighs any benefits. In the absence of treatment with insulin, hypoglycemia in association with CPB is extremely rare and, if encountered, should be judiciously treated and its cause investigated.

- Lactate (0.7–2.5 mmol/l) – elevated serum lactate levels are encountered frequently during prolonged episodes of CPB, particularly if there have been periods of low flow or deep hypothermic circulatory arrest. Treatment of lactic acidosis per se is not usually instituted but increasing values must be seen as a potential indicator of inadequate organ perfusion (see also Chapter 10).

- Acid-base balance – a large proportion of patients develop some degree of acidosis during CPB. Acidosis causes myocardial depression, increased pulmonary vascular resistance, reduces the efficacy of inotropic drugs and increases coagulopathy and should be corrected prior to weaning.

    Increasing or decreasing the sweep gas flow to the oxygenator can readily and rapidly treat respiratory acid-base disorders by altering CO_2 levels as appropriate. Metabolic acidosis commonly results from iatrogenic sodium chloride administration, tissue hypoxia, catecholamine administration and electrolyte imbalance. It often resolves with the increase in flow rate on rewarming but may require treatment

prior to weaning, although there is wide variation in clinical practice with regard to the level of acidosis to treat. Acidosis is generally treated with sodium bicarbonate (see Chapter 10 for more detail). Although cardiac myocytes have effective intracellular buffering mechanisms, the administration of a large volume in a short period may generate paradoxical intracellular acidosis. Clearance of this excess generated carbon dioxide via the oxygenator may take 5–10 minutes. In patients with poor cardiac function, weaning from CPB should not be attempted until the risk of significant paradoxical intracellular acidosis has passed and the excess carbon dioxide has been cleared.

- Hemoglobin – for most patients, the hemoglobin concentration should be above 7.5 g/dl prior to termination of CPB but decisions to transfuse should be based on the clinical situation. Higher Hb levels might be indicated if oxygen delivery is expected to be impaired by a post-CPB low cardiac output state or if bleeding is expected to be an ongoing problem.

Levels

- Reservoir volume – there needs to be sufficient volume in the CPB circuit to fill the heart in order to wean it from CPB. Usually at least 300–500 mls are required to fill the heart. If the reservoir volume is close to the low level sensor it is essential to add additional volume. To minimize crystalloid requirements the surgeon should check the chest and pleural spaces for shed blood and consider using the cardiotomy sucker to retrieve. However, the benefits of direct reinfusion of shed mediastinal blood must be weighed against the risks of adding blood that is likely to be diluted or highly activated with inflammatory mediators. Alternatively shed blood is collected to an autotransfusion device where it is washed and the red blood cells concentrated before administration.

- Bed position and transducer levels – it is common during surgery, and in particular during cross clamp release, for the operating table position to be moved. Prior to weaning, the table should be returned to a neutral position and pressure transducers should be leveled and re-zeroed.

Predicting Difficulty

Occasionally weaning from CPB is difficult and identification of patients who will present a particular challenge allows additional preparations to be made in advance.

Commonly encountered risk factors for difficulty or failure to wean from CPB include:

1. poor preoperative ventricular function
2. urgent and emergency surgery
3. prolonged aortic cross clamp time
4. inadequate myocardial protection
5. incomplete surgical repair or revascularization.

Several strategies may be considered if weaning from CPB is likely to be difficult:

- Inotropes and vasopressors can be commenced at rewarming, ensuring they have cleared the deadspace of administration lines. Some inotropes require a loading dose (e.g. enoximone, milrinone, levosimendan) which should be given after aortic unclamping.

- If sinus rhythm is not established and supraventricular arrhythmias or ventricular irritability are present despite correction of metabolic parameters, anti-arrhythmic treatments should be considered and given in advance of any attempts at weaning from CPB. Direct current cardioversion (DCCV) using paddles directly applied to the heart and low energy at 10–20 J is often successful.

- An IABP may be inserted before the start of surgery in patients with poor ventricular function. Or if an IABP is anticipated, but not inserted, a femoral arterial line may be placed on anesthetic induction to allow rapid insertion of a balloon catheter over a wire in an emergency.

Mechanics of Separation from CPB

As soon as cardiovascular, respiratory and metabolic parameters are within acceptable limits and the patient is adequately rewarmed and ventilated, the perfusionist commences weaning in coordination with the anesthesiologist and surgeon.

Weaning begins with:

- confirming with the anesthesiologist that the patient is adequately ventilated – "happy with ventilation?"

- incrementally occluding the venous return to the CPB circuit, thus allowing the heart to fill with and eject blood, and

- gradually reducing the arterial pump flow to 0.

The order and speed of these actions will depend on the volume in the reservoir, the patient's ventricular function and systemic vascular resistance, the surgery and any risk factors for failure to wean from CPB. Preload, contractility and afterload are assessed as the flow is reduced.

Weaning from CPB may take just a few seconds in a patient with vigorous cardiac activity and typically be taken to "half-flow" and then off CPB. In patients with less promising cardiac function, the weaning process may need to be protracted. This can take up to 30 or more minutes and may include reducing pump flow by as little as 0.5 l every 5–10 minutes. After each new transition TEE evaluation, titration of ventricular volume loading by visual inspection of the RV and/or assessment of direct left atrial pressure or pulmonary artery/pulmonary capillary wedge pressure measurements, optimization of inotropes and vasoconstrictors and assessment of cardiac rhythm should be undertaken. At each stage volume can be added by further occlusion of the venous clamp during "partial bypass" or transient increase in arterial flow; volume can be removed by releasing the venous clamp or decreasing arterial flow. Alternatively, some centers or teams prefer to come off bypass and, if the heart does not sustain adequate cardiac output, go back on bypass and reperfuse the myocardium for a period of time.

The introduction of electronic venous occluders has been beneficial to fine tuning venous occlusion during weaning. The vent and cardiotomy suction may still be working during separation from CPB and the patient will slowly exsanguinate if this blood is not returned. The perfusionist will return the amount gained from vent and suckers to the patient 1:1 unless agreed otherwise.

As cardiac stroke volume progressively increases to a level compatible with physiological circulation, the venous return line is completely occluded, the arterial flow reduced to "off" or "matching vents or suction" and the transition from CPB to "normal" circulation is complete.

Assessment of Cardiac Function and Inotropic Support

Assessment of ventricular contractility and valvular function is vital during weaning. Myocardial contractility can be estimated from observing the heart both directly and with TEE, looking for coordinated muscle contraction generating an acceptable aortic pressure pulsation and arterial blood pressure. Commonly employed quantitative measures of LV function include assessment of cardiac output with thermodilution and stroke volume and ejection fraction assessments by TEE. Any valvular pathology, particularly after repair, needs to be considered at this stage as well.

The pharmacological and mechanical strategies to support the heart during and after weaning from CPB are considered below and are generally guided by institutional practice or individual preference. Inotropic support should ideally be optimized prior to weaning from CPB or during "partial bypass" to enable successful transition from CPB to physiological circulation.

It is worth noting that on initial separation from CPB, cardiac output and/or vascular tone can be low, and thus arterial blood pressure is frequently low. After optimization of preload and rhythm, hypotension is frequently managed with the use of short acting vasoconstrictors. This temporarily increases systemic vascular resistance (SVR), increasing diastolic blood pressure, which increases coronary artery blood flow, and aids myocardial contraction.

Assessment of Afterload

Commonly SVR is low following CPB because of the systemic inflammatory response and hemodilution. Short acting vasoconstrictors (e.g. metaraminol, phenylephrine) are administered during CPB and in the weaning phase; along with the above agents, infusions of norepinephrine or vasopressin may be used to maintain SVR in the weaning and post-CPB periods. The amount of vasopressor used by the perfusionist to maintain blood pressure during CPB may serve as a guide as to whether infusions will be necessary at the weaning stage and beyond.

TEE in Weaning from CPB

There is a wide variation in the use of TEE in adult cardiac surgery, ranging from routine to highly

Table 12.3. Key benefits of TEE during weaning from CPB

Ensure adequate de-airing

Guide ventricular filling

Identify global ventricular dysfunction

Guide inotropic support

Ensure adequate surgical success (e.g. valve size, position and function, paravalvular leaks, residual intracardiac shunts)

Identify regional wall motion abnormalities

Identify pleural and pericardial effusions

Guide insertion and positioning of mechanical support devices

Diagnose aortic dissection after decannulation

selective. Echocardiography during the final stages of CPB can inform on surgical success after valve repair or replacement, new or unresolved wall motion abnormalities, intracardiac shunts and other pathologies that might make the weaning process difficult. It is an excellent guide to de-airing after open chamber surgery (see Figure 12.1). Table 12.3 summarizes the key benefits of using TEE during weaning from CPB.

In the event of failed weaning from CPB, TEE is a useful real-time modality for guiding the placement of mechanical support devices such as intra-aortic balloon pumps, ECMO cannulae and ventricular assist devices.

Reversal of Anticoagulation

Protamine is used to reverse heparin anticoagulation after successful transition from CPB to physiological circulation. Heparin reversal practices vary among centers and are discussed in detail in Chapter 16. Vents and suction must be stopped prior to protamine administration.

Residual Blood Management

It is important to have a blood conservation strategy in cardiac surgery and transfusion of the residual volume in the CPB circuit is part of this. Practice varies among centers and blood can be retransfused directly or processed by cell salvage or ultrafiltration in order to minimize allogenic blood transfusion.

Failure to Wean from CPB

Inadequate hemodynamic performance, when attempting to wean a patient from CPB despite providing optimal conditions, should prompt the team to consider returning to full CPB, particularly if a deterioration is catastrophic or unexpected.

Common conditions leading to failure to wean are:

- surgical complications
- arrhythmias
- vasodilation/hypotension
- ventricular failure
- hypoxia
- bleeding
- residual air escaping from left ventricle into coronary circulation.

Table 12.4 summarizes common and procedure specific problems with weaning from CPB and potential management plans.

Reinstituting CPB should not necessarily be viewed as an adverse event or failure. It will result in a prolongation of the total CPB time, but it allows:

- time for the heart to recover
- escalation of monitoring
- reassessing and possibly optimizing of pharmacological support
- (re)adjustment of hematocrit, acid-base, and electrolytes
- examination of graft and valvular integrity (e.g. kinked coronary bypass grafts, paraprosthetic leaks)
- implementation of mechanical support

Reinstitution of CPB

Whatever the degree of urgency, and even in situations of cardiac massage, adequate anticoagulation needs to be achieved before going back onto CPB and if time permits an ACT should be obtained prior to reinstitution.

To assure preparedness it is common to leave the CPB lines on the table and to keep the circuit primed until at least sternal closure. To facilitate this, the circuit is filled with crystalloid fluid via the venous line while being drained of blood. This still allows retransfusion of the residual blood while keeping the circuit immediately available.

Pharmacological Choices in Weaning from CPB

Administration of inotropes and/or vasopressor infusions may be indicated for successful weaning from CPB. Drugs should be titrated to effect, optimizing blood pressure and heart rate, with patients monitored using an appropriate combination of arterial blood pressure, pulmonary artery catheter, TEE, blood gas analysis and assessments of end-organ perfusion such as urine output. The particular therapeutic regimen will be dictated by the hemodynamic abnormality at hand (e.g. vasodilation versus impaired contractility) along with institutional preferences. Drugs to be considered for acute hemodynamic support during weaning from CPB are:

- Epinephrine – has both alpha and beta-adrenoceptor activity. Epinephrine increases cardiac output by increasing contractility and heart rate and is frequently employed where moderate to severely impaired cardiac contractility is present. At high dose continuous infusion, it may cause considerable vasoconstriction and tachycardia, impair diastolic function and raise serum lactate concentrations.
- Dopamine – binds to dopaminergic receptors and to alpha and beta-adrenergic receptors. It increases cardiac output by increasing heart rate and contractility; however, at higher doses blood pressure may be increased by raising systemic vascular resistance with no increase in cardiac output and may cause dysrhythmias. Dopamine is generally used with more mild impairment of hemodynamic performance.
- Dobutamine – is a synthetic catecholamine with a strong affinity for beta-adrenoceptors and little alpha activity. Contractility and heart rate are increased along with a reduction in systemic vascular resistance, leading to a rise in cardiac output. At higher doses the effects on heart rate and increased oxygen consumption and demand tend to dominate and may limit its usefulness in moderate to severe cardiac failure.
- Milrinone and Enoximone – are often referred to as "inodilators." They are bipyridine phosphodiesterase-III (PDE III) inhibitors, which block the breakdown of intracellular cyclic AMP

119

Table 12.4. Common problems encountered with weaning from CPB in specific operations and suggested management plan

PROCEDURE	ISSUE	PLAN
CABG	Graft issues	Surgical correction
	Myocardial protection	Rest on CPB, inotropes, mechanical support
	Unrecognized valve issue	Surgical correction
	Conduction issues	Pacing
AVR	Myocardial protection	Rest on CPB, inotropes, mechanical support
	Air embolus	Rest on CPB with increased perfusion pressure
	Valve issue – stuck leaflet, paravalular leak, valve upside down	Surgical correction
	Coronary occlusion right or left coronary ostial occlusion	Surgical correction
	Conduction issues	Pacing
MVR	Myocardial protection	Rest on CPB, inotropes, mechanical support
	Air embolus	Rest on CPB with increased perfusion pressure
	Valve issue - stuck leaflet paravalular leak valve upside down stitch around a strut if a tissue valve circumflex artery injury	Surgical correction
	Conduction issues LVOT obstruction (in repair)	Pacing Filling, stop inotropes, slow heart rate, vasoconstriction, surgical intervention
ASD	Myocardial protection	Rest on CPB, inotropes, mechanical support
	Air embolus	Rest on CPB with increased perfusion pressure
	Pulmonary hypertension	Pulmonary vasodilators e.g. phosphodiesterase inhibitors
	Anatomical - Residual shunt Coronary sinus impingement mitral valve issues unrecognized anomalous pulmonary venous drainage	Surgical correction
	Conduction issues	Pacing
VSD	Myocardial protection Poor RV and/or LV	Rest on CPB, inotropes, mechanical support
	Air embolus	Rest on CPB with increased perfusion pressure
	Residual shunt	Surgical correction
	Conduction issues	Pacing

and increase stores of ATP. PDE III inhibitors improve contractility and because they cause pulmonary vasodilatation (in addition to systemic vasodilation) they are commonly used when right heart dysfunction is present. They are associated with a lower incidence of tachycardia and arrhythmia than beta agonists, but they may need to be administered concurrently with a vasoconstrictor to maintain adequate arterial pressure. Cardiac output increases without a significant increase in myocardial oxygen consumption and demand.

- Norepinephrine – has predominantly alpha-adrenergic effects and lesser beta-receptor activity. It causes smooth muscle contraction and vasoconstriction. Norepinephrine may be useful when the SVR is low, to counter the vasodilator effects of phosphodiesterase-III inhibitors, and to manage acute right heart dysfunction. A concern with norepinephrine in high doses is reduced perfusion of the kidneys, gut and extremities, resulting in hypoperfusion or overt ischemia.

- Vasopressin – is also known as anti-diuretic hormone (ADH) or argipressin. It acts on a family of vasopressin receptors in the smooth muscle of vasculature, resulting in vasoconstriction. However, stimulation of the V1 receptors in the coronary and pulmonary vasculature causes release of nitric oxide and vasodilation. The action of vasopressin is independent of adrenoreceptors, and it may be useful in conjunction with norepinephrine for low SVR states.

- Levosimendan – has inodilator properties, mediated by calcium sensitization of troponin C and the opening of potassium channels on the sarcolemma of vascular smooth muscle cells. Levosimendan is also thought to confer cardioprotection via its action on mitochondrial potassium channels in the cardiomyocytes. Hemodynamics are improved without a significant increase in myocardial oxygen consumption. The evidence for improved outcomes is equivocal at best, however, and due to its very high cost levosimendan is generally only be used in selected difficult-to-wean patients.

- Calcium – may be given as a bolus dose in the event of ventricular dilation and poor function immediately on separating from CPB. Calcium has both positive inotropic and vasopressor effects

and may stabilize hemodynamics or improve them in the short term.

- Glyceryl trinitrate – is an organic nitrate that is converted to nitric oxide and promotes both venous and arterial dilation. It may be used post-CPB to control hypertension, decreasing myocardial wall tension and oxygen consumption, and protecting the integrity of vascular suture lines.

- Inhaled pulmonary vasodilators – nitric oxide (NO) is an endogenous smooth muscle relaxant and vasodilator produced by nitric oxide synthase. Inhaled nitric oxide acts as a selective pulmonary vasodilator and is often used in pulmonary hypertension in order to preserve right heart function. Nitric oxide is aerosolized into the inspiratory limb of the breathing circuit and the dose titrated up to a maximum of 40 ppm. The drug is delivered directly to the pulmonary vasculature and has an extremely short half-life, limiting any systemic hypotension. Prolonged exposure to high concentrations of nitric oxide may result in methemoglobinemia and pulmonary edema. The use of alternative inhaled pulmonary vasodilators, such as epoprostenol, iloprost or inhaled milrinone, has gained popularity as first line therapy.

Pharmacological Side Effects

The more potent a pharmacological agent is, the more serious are the potential side effects. Potent vasoconstrictors such as norepinephrine and vasopressin can cause splanchnic vasoconstriction, which can be associated with postoperative gastrointestinal ischemia. Potent inotropes, like epinephrine, increase myocardial oxygen consumption, and can be associated with a difficult-to-treat acidosis. Phosphodiesterase inhibitors, such as enoximone, are potentially arrhythmogenic. Potent chronotropes include dopamine and dobutamine, which can cause reflex tachycardias and arrhythmias.

Mechanical Support in Weaning from CPB

After failure to separate from and returning to CPB, attention is directed to identifying and treating reversible causes, such as inadequacy of surgery, and to optimizing hemodynamics while allowing myocardial recovery. In a small number of cases the ventricular function remains insufficient to maintain adequate organ perfusion, despite appropriate measures. If necessary mechanical therapies are warranted to facilitate separation from CPB. Strategies are discussed briefly here and mechanical support is described in greater detail in Chapter 14.

Intra-aortic balloon pump (IABP) – the most commonly used method of mechanical therapy, intra-aortic balloon counterpulsation is achieved using a balloon-tipped catheter that is positioned within the descending aorta, with the tip just distal to the origin of the left subclavian artery. Inflation of the balloon coincides with diastole, timed with the dichrotic notch on the arterial waveform or the T wave on the ECG. The benefits of arterial counterpulsation lie with the augmented coronary flow and improved myocardial oxygen delivery that occur through increases in diastolic blood pressure from balloon inflation and the decrease in LV afterload that occurs during balloon deflation, thus reducing myocardial oxygen demand while increasing delivery.

Veno-arterial extracorporeal membrane oxygenation (VA ECMO) – is a means of mechanically supporting the heart (and lungs) using a modified CPB circuit, often making use of the existing bypass cannulation. ECMO may continue for a period of days to weeks until myocardial recovery has been achieved or as a bridge to VAD or transplant.

Ventricular assist device (VAD) – may be applied to either one or both ventricles to support a failing heart and preserve organ perfusion. Few data exist to support the use of VAD over ECMO when a patient fails to separate from CPB. The decision to implement either technique should be based on center-specific expertise and experience and specific patient condition. The benefits of VA ECMO over VAD are that the single VA ECMO circuit supports both ventricles and also the lungs and can be more rapidly initiated since cannulae are already in situ and only a change of circuit is required.

Suggested Further Reading

1. Cui Wilson W, Ramsay James G. "Pharmacologic approaches to weaning from cardiopulmonary bypass and extracorporeal membrane oxygenation." *Best Practice & Research Clinical Anaesthesiology* 29.2 (2015): 257–270.

2. Kim Heezoo. "Weaning from cardiopulmonary bypass." *Korean Journal of Anesthesiology* 64.6 (2013): 487.

3. Licker Marc et al. "Clinical review: management of weaning from cardiopulmonary bypass after cardiac surgery." *Annals of Cardiac Anaesthesia* 15.3 (2012): 206.

4. Murkin J M, Arango Murkin M. Near-infrared spectroscopy as an index of brain and tissue oxygenation. *British Journal of Anaesthesia*. 103,suppl1,2009, i3–i13.

5. Totaro R J, Raper R F. Epinephrine-induced lactic acidosis following cardiopulmonary bypass. *Crit Care Med*. October 1997;25(10): 1693–1699.

6. Bernard Francis, Denault André, Babin Denis et al. Diastolic dysfunction is predictive of difficult weaning from cardiopulmonary bypass, *Anesthesia & Analgesia*: February 2001,92(2): 291–298

7. Vakamudi M. Weaning from cardiopulmonary bypass: problems and remedies. *Ann Card Anaesth*. July 2004;7(2): 178–185.

8. Cui WW, Ramsay JG. Pharmacologic approaches to weaning from cardiopulmonary bypass and extracorporeal membrane oxygenation. *Best Pract Res Clin Anaesthesiol*. June 2015;29(2): 257–270.

Intraoperative Mechanical Circulatory Support and Other Uses of Cardiopulmonary Bypass

Mark Buckland and Jessica Underwood

Both cardiopulmonary bypass (CPB) and its "off-spring," extracorporeal membrane oxygenation (ECMO), are forms of mechanical circulatory support (MCS) utilized for short or long-term supplementation of native cardiac and/or respiratory function. As institutions tackle more complex pathologies, the indications for these specialist techniques are becoming increasingly broad. This chapter addresses thoracic surgical requirements for MCS including mediastinal mass and tumor excision, complex MCS techniques employed during thoracic aortic surgery and specialist techniques utilized during donor organ procurement and heart, lung and liver transplantation. Emergent uses of MCS both inside and outside the operating room are also discussed, including endobronchial hemorrhage, extracorporeal cardiopulmonary resuscitation (ECPR) and MCS for treatment of hypothermic circulatory arrest and trauma patients. MCS is also highlighted as a crucial preemptive tool to support patients during induction of anesthesia, whether it be due to difficult airways or risk of pulmonary hypertensive circulatory collapse.

Historically, conventional CPB has been the mechanical circulatory support system of choice, but with evolution of equipment, technique and experience, ECMO has become an almost exclusive "player" in the support realm and is being used more and more in the surgical arena.

Historical Perspective of MCS in Cardiac and Respiratory Failure

Although CPB has been utilized for cardiac surgery since the 1950s, the first successful report of its use as a form of cardiorespiratory support was in 1972 when Hill and colleagues used a heart-lung machine to support a young man, who had developed acute respiratory distress syndrome (ARDS) after repair of a traumatic aortic disruption, for a period of 75 hours. Following this, ECMO was successfully used to support neonates by Bartlett and others in 1975.

These successes led to the enthusiastic application of MCS to provide cardiorespiratory support for a range of indications, but overall results were poor. The therapy became confined to a few expert centers that persisted and developed the techniques, including veno-venous (VV ECMO) and veno-arterial ECMO (VA ECMO). In 2009, the CESAR trial demonstrated clinical efficacy and cost effectiveness of ECMO in the treatment of adult acute respiratory distress syndrome (ARDS), compared with advanced conventional therapy in designated expert centers. Shortly after this, the publication of good results of the use of ECMO in supporting patients effected by the H1N1 influenza pandemic in Australia and New Zealand established MCS as an acceptable and feasible therapy to support patients with severe acute pulmonary failure. The advances in equipment, technique and expertise that led to acceptance of MCS for successful long-term respiratory support have made its use in acute and longer term circulatory support accepted as a standard of care both in and outside the operating room in institutions with appropriate expertise and experience.

MCS Equipment Selection

With ever increasing clinical applications of MCS and a multitude of hardware and consumable options, early communication of the surgical plan is vital, especially in complex procedures, like those on the thoracic aorta, as perfusion equipment needs to be tailored to the style of MCS required (see Table 13.1).

It is worth noting that there may be a number MCS options to achieve the support goals for a given procedure; each of these will have a number of clinical advantages and disadvantages that need to be considered (see Table 13.2).

Table 13.1. Mechanical circulatory support style and perfusion equipment suitability

	Centrifugal pump and heat exchanger	ECMO circuit	Open bypass circuit	Open bypass circuit + specialized add-on circuitry
Left Heart Bypass	Y	Y	Y	Y
Partial Cardiopulmonary Bypass	N	Y	Y	Y
Complete Cardiopulmonary Bypass	N	Y	Y	Y
Complete Cardiopulmonary Bypass with Hypothermic Circulatory Arrest	N	N	Y	Y
Selective Spinal/ Reno-Visceral Hypothermic Perfusion	N	N	N	Y

Table 13.2. Advantages and disadvantages of various perfusion equipment options

Perfusion Equipment	Advantages	Disadvantages
Centrifugal pump with heat exchanger	• Technically simple • Economical • Full heparinization not required • Low prime volume • Temperature control	• Custom tubing pack may be required • Unable to salvage whole blood from the surgical field directly into the circuit, leading to heavy cell saver use and greater likelihood of transfusion • Completely reliant on lungs for oxygenation • Anesthetist is required to give volume and maintain adequate filling • Anesthetist is required to manage blood pressure and administer any drugs • Risk of air embolism in the setting of access cannula dislodgement
ECMO circuit (centrifugal pump, heat exchanger and oxygenator)	• Circuit and hardware readily available in most institutions • Full heparinization not required • Low prime volume • Temperature control • Oxygenator support	• Unable to salvage whole blood from the surgical field directly into the circuit, leading to heavy cell saver use and greater likelihood of transfusion • Anesthetist is required to give volume and maintain adequate filling • Anesthetist is required to manage blood pressure and administer any drugs • Risk of air embolism in the setting of access cannula dislodgement

Table 13.2. (cont.)

Perfusion Equipment	Advantages	Disadvantages
Complete heart-lung machine with open cardiopulmonary bypass circuit	• Circuit and hardware readily available in most institutions • Temperature control • Oxygenator support • Cardiotomy and several other pumps available as sump suckers to salvage whole blood from the surgical field • Reduced requirement for cell saver processing • Complete control of filling • Complete control of blood pressure • Readily able to administer fluids, blood products or pharmacological agents as required • Ability to add additional pumps or circuitry as required • Inclusion of an open reservoir, reduces risk of air embolism in the setting of access cannula dislodgment, assuming level and bubble safety sensors and arterial pump servo-regulation are utilized	• Full heparinization required • Larger priming volume • Greater technical complexity, particularly if selective organ perfusion or hypothermic circulatory arrest is used

Thoracic Surgeries

There are a large number of case reports/series describing a wide range of both diagnostic and therapeutic procedures on non-cardiac thoracic structures that have made use of MCS.

Anterior Mediastinal Masses and Difficult Airways

Anterior mediastinal masses, causing airway or cardiovascular compromise by compression, have always provided a challenge during induction of anesthesia and positioning for surgery. The traditional approach of maintaining spontaneous ventilation and use of fiberoptic intubation is wise but may not guarantee protection from airway compression or circulatory collapse. Several groups have described the use of awake CPB or ECMO in a range of patients with awake peripheral cannulation and initiating circulatory support prior to induction of anesthesia and intubation; the pathologies dealt with included massive intrathoracic goiter, thymoma and teratoma. Most authors make the point that if there is enough concern to consider use of bypass or ECMO support,

then it should be done preemptively rather than as standby with rescue, as it takes at least 5–10 minutes to initiate support, even with experienced hands in the room.

The approach to the difficult airway promulgated by the learned anesthesia societies and colleges worldwide rely on four fundamental techniques – bag-mask ventilation (BMV), supraglottic airways (SGA), tracheal intubation (ETT) and front-of-neck airway. If the obstruction occurs at or lower than the glottis, the above may not be enough to maintain oxygenation. Some have suggested elective use of MCS to maintain gas exchange as the potential fifth option in the non-urgent situation. Several groups have described use of CPB and ECMO (both VA and VV) in the management of lesions causing subtotal obstruction of the airway at or below the glottis. These include creation of end-tracheostomy and resection of invasive thyroid cancer using awake peripheral VA ECMO; bronchoscopy, stenting and tracheostomy for "benign" obstructing tracheal lesions on CPB; use of VV ECMO and high flow nasal oxygen for debridement of distal airway melanoma metastases; and bronchoscopic laser resection of tracheal papillomatosis, with awake VV ECMO established prior to induction. Both CPB and ECMO have also been used to support pediatric tracheal reconstruction for congenital tracheal stenosis. Both support techniques have pros and cons, but overall results and outcomes are comparable.

Thoracic and Abdominal Tumor Surgery

A number of groups have reported case series using CPB for surgical resection of locally advanced thoracic malignancies, particularly where the tumor involves chambers of the heart or great vessels. These show that the use of CPB is associated with reasonable early morbidity and mortality. The importance of patient selection is key with better long-term results dependent on shorter bypass times, the nature of the tumor and the extent of lung resection.

Renal cell carcinomas with tumor thrombi invading the inferior vena cava (IVC) have a poor prognosis; however, if the tumor can be resected in its entirety via radical nephrectomy and IVC thrombectomy, overall survival is reasonable. In situations where the tumor thrombus extends into the retrohepatic or supra-diaphragmatic IVC or into the right atrium (RA), CPB can be used with standard arterial cannulation and venous drainage via the superior vena cava (SVC) and the IVC below the tumor thrombus, enabling en-bloc tumor removal. In circumstances where the thrombus extends beyond the RA into the pulmonary artery (PA) it is possible to cool the patient to 18–20°C and remove it under deep hypothermic circulatory arrest (DHCA).

Thoracic Aortic Surgery

In recent years, treatment for aneurysms of the descending thoracic aorta (segments distal to the left subclavian artery to the diaphragm) and thoracoabdominal aorta (segments distal to the left subclavian artery to the iliac arteries) has focused on endovascular stent-graft repairs. Endovascular treatment has the obvious appeal of a minimal access approach and a reduced average mortality rate (5.8%) compared to open surgery (13.9%). However, it is not without its limitations, including reduced suitability with increased complexity and extent of disease, anatomic confounders such as aortic angulation and tortuosity, landing zone inadequacy and risk of endoleak leading to reintervention. Open surgical repair remains an indispensable treatment modality, particularly in the setting of complex pathologies.

Over time several adjunct therapies have been adopted to address the major challenges associated with open surgical repair – hemodynamic instability and protection from spinal cord and reno-visceral malperfusion. Arguably one of the greatest protectors against hypoperfusion and hemodynamic instability throughout the procedure is assistance provided by MCS.

In its simplest form, distal aortic perfusion preserves blood flow to the lower extremities and vital organs during fashioning of the proximal anastomosis. In particular, the inherently vulnerable spinal cord and kidneys can be protected from ischemic injury by maintaining blood flow to the renal and intercostal arteries, as well as perfusion via collateral circulations. A 2012 Cochrane Review found evidence from observational studies suggesting that distal aortic perfusion during open thoracoabdominal aortic aneurysm repair reduces the incidence of neurological deficits, with the greatest benefits seen in Crawford extent II aneurysms. The review however did note a, likely ethically-driven, lack of randomized controlled trials comparing open surgical repair with or without distal perfusion, as the use of MCS has become an accepted prophylactic strategy used to combat ischemic complications.

MCS may be utilized in a variety of forms during open surgical repair including, but not limited to, intermittent or continuous, selective hypothermic perfusion, distal aortic perfusion via left heart bypass or partial cardiopulmonary bypass and complete cardiopulmonary bypass, often including deep or profound hypothermic circulatory arrest (Table 13.1). The techniques employed in a given case depend on the extent of disease, operative plan and surgical preference.

Left Heart Bypass

Left heart bypass can be achieved via pulmonary vein or left atrial access cannulation and femoral arterial or distal aortic return cannulation (see Figure 13.1). Some left atrial filling is maintained throughout the systematic clamping of the thoracic descending and thoracoabdominal aorta to allow proximal perfusion via left ventricular ejection, while distal perfusion is provided by the femoral arterial or distal aortic return cannula. The perfusion and anesthetic teams work to ensure that proximal and distal perfusion pressures, measured by way of radial and femoral arterial lines, are maintained in equilibrium throughout the procedure and to prevent accidental emptying of the left atrium during the procedure. Proximal perfusion is being provided by

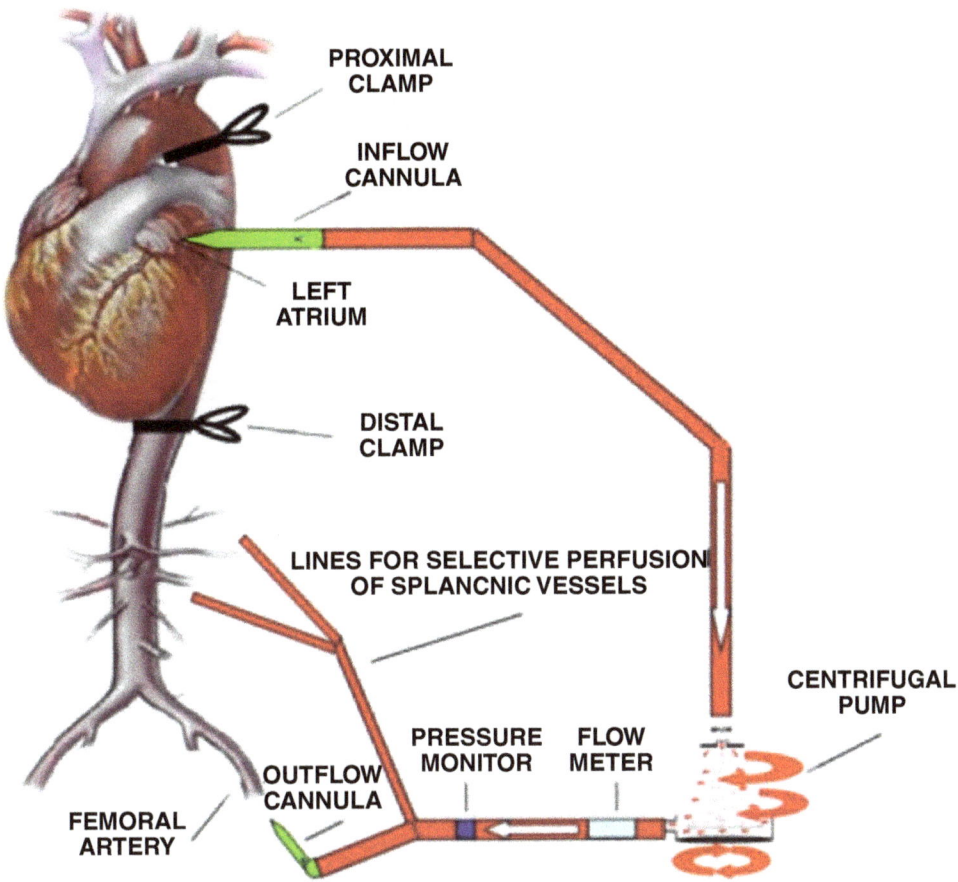

PROXIMAL CLAMP

INFLOW CANNULA

LEFT ATRIUM

DISTAL CLAMP

LINES FOR SELECTIVE PERFUSION OF SPLANCNIC VESSELS

CENTRIFUGAL PUMP

PRESSURE MONITOR

FLOW METER

OUTFLOW CANNULA

FEMORAL ARTERY

Figure 13.1 Left heart bypass: inflow cannula in left pulmonary vein or in left atrium and return to femoral artery or distal aorta (it is possible to incorporate an oxygenator in this circuit for additional support). (De Simone F, De Luca M. Left Heart Bypass (Ch24) in *Thoraco-Abdominal Aorta: Surgical and Anesthetic Management.* R. Chiesa et al. (eds.) © Springer-Verlag Italia 2011.)

the heart and it is therefore important to avoid moderate–deep hypothermia in order to prevent temperature related arrhythmias. In the instance where aortic cross clamping at the distal aortic arch is not possible due to atherosclerotic plaque or further aneurysmal tissue, complete cardiopulmonary bypass is likely to be the chosen modality of mechanical circulatory support to allow for DHCA during open proximal anastomosis, with the option to continue perfusing tissues distal to the aortic cross clamp.

Partial or Complete Cardiopulmonary Bypass

Partial or complete cardiopulmonary bypass is often achieved via femoral venous access cannulation and femoral arterial or distal aortic return cannulation. This setup affords the surgical team the ability to utilize the full possibility of perfusion techniques, including hypothermia, circulatory arrest, the ability

to turn off ventilation to one or both lungs and rely on the extracorporeal oxygenator, as well as selective spinal and reno-visceral perfusion. These perfusion techniques provide superior surgical access, visibility and flexibility with the operative plan, as well as the ability to perform the procedure with reduced time pressure, which is evoked by the known risks associated with prolonged ischemic clamp time in the absence of hypothermia or selective perfusion.

Selective Spinal and Reno-visceral Perfusion

Matalanis et al are pioneering the "branch first" surgical approach in tackling Crawford extent II thoracoabdominal aneurysms in an attempt to maximize the benefits provided by MCS and to provide near continuous reno-vascular perfusion (see Figure 13.2a and b). In this approach, partial bypass is instituted via femoral-femoral cannulation, using an open

127

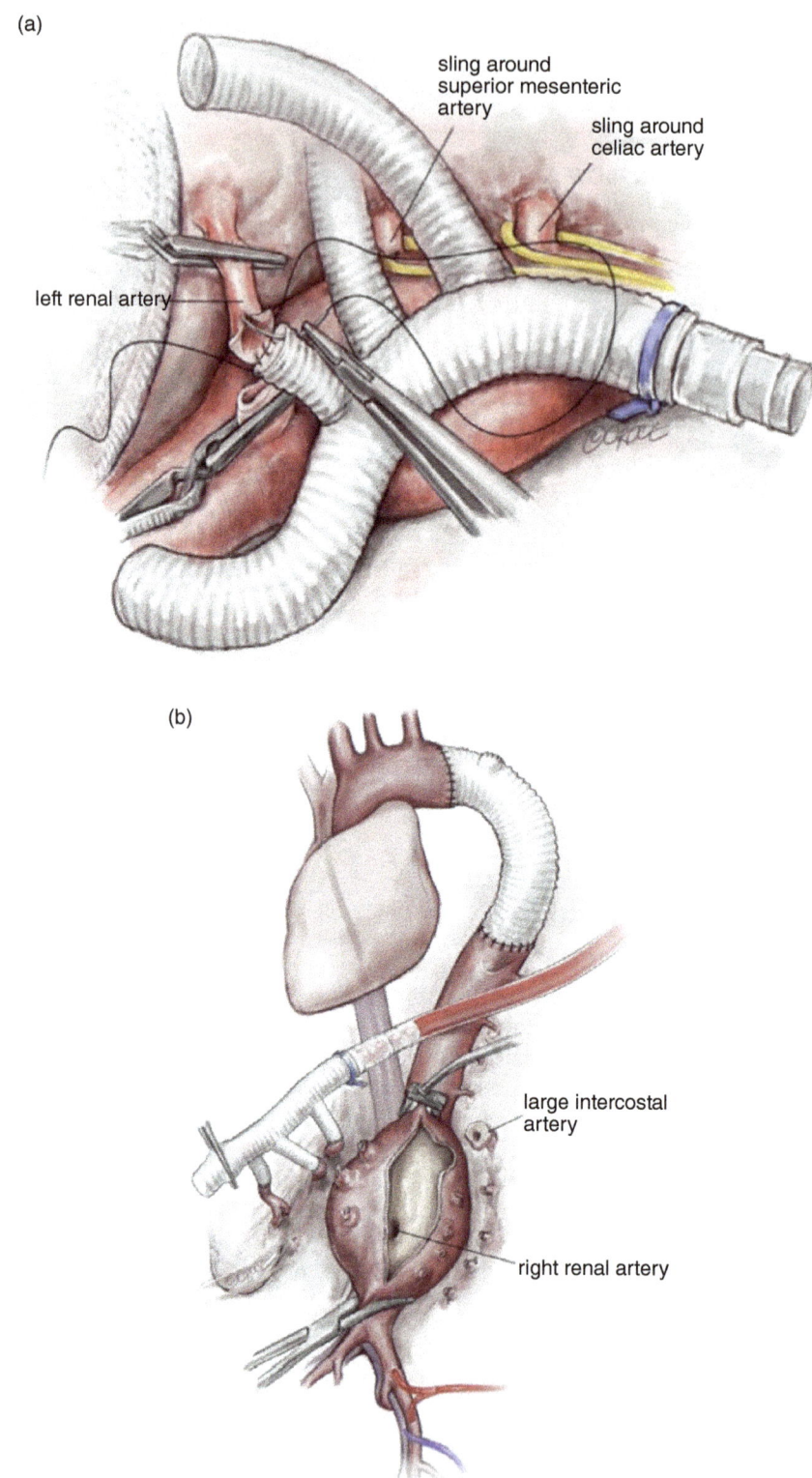

(a)

sling around
superior mesenteric
artery

sling around
celiac artery

left renal artery

(b)

large intercostal
artery

right renal artery

Figure 13.2 Branch first approach to thoraco-abdominal aneurysm repair. (a) Sequential debranching and perfusion of reno-visceral vessels using a trifurcated graft with perfusion limb. (b) Clutter-free access to the abdominal aorta, with left renal, SMA, coeliac trunk being perfused by the graft and smaller lumbar arteries already ligated, allowing access to aortic pathology. (Reproduced with kind permissions from Matalanis and Ch'ng, *Semin Thorac Cardiovasc Surg* 2020; 31.4:627–872.)

bypass circuit with specialized add-on circuitry prepared for selective reno-visceral perfusion using an additional roller pump, and intercostal artery perfusion using the cardioplegia pump. This technique provides complete mechanical circulatory support flexibility including systemic and selective temperature control, partial or complete cardiopulmonary bypass, selective perfusion and the option of hypothermic circulatory arrest if required.

Circulatory Support during Donor Organ Procurement

Organ Donation for Heart Transplantation

Heart procurement after the cessation of cardiac activity was utilized for the first and other early cardiac transplants, as brain death criteria and legislation were not widely established until the early to mid-eighties. With revised legislation and commercial availability of specialized MCS devices some groups have revived the donation after cardiac death (DCD) heart transplant pathway. The first report of three successful cases of orthotopic cardiac transplantation using hearts from DCD was published in 2014. Promising outcomes have helped spread this technique and globally its uptake is increasing rapidly.

DCD donation involves either direct procurement and perfusion, direct procurement and cold storage or normothermic regional perfusion (NRP) (see Figure 13.3).

Direct procurement and perfusion (DPP) – involves prompt transfer of the donor to the operating room after death has been declared, with expeditious sternotomy, administration of cold cardioplegia and removal of the heart following standard surgical technique. The organ is then connected to the Transmedics Organ Care System (OCS™) (see Figure 13.4) and perfused at normothermia with a mixture of a priming solution and 1.5 liters of heparinized donor blood. The flow rate is initially set at 1 l/min and adjusted to maintain a mean aortic pressure of 65–90 mmHg, coronary blood flow of 650–900 ml/min and a heart rate of 65–100 beats/min. The suitability of the reanimated heart for transplantation is assessed functionally, via macroscopic assessment, and biochemically with serial lactate measurements. The design of the device also allows epicardial echocardiography in an aseptic manner.

Normothermic Regional Perfusion (NRP) – also involves prompt sternotomy after declaration of death followed by heparinizing via the right atrium and pulmonary artery and clamping of the innominate, left carotid and left subclavian arteries to ensure that cerebral circulation cannot be restored. MCS is instituted via right atrial access and an aortic return cannula. Following restoration of mechanical ventilation, cardiac reanimation and a period of reperfusion, MCS is weaned. Suitability of the reanimated heart for transplantation is assessed functionally via transesophageal echocardiogram and thermodilution cardiac output measurements. If found suitable the donor heart is prepared for transport to the recipient hospital. These hearts are then given cold cardioplegia, procured and transported using either the OCS system or conventional cold storage.

Organ Donation for Lung Transplantation

The lung transplant community were much earlier adopters of the DCD pathway, largely due to fewer ethical hurdles and the decreased vulnerability of the lungs to warm ischemia, allowing a simple retrieval and transportation strategy utilizing pneumoplegic cold storage. The International Society for Heart and Lung Transplantation (ISHLT) DCD Registry has reported comparable 5-year survival rates, of 63% and 61%, between DCD and donation after brainstem death (DBD) lung donor recipients, respectively. With a large number of lung donor offers available, efforts have been focusing on increasing the percentage of organs that can be accepted as suitable for transplantation by using pre-transplant, normothermic, ex vivo lung perfusion (EVLP).

EVLP allows explanted donor lungs to be perfused and ventilated in order to thoroughly assess their suitability for transplantation prior to implant. This is particularly useful in marginal organs which sit outside an institution's standard donor organ acceptance criteria. Not only can marginal organs be assessed during EVLP, but they can potentially be reconditioned using various resuscitative maneuvers, rescuing and restoring donor organs that would have otherwise been discarded.

The XVIVO system (Figure 13.5) is usually located at the recipient hospital for reanimation and assessment of distantly retrieved, marginal donor lungs prior to implant. The explanted lungs, which

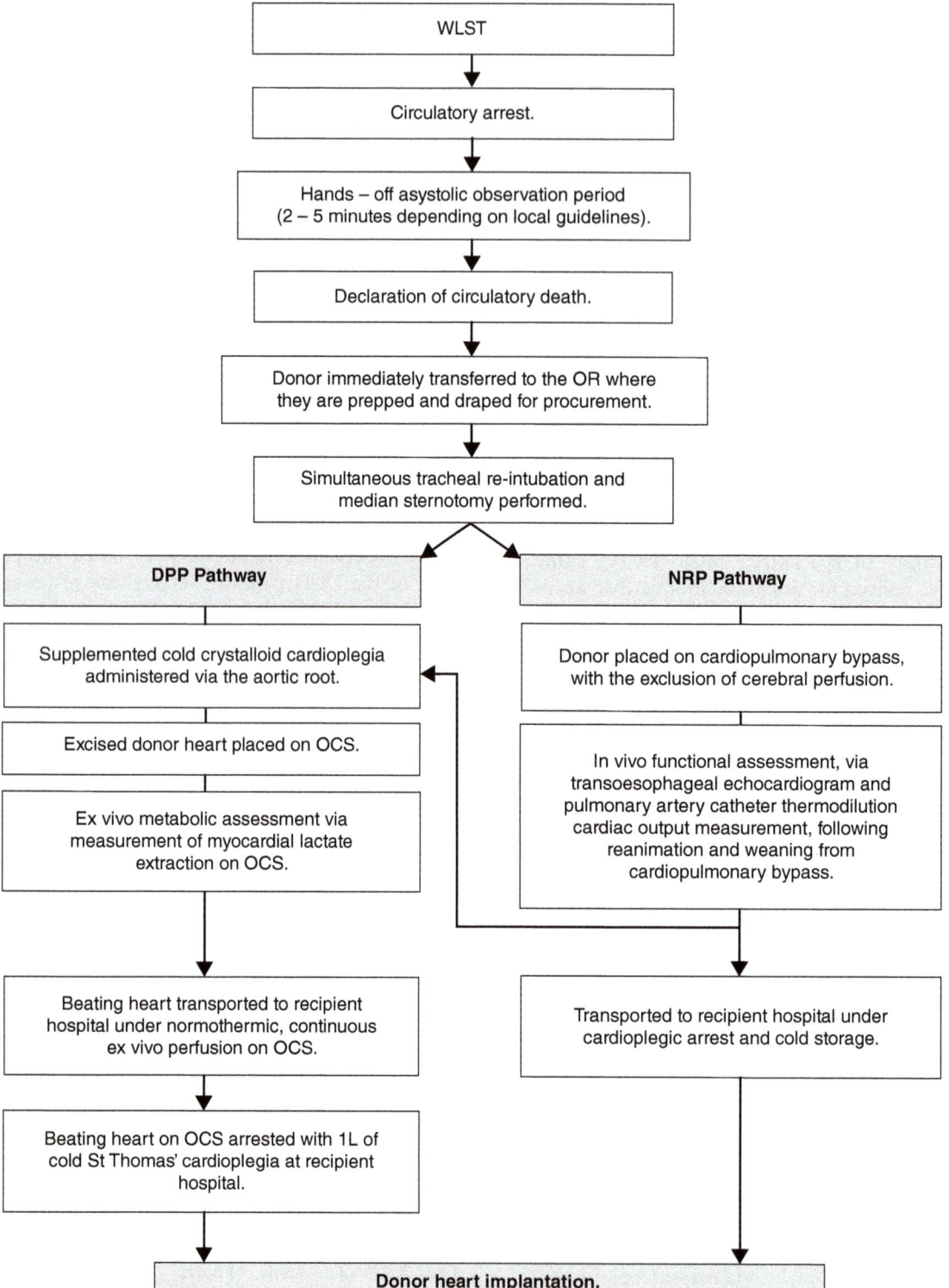

Figure 13.3 Donation after circulatory death organ procurement pathway for heart transplantation.

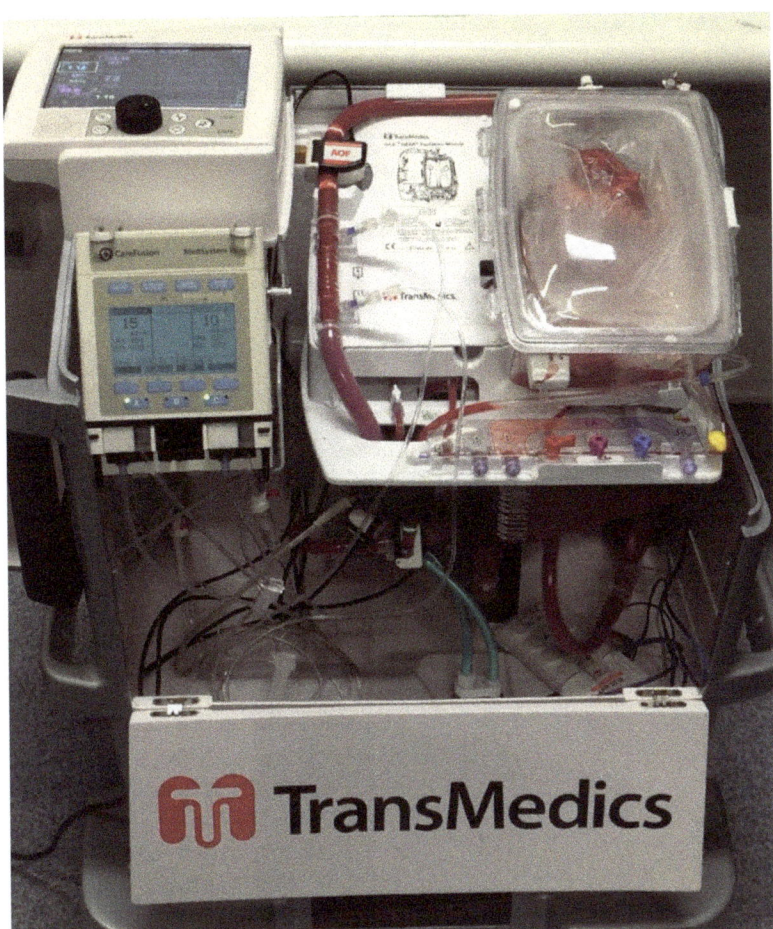

Figure 13.4 TransMedics Organ Care System with heart in situ on rig.

have been flushed with cold Perfadex solution, sit inside a sterile dome, connected to a mechanical ventilator and a perfusion circuit, which are incorporated into the device. The perfusion circuit priming solution is two liters of acellular, manufacturer-supplied Steen solution, supplemented with heparin, methylprednisolone and imipenem antibacterial agent. During operation, perfusate, oxygenated by the mechanically ventilated lungs, drains from a left atrial pulmonary vein cuff cannula into a hard-shell reservoir. The perfusate is then pumped via a centrifugal pump from the reservoir through a gas exchange membrane, which is supplied with a specialized sweep gas, containing 6% oxygen, 8% carbon dioxide and 86% nitrogen, so that deoxygenation of the perfusate occurs due to the low oxygen concentration. The gas exchange membrane also contains a heat exchanger to enable temperature control of the perfusate. From the gas exchange membrane, the deoxygenated perfusate

subsequently passes through a leukocyte depleting filter to the pulmonary artery return cannula for reoxygenation in the donor lungs. Lungs usually remain on the EVLP system for 4–6 hours, with hourly recruitment maneuvers and partial exchange of the perfusate solution to ensure provision of adequate metabolites. If the lungs are deemed viable for transplantation following functional assessment, they are cooled, flushed with cold Perfadex solution and are kept under cold storage until implant.

To date EVLP is yielding promising results. A recent multicenter US study (the NOVEL trial) comparing transplants utilizing organs that met standard procurement criteria, with those utilizing marginal donor lungs that underwent pre-transplantation EVLP, found comparable early survival.

A portable lung Transmedics OCS was introduced relatively recently; clinical reviews have commenced but are still in their infancy.

Mark Buckland and Jessica Underwood

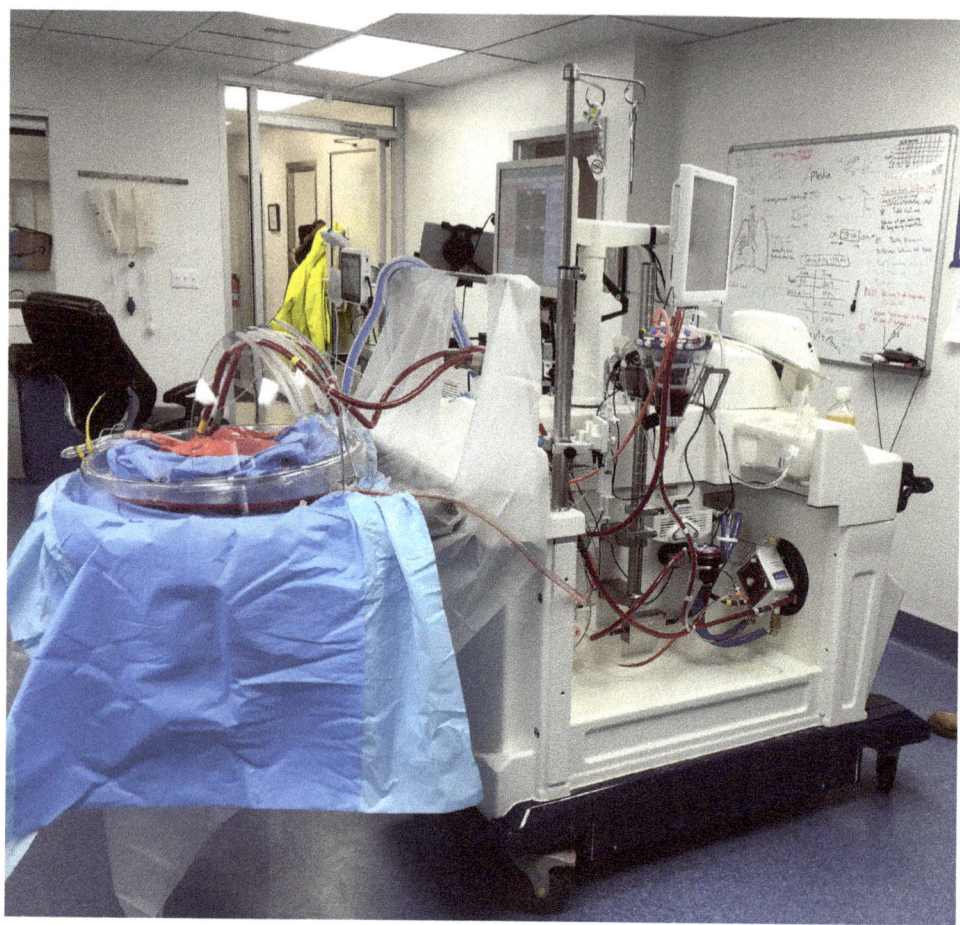

Figure 13.5 XVIVO lung perfusion system.

Circulatory Support during Organ Implant

Heart and Heart-Lung Transplantation

That standard cardiopulmonary bypass needs to be used for both heart and en bloc heart-lung transplants is obvious. The variations of the standard central bi-caval and aortic cannulation will be dependent on the indications for transplant, whether there have been any previous surgeries including ventricular assist device (VAD) insertion (see also Chapter 14) and whether the recipient is on ECMO at the time of transplant. These may include putting a "Y" in the venous line to allow for SVC cannulation, as well as femoral venous and arterial cannulation. Peripheral cannulation may occur with or without commencement of bypass prior to sternotomy or awake commencement of bypass prior to induction of anesthesia, particularly in patients with severe

pulmonary arterial hypertension (PAH) undergoing heart-lung transplantation. During initiation of awake bypass, the surgical team is scrubbed, patient prepped and draped, peripheral cannulae inserted with local anesthetic, and bypass slowly commenced. Following induction of anesthesia, the venous cannula position is optimized using transesophageal echocardiographic guidance, to optimize flows.

The subsequent surgery and bypass management follow the principles discussed in the rest of this book.

Lung Transplantation

Single or bilateral lung transplantation can be performed using sequential one lung ventilation (OLV) or with extracorporeal circulatory support. Practice varies widely across the world with some high volume units utilizing MCS in only 20% of cases, others for almost all. There seems to be a consensus among transplant centers that the sickest patients should be put on MCS electively. These include:

- all cases of primary PAH,
- other types of pulmonary hypertension when the pulmonary artery pressures approach or exceed systemic blood pressure,
- severely compromised right ventricular function,
- if there is need to correct a coexistent cardiac problem (such as valve or coronary lesions) and
- when the patient is on preexisting MCS.

Both CPB and VA ECMO are used; both are able to replace or support the functions of the heart and lungs. The primary difference between the two is the absence of a venous reservoir and the inability to suction spilled blood from the operative area in ECMO systems and the potential to run at much lower levels of anticoagulation, particularly if heparin bonded circuit components are used in ECMO (see also Table 13.2).

Two meta-analyses using almost the same pool of papers came to the conclusions that there may be some advantage in using ECMO compared with CPB, but there was no significant difference in long-term outcomes and that further randomized trials were needed.

Liver Transplantation

MCS may be utilized during liver transplantation, either as a standby hemodynamic rescue option or electively employed to provide hepatoportal circulatory decompression and hemodynamic stability. MCS largely achieves these goals by ensuring adequate systemic venous return, which may be compromised secondary to surgically-induced IVC obstruction. Assisted return of blood distal to the hepatic vessels enables maintenance of right atrial filling pressures, allowing the heart and lungs to provide adequate cardiorespiratory function.

Classic liver transplantation involved complete cross clamping and replacement of the retrohepatic IVC, thus the use of MCS was far more common. In modern "piggy-back" hepatic transplant, the retrohepatic IVC is preserved and only partially cross clamped, reducing the need for MCS.

Today, in most high volume units, MCS is reserved for patients with a high Model of End-stage Liver Disease (MELD) score, as this is where it may have the greatest benefits in reducing adverse renal, respiratory and hemodynamic outcomes.

Cannulation is usually percutaneous via a short femoral venous cannula, with or without direct cannulation of the portal vein in cases of persistent portal hypertension, with return via the percutaneously cannulated internal jugular or axillary vein. Although a simple centrifugal pump could be utilized, most units use a complete ECMO style MCS circuit with integrated heat exchanger and oxygenator. This has the advantages of

- allowing maintenance of body temperature,
- potential to assist oxygenation and
- "tip to tip" heparin bonding of all circuit components, avoiding heparinization in what historically has been a notoriously "bloody" procedure.

Emergent or Bail-out Applications of MCS

Perioperative

Cardiac teams have cause to heed and invoke the late Norman Shumway's second law – "the pump is your friend" – to take advantage of the hemodynamic stability and optimized gas exchange that CPB can provide when intraoperative problems occur. In all of the operations discussed above, case reports and series exist where MCS was not used initially but was employed to bail out of a deteriorating situation. As Table 13.2 shows, CPB requires full anticoagulation; VA ECMO on the other hand enables the same level of hemodynamic and gas exchange support with little or no anticoagulation, at least in the short term. One of the best demonstrations is VA ECMO support in case of massive endobronchial hemorrhage after pulmonary endarterectomy for chronic thromboembolic pulmonary hypertension. Short-term VA ECMO after weaning from CPB and heparin reversal enables effective resolution of this feared complication with 87% long-term survival.

Outside the Operating Room

Cardiogenic shock is probably the biggest indication for using MCS outside the operating room, with acute myocardial infarction by far the commonest cause. Other common indications include acute myocarditis and acute decompensation of chronic heart failure. MCS in the form of VA ECMO can provide complete support, enabling stabilization of the clinical situation and a bridge to decision making.

133

Three indications for emergent MCS warrant special mention:

- ECPR – describes the use of extracorporeal technology in patients who suffered a cardiac arrest and who are proving refractory to standard advanced cardiac life support (ACLS) measures. The CHEER trial from 2015 demonstrated feasibility and reasonable outcomes in patients who suffered >30 minutes refractory cardiac arrest, in or out of hospital, that were managed by a combination of mechanical CPR and VA ECMO. Twenty-four of 26 eligible patients were established on ECMO within a median time of 56 minutes from collapse. Survival to hospital discharge with good neurological recovery occurred in 14/26 (54%) of patients. Factors associated with poor outcome included age >65, unwitnessed arrest, asystole, terminal illness, known preexisting severe neurological injury, no flow, i.e. no effective extracorporeal circulation (ECC) > 10 minutes, and lactate > 18 mmol/l on ECC initiation. Other case series using a similar approach have achieved much more modest outcomes, fanning the discussion who should be offered this costly and resource-intensive therapy.

- Accidental hypothermic cardiac arrest (HCA) – the cardiovascular effects of hypothermia are well known to anyone involved in management of cardiac surgery and CPB. As the core temperature falls below 30°C cardiac activity and rhythm are affected, at <28°C ventricular fibrillation is common, vasoconstrictive failure and then asystole occur at around 20°C. Accidental hypothermia – i.e. core temperature <35°C – is thought to cause approximately 1500 deaths per annum in North America alone. It is normally associated with colder climates involving snow and icy bodies of water, but can also occur in more moderate climates, where exposure, intoxication and other cofactors play a role. A clinical staging guide – the Swiss Staging System – is used in the field to plan and prioritize management (see Table 13.3). In patients with HT IV (hypothermic cardiac arrest) and no overt signs of life, the dilemma is differentiating between actual death and potential viability.

The results of several clinical series have led to the notion that "no one is dead until warm and dead" and thus most victims are rescued with basic and advanced cardiac life support treatment

Table 13.3. Staging guide of accidental hypothermia

Stages	Clinical findings	Core temperature (°C)
Hypothermia I [mild] HTI	Conscious, shivering	35–32°C
Hypothermia II [moderate] HTII	Impaired consciousness, may or may not be shivering	<32–28°C
Hypothermia III [severe] HTIII	Unconscious, vital signs present	<28°C
Hypothermia IV [severe] HT IV	Apparent death, vital signs absent	Variable

before initiation of MCS at the earliest opportunity. This most commonly involves VA ECMO via femoral arterial and venous cannulation, providing immediate restoration of circulation and gas exchange as well as enabling rapid rewarming. Most groups recommended increasing flows gradually with the initial circuit temperature about the same as that of the patient. Rewarming should occur at a rate of between 1–4°C per hour to a target temperature > 32°C and continue until a stable cardiac rhythm with adequate perfusion and gas exchange is established and supported with modern post cardiac arrest management. Withdrawal of MCS should be considered if there is no return of spontaneous circulation (ROSC) at 32–35°C.

Most management guides, such as ICAR MEDCOM or the Bernese Hypothermia Algorithm (see Figure 13.6), endorse this approach unless there are obvious signs of irreversible death.

A recent individual patient data meta-analysis of over 650 MCS treated cases of HCA showed a mean overall survival rate of 46%, with 40.3% having good neurological outcomes. This compares very favorably with a survival rate of 10–37% in non MCS treated HCA victims. Attempts to develop a more reliable outcome prediction scoring system led to the HOPE score (Hypothermia Outcome Prediction after ECLS) based on gender, asphyxia related mechanism of arrest, age, potassium level, duration of CPR and temperature. The score has subsequently been

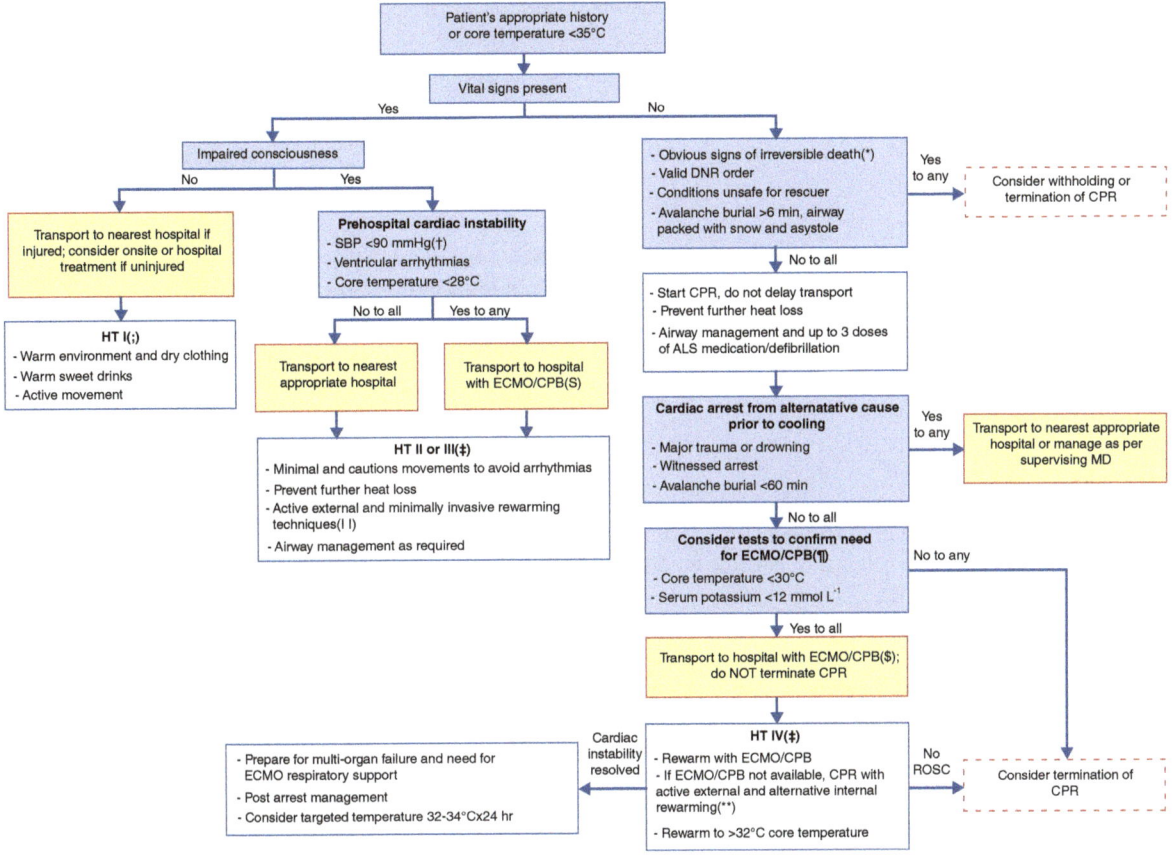

Figure 13.6 Management in Accidental Hypothermia. (*) Decapitation; truncal transection; whole body decomposed or whole body frozen solid (chest wall not compressible). (†) SBP <90 mmHg is a reasonable prehospital estimate of cardiac instability but for in-hospital decisions, the minimum sufficient circulation for a deeply hypothermic patient (e.g. <28°C) has not been defined. (‡) Swiss staging of accidental hypothermia. In remote areas, transport decisions should balance the risk of increased transport time with the potential benefit of treatment in an ECLS center. (‖) Warm environment, chemical, electrical, or forced air heating packs or blankets, and warm IV fluids (38–42°C). In case of cardiac instability refractory to medical management, consider rewarming with ECLS. If the decision is made to stop at an intermediate hospital to measure serum potassium, a hospital en route toward the ECLS center should be chosen. CPR denotes cardiopulmonary resuscitation, DNR do-not-resuscitate, ECLS extracorporeal life support, HT hypothermia, MD medical doctor, ROSC return of spontaneous circulation, SBP systolic blood pressure.

validated as a predictive tool and may be helpful in the triage of whether or not to use MCS rewarming in the HCA patient and is available online (www.hypothermiascore.org).

- ECLS in trauma patients – The use of VA ECMO to provide circulatory support to patients with acute traumatic cardiac arrest or cardiogenic shock presenting to hospital has been reported in several case series, but survival rates of 14–20% have been unimpressive.

Outside of the above circumstances there is evidence that MCS for respiratory or circulatory failure developing in trauma patients, during or after stabilization in hospital, is an effective option. A number of retrospective reviews,

including a national trauma database, a systematic review of published series of MCS in trauma victims and a review of trauma patients in the ELSO registry, showed an overall survival to discharge of between 50 and 79%.

A review of ECMO support in traumatic injury from five ECMO centers in the United Kingdom identified 52 patients with an overall mortality of 15%. Forty of the patients had surgical procedures prior to ECMO. The authors found an overall incidence of bleeding complications of 50% but no difference in incidence between those receiving and not receiving anticoagulation, and only four patients requiring return to the OR. They concluded that ECMO does not appear to worsen traumatic injury despite use of anticoagulation.

Table 13.4. Methods of combining continuous renal replacement therapy with extracorporeal life support

Combination CRRT & ECLS	Type	Advantages	Disadvantages/risks
Integrated approach	In-line haemofilter	Easy setup Low cost	Less precise ultrafiltration & limited solute clearance Flow turbulence and risk of hemolysis
	Integration of CRRT device in ECMO circuit	Both ultrafiltration and solute clearance Mode of solute clearance not restricted Control of ultrafiltration No need for separate vascular access or anticoagulation	Potential exposure of CRRT device to excessive pressure Risk of air entrapment Turbulent flow and hemolysis Shunt within ECLS circuit Thrombosis risk on extra circuit connectors
	Connection of CRRT device to oxygenator	Control of ultrafiltration Pressure in safe range of CRRT device	Potential of interfering with oxygenator
Parallel systems	Separate CRRT and ECLS circuits	Provision of solute and ultrafiltration clearance Mode of solute clearance not restricted Precise control over fluid removal A degree of "independence" from ECLS in terms of coagulation management and circuit changes	Need for separate vascular access Two extracorporeal circuits to be managed Higher extracorporeal blood volume

Organ Support during ECLS

Patients receiving ECLS are still at risk of running into problems with other organ systems. This can be due to the primary disease process, or because of exposure to ECLS and its circuit. The most vulnerable organs, with greatest impact of their failure, are the kidneys. The incidence of acute kidney injury (AKI) can be as high as 85% in patients on ECLS, is most often multifactorial in nature and has significant effect on fluid management and outcome. Renal replacement therapy (RRT) should be considered even though it represents a significant increase in the complexity of care. In most circumstances, this is done continuously (CRRT).

Broadly speaking there are two ways to do this; a parallel system with separate CRRT and ECLS circuits or an integrated approach with either a hemofilter in-line or a CRRT device "plumbed" into the ECMO circuit. Each of these approaches have a number of advantages/disadvantages as described in Table 13.4 and, while a detailed discussion is beyond the scope of this chapter, a number of points need be made.

A parallel system requires separate cannulation and managing two extracorporeal circuits. The integrated approach with in-line hemofilter, while easier and less expensive, offers less precise filtration and an increased risk of hemolysis. The CRRT device can be "plumbed" into the ECLS circuit in a number of places each with pros and cons. These devices offer the most flexibility in control of the filtration process but are characteristically "low pressure" systems and need modification to be incorporated in the relatively increased pressures of an ECLS circuit. A number of approaches used include incorporating some type of "reduction" device on the inflow or simply adjusting the pressure alarm limits in suitable CRRT systems. It is worth noting that any integrated CRRT system will lead to a shunt within the ECLS circuit but this is usually less than 5%. Some centers routinely have the CRRT drainage and return between the pump and oxygenator of the circuit with pressure alarms on the CRRT system adjusted appropriately; other centers vary, with perhaps the major determinant being local expertise of staff and availability of the various systems.

Suggested Further Reading

1. Surman TL, Worthington MG, Nadal JM. Cardiopulmonary bypass in non-cardiac surgery. *Heart Lung Circ* 2019; 28: 959–969.

2. Slinger P, Karsli C. Management of the patient with a large anterior mediastinal mass: recurring myths. *Curr Opin Anaesthesiol* 2007; 20: 1–3.

3. Arif R, Eichorn F, Kallenbach K et al. Resection of thoracic malignancies infiltrating cardiac structures with use of cardiopulmonary bypass. *J Cardiothor Surg* 2015; 10: 87–94.

4. Hsu C, Kwan G, Van Driel M et al. Distal aortic perfusion during thoracoabdominal aneurysm repair for prevention of paraplegia. *Cochrane Database Syst Rev* 2012; 3: CD008197.

5. Matalanis G, Ch'ng S. Thoracoabdominal aortic aneurysm – The branch first technique. *Semin Thorac Cardiovasc Surg* 2020; 31.4: 627–872.

6. Page A, Messer S. Large SR heart transplantation from donation after circulatory determined death. *Ann Cardiothorac Surg.* 2018;7(1): 75–81.

7. Van Raemdonck D, Keshavjee S, Levvey B et al. Donation after circulatory death in lung transplantation – Five-year follow-up from ISHLT registry. *J Heart Lung Transplant* 2019; 38: 1235–1245.

8. Kiziltug H, Falter F. Circulatory support during lung transplantation. *Curr Opin Anaesthesiol* 2020; 33: 37–42.

9. Czigany Z, Scherer M, Pratschke J et al. Technical aspects of orthotopic liver transplantation – A survey-based study within the Eurotransplant, Swisstransplant, Scandiatransplant and British transplantation society networks. *J Gastrointest Surg* 2019; 23: 529–537.

10. Stub D, Bernard S, Pellegrino V et al. Refractory cardiac arrest treated with mechanical CPR, hypothermia, ECMO and early reperfusion (the CHEER trial). *Resuscitation* 86; 2015: 88–94.

11. Paal P, Gordon L, Strapazzon G et al. International Commission for Mountain Emergency medicine (ICAR MEDCOM): accidental hypothermia – an update. *Scan J of Trauma Resus Emerg Med* 2016; 24: 111.

12. Kruitt N, Prusak M, Miller M et al. Assessment of safety and bleeding risk in the use of extracorporeal membrane oxygenation for multitrauma patients: a multicenter review. *J Trauma Acute Care Surg* 2019; 86: 967–973.

13. Ostermann M, Connor M, Kashani K. Continuous renal replacement therapy during extracorporeal membrane oxygenation: why, when and how? *Curr Opin Crit Care* 2018, 24: 493–503.

Mechanical Circulatory Support

Jason M Ali, Ayyaz Ali and Yasir Abu-Omar

Over the last decade there has been a significant increase in the utilization of mechanical circulatory support (MCS) devices. Traditionally, MCS was reserved as a "bridge to transplantation" primarily for patients with end-stage heart failure who were deemed candidates for transplantation. Nowadays, advanced MCS devices are commonplace in the cardiothoracic intensive care. The indications for their use have broadened to include the prophylactic use in high-risk percutaneous coronary interventions or surgery, as an adjunct to cardiopulmonary resuscitation (ECPR, see also Chapter 13) and as part of the routine management of intractable cardiogenic shock.

There are several forms of MCS that are typically classified as either temporary or durable and will be discussed in this chapter. Temporary MCS devices (Table 14.1) include the intra-aortic balloon pump (IABP), the Impella (Abiomed), the TandemHeart system (CardiacAssist), veno-arterial extracorporeal membrane oxygenation (VA-ECMO) and temporary ventricular assist devices (VAD). These devices are typically used in the context of acute, intractable cardiogenic shock from a range of etiologies including myocardial infarction, post-cardiotomy failure, myocarditis and acute deterioration in patients with end-stage cardiac failure. Durable MCS devices are the implantable left and right VADs. These devices are most commonly used as either a bridge to transplantation/candidacy or as destination therapy, in patients with end-stage cardiac failure.

Intra-aortic Balloon Pump

The IABP is the commonest form of mechanical support utilized in cardiac practice. Its first use was in the 1960s following the work of Kantrowitz who identified that "diastolic augmentation" could be utilized to improve myocardial oxygenation and thus ventricular performance (Table 14.2). The IABP comprises a drive console with a pump and a double-lumen balloon catheter that is typically introduced percutaneously into the femoral artery. The tip of the balloon is ideally positioned just distal to the left subclavian artery to reduce the risk of occluding the cerebral arteries proximally and abdominal visceral arteries distally (see Figure 14.1). One lumen is used for pressure monitoring, helium is delivered into and removed from the balloon through the other one. Helium is used due to its low viscosity (permitting rapid transfer) and high blood solubility (reducing the impact of gas embolism should the balloon rupture). If there is no contraindication patients should receive therapeutic anticoagulation to reduce the risk of thromboembolic events. Distal limb perfusion must be examined regularly, and distal pulses checked either by palpation or with a handheld Doppler probe. The leg should be checked regularly for the development of compartment syndrome.

The hemodynamic effects of the IABP (see Table 14.3) depend upon the counterpulsation that results from balloon inflation and deflation at precise points in the cardiac cycle which are controlled by the drive console, using either pressure or electrocardiogram triggers. Figure 14.2 shows how the balloon inflation is timed to occur immediately after aortic valve closure resulting in augmentation of the diastolic pressure ("diastolic augmentation"). This results in increased coronary artery perfusion and therefore improved myocardial oxygen delivery. Balloon deflation is timed to occur immediately prior to the opening of the aortic valve, creating a vacuum effect leading to reduced afterload which leads to reduced myocardial stroke work and oxygen demand. The reduced afterload can additionally increase cardiac output, although this increase is believed to be small (0.5–1 liter/minute at most), and of course is dependent upon the ventricular function.

Table 14.1. Comparison of temporary mechanical circulatory support devices

	Intra-aortic balloon pump	Impella	TandemHeart	Veno-arterial ECMO	Central ventricular assist device
Pump mechanism	Pneumatic	Axial	Axial	Centrifugal	Centrifugal
Insertion technique	Descending aorta via femoral artery	Into left ventricle retrogradely via femoral artery and through aortic valve	Cannula into left atrium. Inserted through femoral vein with trans-septal puncture	Peripheral (e.g. femoral artery and vein cannulation) or central (right atrial and ascending aorta cannulation)	Central cannulation (left atrial and ascending aorta)
Risk of limb ischemia	+	++	++	+++ (if peripheral)	-
Anticoagulation	+	++	++	+++	+++
Hemolysis	+	++	++	++	++
Hemodynamic support					
– **Cardiac output increase**	0.5–1 L/min	2.5 or 5.5 L/min	4 L/min	>4.5 L/min	>4.5 L/min
– **Afterload**	Reduced	Unchanged	Increased	Increased	Increased
– **LV preload**	Slightly reduced	Slightly reduced	Reduced	Reduced	Reduced
– **LV stroke volume**	Slight increase	Reduced	Reduced	Reduced	Reduced
– **Coronary perfusion**	Slight increase	Unknown	Unknown	Unknown	Unknown
– **Systemic perfusion**	Little change	Improved	Improved	Improved	Improved

Management of the Patient with IABP

The frequency and magnitude of balloon augmentation can be controlled via the balloon pump console. The inflation ratio refers to the number of balloon inflations to the number of QRS complexes and can be set at 1:1, 1:2 or 1:3. The magnitude of augmentation can range from 10% to 100%. During normal use, maximal IABP support is provided with a 1:1 inflation ratio at 100% augmentation. The timing of the inflation/deflation triggers should be checked regularly and adjusted when required to optimize the support provided. Current consoles have an "auto-pilot" mode which uses an algorithm to automatically select the best ECG lead and trigger source to optimize the inflation and deflation timing.

The effectiveness of IABP augmentation is diminished when there is excessive tachycardia (>120 bpm) or when the cardiac rhythm is irregular e.g. atrial fibrillation. If the cardiac index is maintained above 2.2 l/min/m^2 with acceptable preload (pulmonary capillary wedge pressure <15 mmHg), attempts can be made to wean the IABP. Firstly, augmentation is reduced to 50% for 2–4 hours. The inflation ratio is then reduced from 1:1 to 1:2 for another 2–4 hours and then to 1:3 before the balloon catheter is removed. The IABP must be switched off and the catheter completely deflated just prior to removal. Heparin infusion should be discontinued at the start of the weaning process so that coagulation is normalized by the time the catheter is ready for removal.

Complications of IABP Use

The incidence of complications in patients with an IABP is 7%, with major complications occurring in 2.6%. IABP-related mortality is estimated to be 0.5%. The commonest complications are vascular and include limb ischemia and vascular trauma (dissection or laceration) leading to false aneurysm, hematoma or hemorrhage. Incorrectly sized IABP catheters can lead to compromised abdominal visceral perfusion. Non-vascular complications include cerebrovascular accident, thrombocytopenia from platelet deposition on the balloon and mechanical disruption, hemolysis, infection and complications of immobility in cases of prolonged therapy due to the requirement to be bedbound. Balloon rupture is a rare but serious complication that can result in gas embolism.

Table 14.2. Indications for intra-aortic balloon pump

Ischemic myocardium	o Unstable angina despite maximal medical therapy
	o Ischemia-induced ventricular arrhythmia
	o Elective support in high-risk percutaneous coronary interventions
Structural complications of acute myocardial infarction	o Ventricular septal defect
	o Acute mitral valve regurgitation
Cardiogenic shock	o Post myocardial infarction
	o Acute myocarditis
	o Acute deterioration of chronic heart failure
	o Post-cardiotomy
	o Primary graft failure of the donor heart following heart transplant

Extracorporeal Membrane Oxygenation (ECMO)

ECMO is an advanced form of temporary life support that can be utilized to aid respiratory and/or cardiac function. It evolved from CPB technology and has been in use since the 1970s. When support of respiratory function alone is required, the oxygenated blood is returned to the venous circulation (veno-venous ECMO or VV-ECMO), relying on intrinsic cardiac function. When circulatory support is required in addition to gas exchange, the oxygenated blood is reinfused into the systemic arterial circulation (veno-arterial ECMO or VA-ECMO).

Circuit Design

Many circuit configurations can be constructed for VA-ECMO. The common components include a venous cannula which drains deoxygenated blood through heparin-bonded tubing to a membrane oxygenator and then via a non-pulsatile centrifugal pump to an arterial cannula. Cannulation for VA-ECMO can be peripheral, typically with femoral venous drainage and femoral arterial return (see Figure 14.3); or central with right atrial venous drainage and ascending aorta return (see Figure 14.4). The

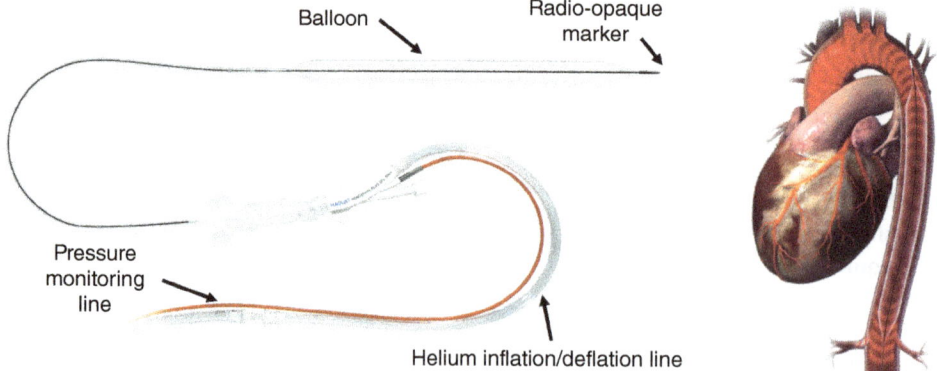

Figure 14.1 Intra-aortic balloon pump catheter and optimal position in the aorta. (Reprinted with the permission of Maquet.)

Table 14.3. Physiological effects of the intra-aortic balloon pump

Balloon deflation during ventricular systole	o Reduces left ventricular afterload
	o Reduces peak LV wall stress and LV stroke work
	o Decreases myocardial oxygen demand
	o Reduces mitral valve regurgitation
	o Increases LV ejection fraction
Balloon inflation during ventricular diastole	o Increases coronary perfusion pressure
	o Augments coronary blood flow
	o Improves myocardial oxygen delivery
	o Improves end-organ perfusion e.g. kidneys, liver, etc.
Overall effects	o Augments cardiac output
	o Reduces pulmonary capillary wedge pressure
	o Relieves pulmonary congestion and tendency for edema

patient must be therapeutically anticoagulated to minimize the risk of thrombosis/thromboembolism.

Indications

The use of VA-ECMO and other advanced mechanical circulatory support devices is generally indicated in patients with refractory cardiogenic shock despite maximal inotropic support and use of an IABP. The goal is to prevent development of end-organ injury, facilitating myocardial recovery or evaluation of further therapeutic decisions (see also Chapter 13). The common indications are summarized in Table 14.4.

Contraindications

Commencing VA-ECMO is a major decision and ideally it should be made with multidisciplinary involvement of cardiologists, cardiothoracic surgeons and specialist anesthesiologists or intensivists. VA-ECMO should only be used in patients in whom there is anticipated early recovery or when it is being used as a bridge to more definitive management, for example transplantation or long-term VAD support ("bridge to decision"). Therefore, ECMO is contraindicated in patients with non-recoverable cardiac failure who are not candidates for transplantation or VAD implantation due to other significant

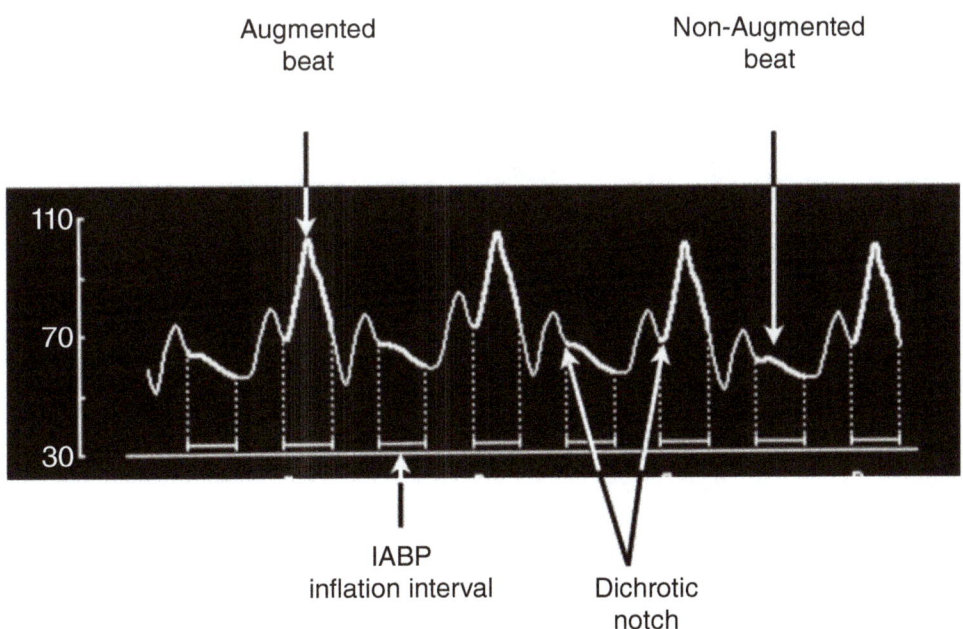

Augmented beat

Non-Augmented beat

IABP inflation interval

Dichrotic notch

Figure 14.2 Aortic pressure trace with IABP inflation set to 1:2. The IABP inflation interval has been highlighted to show balloon inflation at the dichrotic notch and deflation just before cardiac systole. (Reproduced from *Core Topics in Cardiothoracic Critical Care.*)

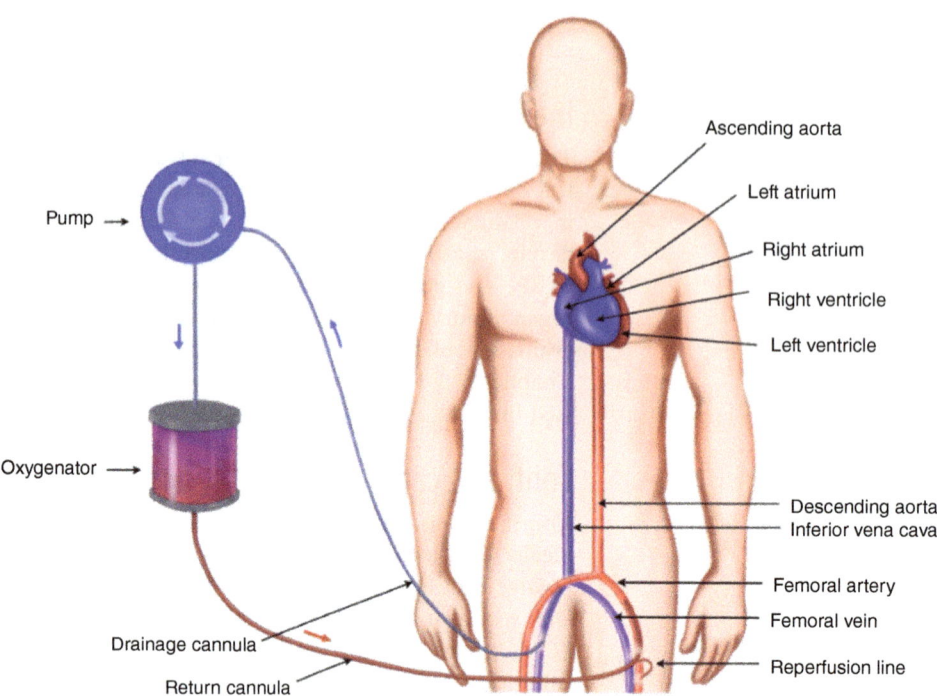

Figure 14.3 Peripheral ECMO. The blood is drained from a large vein, typically IVC, using femoral access. It is then pumped through an oxygenator and returned to the patient into the femoral artery in a retrograde fashion. Reperfusion line from inflow cannula is inserted into the distal femoral artery to provide distal limb perfusion. (Reproduced from Core Topics in Cardiothoracic Critical Care.)

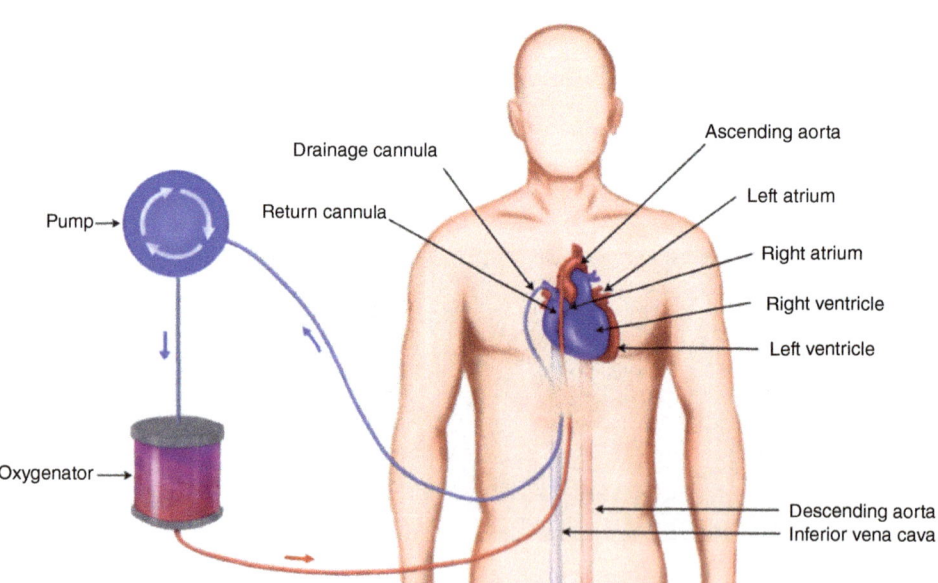

Figure 14.4 Central ECMO diagram: Using open chest the blood is drained via a cannula from a central vein (IVC or SVC) or right atrium. It is pumped through an oxygenator and returned through an arterial cannula into the ascending aorta. The chest can be left open for a short while, or the cannulae can be tunneled under the skin and chest closed. (Reproduced from Core Topics in Cardiothoracic Critical Care.)

Table 14.4. Indications for cardiac VA-ECMO

Acute myocardial infarction with cardiogenic shock/ arrest

Fulminant myocarditis

Acute exacerbations of chronic heart failure

Cardiac failure due to intractable arrhythmias

Post-cardiotomy cardiac failure

Primary graft failure following cardiac transplantation

Acute heart failure secondary to drug toxicity

Post cardiac arrest (as part of Advanced Life Support)

Table 14.5. Complication rates of cardiac VA-ECMO

Complication	Incidence (%)
Acute kidney injury	55.6
Renal replacement therapy	46.0
Re-thoracotomy for bleeding or tamponade in post-cardiotomy patients	41.9
Major or significant bleeding	40.8
Significant infection	30.4
Lower extremity ischemia	16.9
Neurological complications	13.9
Fasciotomy or compartment syndrome	10.3
Stroke	5.9
Lower extremity amputation	4.7

comorbidities. Relative contraindications to VA-ECMO include the presence of severe aortic regurgitation, aortic dissection, contraindications to therapeutic anticoagulation (such as active bleeding, a hemorrhagic intracranial event), pre-existing multi-organ failure and patients who have been mechanically ventilated for >10–14 days.

Complications

ECMO comes with significant associated morbidity. The major complications are thrombotic and hemorrhagic in nature and highlight the difficult balancing act between ensuring adequate anticoagulation and causing excess bleeding on the one hand and unwanted thrombotic risk on the other. Patients on ECMO mostly have very restricted mobility, similar to those with IABP and are likely to suffer similar complications. Tunneling lines through the chest wall, allowing formal chest closure, gives patients on central VA-ECMO the benefit of increased mobility, reducing the number of thromboembolic complications and minimizing deconditioning while on support.

The Harlequin syndrome describes a differential cyanosis associated with peripheral VA-ECMO. Oxygenated blood is pumped retrograde through the descending aorta into the ascending aorta to perfuse the coronary arteries and cerebral vessels; native ventilation can often be inadequate and the blood exiting the left ventricle will be relatively deoxygenated. If there is native left ventricular output there will be a "mixing zone" where ejected native, poorly oxygenated anterograde and highly oxygenated retrograde blood meet. Any vascular bed proximal to the mixing zone receives blood with poor oxygen content from the native cardiac output, leading to local hypoxemia mainly in the coronary and cerebral circulation. Monitoring of cerebral saturations and right radial artery blood gases can be indicative of this differential cyanosis.

A recent meta-analysis has summarized the complications of VA-ECMO (see Table 14.5).

Clinical Outcomes

Survival of patients supported with VA-ECMO is dependent on a range of factors including the underlying diagnosis and the presence of end-organ injury prior to commencement. The Extracorporeal Life Support Organization (ELSO) registry reports that 62% of adult patients treated for all indications with VA-ECMO survive extracorporeal life support, with 45% surviving to hospital discharge or transfer.

Managing Patients on VA-ECMO

Patients supported with VA-ECMO will be managed in an intensive care unit by multidisciplinary specialists. ECMO support should be titrated to clinical targets, which may include:

- arterial oxygen saturations >90%
- venous oxygen saturations >70%
- adequate tissue perfusion – as judged by end-organ function (urinary output, gut function, cerebral function) and lactate levels.

Pumping blood into the arterial system during VA-ECMO alters loading conditions and can worsen LV function. It is imperative that any remaining native cardiac stroke volume is assessed and maintained to avoid complications of left ventricular stasis and distension, pulmonary hypertension or intracardiac thrombus formation. Echocardiography is a useful tool to inform on the cardiac volume status, to guide concomitant inotrope and IABP use and to inform about recovery of cardiac function. Persistent ventricular distension and pulmonary hypertension will need to be managed with LV venting via the left ventricular apex, or trans-septally via the atrium.

Anticoagulation must be monitored to prevent circuit thrombosis and embolism, which could be fatal. For patients receiving unfractionated heparin an activated clotting time (ACT) of 180–210 seconds or an APR (normalized aPTT) of 1.8–2.2 are recommended.

Mechanical ventilation is usually conducted with lung protection in mind. Reduction in the ventilator support is often accompanied by increased venous return and cardiac output. When cardiac recovery occurs and increasing amounts of blood are ejected from the right ventricle, increased ventilation may be necessary to prevent deoxygenated blood from reaching the left atrium.

Weaning VA-ECMO

It is important to develop an individualized weaning strategy for each patient. VA-ECMO support will only be possible for 1–2 weeks and can therefore ever only be a temporary measure to support the recovery of heart function or a bridge to another treatment. Some patients cannot be weaned off support and may be candidates for urgent cardiac transplantation or, if no donor organ becomes available in a timely enough manner, a planned VAD implant.

Once adequate recovery is thought to have occurred, an attempt to wean off ECMO can be made. This is usually accomplished by daily incremental reduction in flow by approximately 0.5 L, until the ECMO support is only 1.5–2.0 l/min. During this time, careful assessment of end-organ function is vital. Most patients will require additional inotropic support. Final decannulation usually occurs in the operating room as formal vessel repair for peripheral cannulation, and chest closure for central cannulation will be necessary.

Ventricular Assist Devices

A number of different devices are available. They differ by the intended duration of support (temporary versus long-term) and by the method of implantation (percutaneous, central and implantable).

Indications for VAD

VADs have a broad range of applications, the common indications include:

Bridge to Recovery: In some cases of post-cardiotomy shock and fulminant myocarditis, VAD therapy can provide a period of circulatory support until cardiac function recovers after which the VAD can be weaned and removed, a process known as *"bridge to recovery."*

Bridge to Transplant: Occasionally, a VAD is utilized for patients with deteriorating cardiac function or end-organ function while waiting for a heart transplant. Here the VAD is used to buy time for the patient until a suitable donor heart can be found, a process called *"bridge to transplant"* or BTT.

Bridge to Candidacy: This third indication involves patients who would otherwise be transplant candidates except for one or more serious, but potentially reversible, complications of advanced heart failure, such as pulmonary hypertension or renal dysfunction. Unless reversed, such complication(s) prevent transplantation and these patients will invariably die from their heart failure. Pulmonary vascular resistance elevated due to left ventricular failure and pulmonary venous congestion often revert to normal levels with mechanical unloading of the left ventricle; renal or hepatic dysfunction due to chronic low cardiac output can often be reversed with improved systemic perfusion. An implantable VAD can often achieve both over time.

Destination Therapy: An implantable VAD can be offered as permanent support for selected patients with advanced heart failure who are not transplant candidates and are unlikely ever to become candidates. The boundary between "bridge to candidacy" and "destination therapy" is often blurred.

The VAD Decision-Making Process

The key decisions include:
- which patient to support with a VAD
- when to insert a VAD

- whether the patient requires a left ventricular VAD (LVAD) alone or biventricular VAD devices (BiVAD)
- which VAD system to use.

These are often difficult to make and are influenced by a number of factors including the acuity of onset, the severity of heart failure, patient comorbidities, expected transplant waiting times, device and resource availability and institutional experience.

Up until a few years ago, patients with heart failure were mostly stratified according to the New York Heart Association (NYHA) classification. Although this provides an assessment of patients' functional status, Class IV heart failure symptoms include a very broad spectrum ranging from those who are stable on oral therapy to those who may be pre-terminal on maximal inotropic support. As the treatment strategy varies with the severity of heart failure a further sub-classification of patients with advanced heart failure became necessary.

The Interagency Registry of Mechanically Assisted Circulatory Support (INTERMACS) was established as a mandatory registry for all patients receiving an implantable mechanical circulatory support device (MCSD) in the USA. Based on patient characteristics at the time of device implantation and outcome analysis, seven profiles have been defined to further stratify patients in advanced heart failure, with Profile 1 being the most severely ill. NHYA Class IV patients are now sub-divided into Profiles 1–6 while those in NYHA Class IIIb are described as Profile 7 (see Table 14.6).

Types of Ventricular Assist Devices

Technical developments in mechanical circulatory support have progressed rapidly over the last 20 years. There is now a large range of systems available for clinical use. These can be classified into temporary systems and long-term systems. The earliest *"first generation"* devices were based on a volume displacement mechanism and generated pulsatile blood flow. These devices were bulky in design, noisy in operation, often were extracorporeal and had limited durability. Most of the newer devices have moved to rotary blood pump technology with a single moving part. They can either be of an axial flow design or have a centrifugal configuration. Implantable LVADs with mechanical bearings are referred to as *"second generation,"* while those with magnetic levitation or hydrodynamic bearings are referred to as *"third*

Table 14.6. INTERMACS Level of limitation at time of implant

INTERMACS Profile	Description	Time Frame for Definitive Intervention
Profile 1	Critical cardiogenic shock	Emergency intervention within hours
Profile 2	Progressive decline	Urgent intervention within days
Profile 3	Stable but inotrope dependent	Elective intervention within days/weeks
Profile 4	Resting symptoms	Elective intervention within months
Profile 5	Exertion intolerant	Variable urgency, maintain nutrition and organ function
Profile 6	Exertion limited	Variable urgency, maintain nutrition and organ function
Profile 7	Advanced NYHA III	Transplant or MCSD may not be currently indicated

generation." Continuous flow devices are generally more compact, silent in operation and more durable. Dimensions and weight have decreased significantly, all modern devices are fully implantable and obviously require normal lung function.

Percutaneous Temporary Ventricular Assist Devices

TandemHeart – The TandemHeart system (CardiacAssist) is an extracorporeal axial flow pump. The TandemHeart works by contributing blood flow to the aorta, working in parallel – or "tandem" – to the LV. The venous inflow cannula is inserted percutaneously into the femoral vein, advanced into the right atrium and finally placed transeptally into the left atrium. It is connected to a centrifugal pump which provides up to 4 l/minute flow to an arterial outflow cannula in the femoral artery, effectively bypassing the LV. Offloading blood from the left atrium reduces LV preload, wall stress and therefore oxygen demand. This facilitates increased cardiac output and systemic perfusion pressures. A continuous infusion of heparinized saline flows

145

Table 14.7. Summary of complication rates of temporary percutaneous mechanical circulatory support devices

Complication	Impella (%)	TandemHeart (%)
Major bleeding	0.05–54	53–59
Access site bleeding	2–40	8–53
Hemolysis	10–46	5.3
Cerebrovascular accident	2.4–6.3	–
Limb ischemia	0.07–10	3.4–11
Vascular injury requiring surgery	1.3–2	0.85–13
Access site infection	1.1	16
Sepsis	0.16–19	29.9
Device migration	0.05–23	8
Device malfunction	0.16–17	–

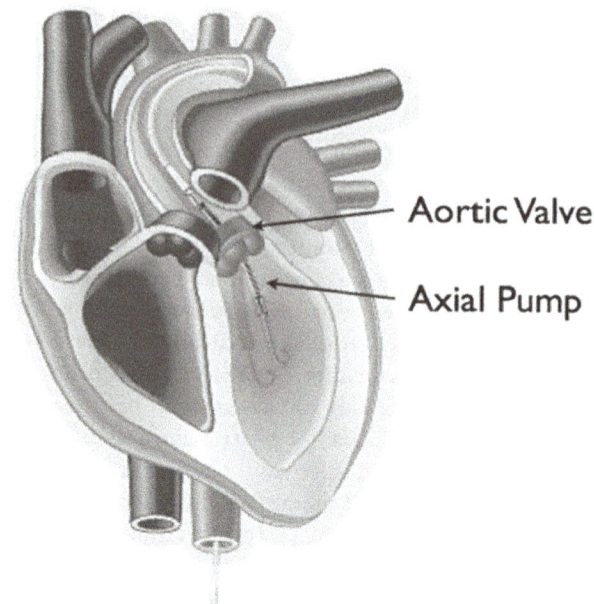

Aortic Valve

Axial Pump

Figure 14.5 Diagram showing an Impella device advanced retrogradely into the left ventricle via the aorta. (Reproduced from Core Topics in Cardiothoracic Critical Care.)

into the lower chamber of the pump, providing lubrication and cooling and prevents thrombus formation.

The most common indications include the treatment of acute myocardial infarction complicated by cardiogenic shock and to facilitate high-risk PCI. With increasing experience, the indications broadened to include acute decompensation of end-stage heart failure, post-cardiotomy cardiogenic shock, and to facilitate off-pump coronary bypass surgery in high-risk patients. The requirement for and the technical challenge of a trans-septal puncture has limited its widespread uptake.

Impaired right ventricular function and severe aortic regurgitation are specific contraindications to the use of the TandemHeart. Additionally, severe peripheral vascular disease may preclude percutaneous cannula placement. Patients must be anticoagulated to reduce the risk of thromboembolism. Complications associated with trans-septal puncture are an important limitation of this device. If the inflow catheter is dislodged into the right atrium, a large right to left shunt can develop (see Table 14.7).

Impella – The Impella (Abiomed) is a non-pulsatile axial flow Archimedes screw pump designed to propel blood into the ascending aorta in series with the LV (see Figure 14.5). The device is introduced to the left ventricle retrogradely through the femoral artery or through the axillary artery. Blood from the

LV is sucked into the inlet area near the tip of the device and is delivered into the aortic root through the outlet, thus offloading the left ventricle. The device comes in various sizes and can provide flow of up to 5 l/min.

The physiological effects, indications and contraindications are essentially the same as for the TandemHeart. The absence of the requirement for a trans-septal puncture has led to the Impella becoming the preferred device in many centers. The recently approved Impella RP has been designed to provide right ventricular support.

Similar to the TandemHeart, the Impella's ability to increase cardiac output is superior to that of the IABP. The main complications for both devices are summarized in Table 14.7.

Central Ventricular Assist Devices

For patients with refractory cardiogenic shock despite IABP therapy, an alternative to VA-ECMO is the use of a temporary central VAD. In general, it is preferable to cannulate the ventricle directly as VAD inflow because this configuration provides superior ventricular decompression, avoids ventricular stasis and affords higher flow rates. Biatrial cannulation is

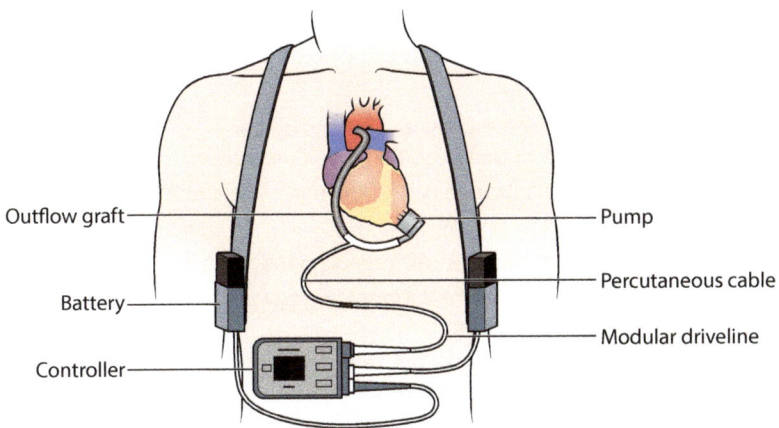

Outflow graft

Battery

Controller

Pump

Percutaneous cable

Modular driveline

preferred when recovery is expected and there is residual ventricular function.

The output of an LVAD is dependent on adequate right ventricular function. Likewise, an RVAD can only provide benefit if the native left ventricle can generate enough stroke work to cope with the pulmonary blood flow produced by the RVAD. If both native ventricles are failing, two VADs are required in order to provide biventricular assistance to support the circulation (BiVAD).

One commonly used system is the Levitronix CentriMag. The CentriMag is a continuous flow extracorporeal system comprising of a single-use polycarbonate centrifugal pump with a magnetically levitated impeller, a motor and a primary drive console, similar to VA-ECMO (see Figure 14.4). It is intended for short-term left, right or biventricular support of up to 30 days duration. The pump is designed to minimize friction and heat generation, and to reduce shear forces on blood cells thus preventing hemolysis. It achieves rotation without friction or wear at speeds of 1500–5500 rpm, providing flow rates of 5.0–6.0 l/minute.

The inflow and outflow cannulae can be rapidly inserted into the beating heart and great vessels with or without cardiopulmonary bypass. Other clinical equipment such as a membrane oxygenator or hemofilter can be spliced into the system. Although patients supported with the CentriMag are kept on the intensive care unit, they can be carefully mobilized and can undergo physiotherapy. Because of its simplicity and versatility, the CentriMag has become one of the most widely adopted temporary MCS device.

The most frequently implanted third generation LVADs include the HeartWare HVAD (Medtronic, Minneapolis, MN, USA) and the HeartMate 3 (Abbott, St Paul, MN, USA [see Figure 14.6]). The HeartWare is a centrifugal pump and the HeartMate 3 has a fully magnetically levitated, self-centering rotor. Both are designed for full intrapericardial implantation obviating the need for creation of a "pump pocket." Although implantation often involves a full sternotomy and cardiopulmonary bypass, minimally invasive and off-pump techniques have been successfully utilized.

These devices are used for LV support, bypassing and offloading it while allowing it to contract with significantly reduced work. The cannulation strategy can protect against LV distension which can occur with VA-ECMO if the LV is not vented. Offloading the LV will result in a reduction in the RV afterload and usually improves RV function.

RV failure has been reported in 5–44% in patients after LVAD implantation. It can be very difficult to predict preoperatively and may be severe enough to require additional, usually temporary, right ventricular mechanical support. RV failure can be precipitated by previously undetected or underestimated elevated pulmonary vascular resistance (PVR) and/or excessive LVAD flow rate. It is prudent to limit the LVAD flow rate in the first few days in order to avoid overwhelming the RV or shifting the ventricular septum to the left and distorting RV dynamics.

The indications for LVAD therapy are well-defined and are very similar to those for VA-ECMO. In some countries durable, implantable LVADs are increasingly being utilized as a destination therapy for selected patients and this is likely to become the commonest indication in the future. A total artificial heart can be used as an alternative to two implantable VADs in patients with severe biventricular failure in need of mechanical support and in some specialist centers as a bridge to transplantation in these cases.

VAD Patient Management

Patients requiring a VAD implant are probably among the highest risk patients to undergo cardiac surgery. They have severe heart failure and are either in impending or established end-organ failure. A low cardiac output state coupled with systemic venous congestion result in compromised organ perfusion. The kidneys become refractory to diuretic therapy and hepatic dysfunction manifests as coagulation abnormalities. The lungs are stiff from pulmonary congestion increasing the work of breathing and many patients are grossly fluid overloaded. They are often on multiple inotropes, supported with an IABP and dependent on renal replacement therapy by the time they arrive in the operating room for VAD placement.

Perioperative Management

The perioperative strategy should be aimed at minimizing further insult to these sick patients during VAD implant-ation, targeting those areas that are known to result in serious morbidities and mortality. Postoperative hemor-rhage is the most commonly encountered complication apart from right ventricular failure.

Broad-spectrum prophylactic antibiotics and anti-fungal agents are administered at induction of anes-thesia. Transesophageal echocardiography (TEE) is used to confirm an intracardiac thrombus, aortic valve competence and exclude the presence of a patent fora-men ovale or an atrial septal defect. If present, they require surgical closure at the time of VAD implant in order to prevent a right to left shunt following decom-pression of the left-sided chambers. If CPB is used, the lungs can be kept ventilated throughout the bypass period, often with the addition of nitric oxide at 5–10 parts per million (ppm) or inhaled epoprostenol to reduce PVR as much as possible. The VAD cannulae are implanted into a beating heart, avoiding aortic cross-clamping and cardiac ischemia. The pericardial space is flooded with carbon dioxide to displace air, allowing gas entrained into the cardiac chambers to dissolve more readily. The right ventricle is supported

Table 14.8. Perioperative LVAD patient management

Broad-spectrum prophylactic antibiotics and antifungal agents

Transesophageal echocardiography
- ○ Confirm aortic valve competence
- ○ Exclude patent foramen ovale and ASD
- ○ Confirm deairing
- ○ Check LVAD cannula position
- ○ Confirm decompression of LA and LV during LVAD support
- ○ Monitor right ventricular and tricuspid valve function when weaning from CPB
- ○ Assess the inter atrial septum and adjust flows to maintain central position

If using cardiopulmonary bypass:
- ○ Normothermic CPB
- ○ Continuous ventilation of the lungs with nitric oxide at 10 ppm
- ○ Filtration on CPB and maintain
  - ▪ Hb > 100 g/L
  - ▪ Base excess ± 2 mEq
- ○ No aortic cross-clamp during VAD cannulae implant
- ○ Pericardial CO_2

Appropriate inotropic support for right ventricle

Vasopressor infusion to maintain SVR

with inotropes as required and the heart rate is opti-mized with temporary pacing at 90–100 bpm; systemic vascular resistance is maintained between 800 and 1000 $dyne.sec.cm^{-5}$ with a continuous infusion of vasopressors. TEE is used to confirm good positioning of the ventricular outflow cannula and to guide deair-ing of the heart before transitioning from CPB (if used) to VAD.

The perioperative management strategy is sum-marized in Table 14.8.

Postoperative Management

Careful hemostasis at the end of the VAD implant is crucial. The percutaneous cannulae (in the case of temporary VAD) or driveline (with durable LVAD) must be secured to minimize movement and trauma to the exit site(s). This is the best way to encourage tissue healing onto the driveline and minimize exit site infections.

Once returned to the intensive care unit, VAD patients must be closely monitored for early complications. Right ventricular function often remains precarious in the first few days following LVAD implantation.

Anticoagulation is device and unit specific but is typically omitted in the first 24 hours and only introduced when the patient has stopped bleeding.

Rising right atrial pressure coupled with a fall in pump flow are signs of either tamponade or impending RV failure. Both can be confirmed with TEE. In the case of RV failure, it will demonstrate full right-sided cardiac chambers with empty left-sided chambers. The atrial and ventricular septa are seen to bulge toward the left and often there is tricuspid valve regurgitation. Immediate treatment consists of not increasing the preload further with more volume and a combination of inotropic support for the RV and pulmonary vasodilators. If the situation does not respond rapidly to these measures, early consideration should be given to the addition of a RVAD which can be achieved using a variety of percutaneous or surgical techniques.

Complications

The early complications of temporary and durable VADs are similar and include bleeding, RV failure, renal failure, infection or thrombosis. The incidence of complications has reduced significantly with increased experience and evolution of the devices, leading to the increased utilization of LVAD as a destination therapy. Ongoing device development aims to further reduce the incidence of associated complications.

Suggested Further Reading

1. Hajjar LA, Teboul J-L. Mechanical circulatory support devices for cardiogenic shock: state of the art. Critical care. *BioMed Central*; March 9, 2019;23(1):76–110.

2. Schramm R, Morshuis M, Schoenbrodt M et al. Current perspectives on mechanical circulatory support. *Eur J Cardiothorac Surg*. June 1, 2019;55(Supplement_1):i31–37.

3. Ali J, Vuylsteke A. Extracorporeal membrane oxygenation: indications, technique and contemporary outcomes. *Heart*. September, 2019;105 (18):1437–1443.

4. Cheng R, Hachamovitch R, Kittleson M et al. Complications of extracorporeal membrane oxygenation for treatment of cardiogenic shock and cardiac arrest: a meta-analysis of 1,866 adult patients. *Ann Thorac Surg*. 2013 ed. February, 2014;97 (2):610–616.

5. Glazier JJ, Kaki A. The Impella device: historical background, clinical applications and future directions. *Int J Angiol. Thieme Medical Publishers*; June, 2019;28 (2):118–123.

6. Thiele H, Jobs A, Ouweneel DM et al. Percutaneous short-term active mechanical support devices in cardiogenic shock: a systematic review and collaborative meta-analysis of randomized trials. *European heart journal*. December 14, 2017;38(47):3523–3531.

7. Subramaniam AV, Barsness GW, Vallabhajosyula S et al. Complications of temporary percutaneous mechanical circulatory support for cardiogenic shock: an appraisal of contemporary literature. *Cardiol Ther. Springer Healthcare*; December, 2019;8(2):211–228.

8. Borisenko O, Wylie G, Payne J et al. Thoratec CentriMag for temporary treatment of refractory cardiogenic shock or severe cardiopulmonary insufficiency: a systematic literature review and meta-analysis of observational studies. *ASAIO J*. September, 2014 ;60(5):487–497.

9. Nagpal AD, Singal RK, Arora RC et al. Temporary mechanical circulatory support in cardiac critical care: a state of the art review and algorithm for device selection. *Can J Cardiol*. January, 2017;33(1):110–118.

10. Kirklin JK, Pagani FD, Kormos RL et al. Eighth annual INTERMACS report: special focus on framing the impact of adverse events. *The Journal of Heart and Lung Transplantation : the official publication of the International Society for Heart Transplantation*. October, 2017;36(10):1080–1086.

Cardiopulmonary Bypass for Pediatric Cardiac Surgery

Joseph J Sistino and Timothy J Jones

The outcomes following surgery for congenital heart disease have improved significantly in recent decades. This has enabled a move from palliative surgical procedures to primary surgical repair in the neonatal period, operating on younger and smaller patients. With earlier repair and more successful outcomes, the majority of children are surviving into adulthood. These developments have in part been due to advances made in our understanding and techniques of cardiopulmonary bypass (CPB).

Cardiopulmonary bypass in patients with congenital heart disease has become increasingly specialized with the choice of circuit setup, priming, cannulation strategies and CPB conduct being tailored to the individual patient and procedure. Pediatric perfusionists must have specialized knowledge related to pediatric physiology and congenital heart disease as well as the ability to utilize perfusion circuits adapted to a wide range of patient sizes. Pediatric perfusion cases can sometimes be very long due to the complexity of the cardiac repairs. Today, there is a large percentage of reoperations and an increasing number of adult congenital operations. As these patients grow older, they need revisions to accommodate their increased cardiac outputs. As the mortality rates have fallen, focus is now on delivering optimal perfusion to reduce associated morbidity.

Over the past 40 years, the trend has been to perform more complex, corrective and fewer palliative procedures on younger and smaller patients. Today, more than 50% of pediatric open-heart operations are performed in infants less than one year of age with more than 20% of all pediatric heart procedures performed during the first month of life. More than 90% of children with congenital heart disease are surviving into adulthood and there are now more adults living with congenital heart disease than children.

Major Differences between the Pediatric and Adult Cardiac Patients

There are some major differences between these two groups of patients. From a physiological standpoint, the metabolic rate for an infant per kilogram of body weight is approximately double that of an adult. Therefore, greater oxygen delivery is required per unit of body weight or surface area. At birth, the pulmonary and systemic vascular resistance are the same and very labile, meaning they can be manipulated to readily increase or decrease pulmonary or systemic blood flow. Pulmonary vascular resistance decreases exponentially over the first few months of life.

In neonates with single ventricles, common arterial trunks or large septal defects a critical balance needs to be maintained between the systemic and pulmonary circulations. To ensure surgical visibility and protect the cerebral circulation, hypothermia is often used to permit reduced blood flow by decreasing oxygen requirements. The small patient size and blood volume make minimizing hemodilution a challenge. There is increased surface area contact due to the size of the perfusion circuit relative to the patient, which exacerbates the systemic inflammatory response to CPB.

Specific Pathophysiology That Affects Cardiopulmonary Bypass

There are several conditions that are more common in pediatric patients than adults and which need consideration during CPB. They include systemic to pulmonary shunts, which at the onset of bypass can produce flooding of the pulmonary circulation, while severely reducing systemic blood flow. Common examples of these shunts are a patent ductus arteriosus, a modified Blalock-Taussig shunt and central shunts. These shunts should be occluded at the onset of bypass to reduce pulmonary blood flow. Another source of systemic to pulmonary shunts are bronchial artery collaterals. Bronchial arteries normally carry about 2% of the cardiac output to supply the lung parenchyma with oxygenated blood. In certain conditions associated with severely reduced pulmonary blood flow, the collaterals expand to increase blood flow to the lungs in order to increase oxygenation. The net effect is reduced systemic blood flow on CPB unless the pump flow is increased to compensate. Another common problem is that of anomalous venous drainage. The most common type is a left superior vena cava (SVC) draining into the coronary sinus. This may require additional cannulation or venting of the coronary sinus and may alter plans for retrograde cardioplegia.

Many patients are cyanotic resulting in an increased red cell mass, significant collateral vessel formation and sensitivity to high oxygen levels, which can produce oxygen free radicals and reperfusion injury. At the onset of bypass of these patients, oxygen levels should be carefully maintained at a normal level to prevent exposure to hyperoxia, which is associated with poorer cardiac outcomes and increased severity of ischemia/reperfusion injury.

Myocardial Protection in the Immature Myocardium

Myocardial protection in the immature myocardium is very different than in the adult. Compared with the adult heart, there are fewer myocytes, fewer mature mitochondria and an increased water content. This is due to the increased number of capillaries which are needed for the heart to grow at a rapid rate over the next year. The primary source of energy for the neonatal heart is glucose, not fatty acids which become the primary fuel at around two years of age and into adulthood. The neonatal heart tolerates ischemia better because there are fewer contractile elements and mitochondria as well as decreased levels of ATPase. Studies have shown that the neonatal heart can tolerate ischemia for up to one hour with good recovery.

Another important consideration for the perfusionist, related to myocardial protection and recovery, is calcium control as there is less sarcoplasmic reticulum in the immature heart. The immature heart is therefore more dependent on circulating ionized calcium levels to maintain good contractility. However, increased ionized calcium levels during cardioplegic arrest can contribute to higher intracellular calcium levels and reperfusion injury. The perfusionist should maintain low normal ionized calcium levels during arrest and only increase ionized calcium levels following cross-clamp release to ensure optimal contractility.

The immature heart has limited contractile reserve, making the cardiac output more dependent on the heart rate rather than the stroke volume. The immature heart is also more susceptible to preload and afterload changes. There is also less independence of the ventricles, meaning that biventricular failure is more common than either isolated right or left ventricular failure. These factors all need to be considered when protecting the myocardium and when weaning a neonate from CPB.

There are several solutions currently being used for cardioplegia; the most popular are del Nido and HTK (also known as Bretschneider solution or Custodiol). Both solutions are depolarizing, del Nido uses potassium and lidocaine while HTK uses low-sodium. Both solutions have buffers and other components to protect the myocardium (see also Chapter 11).

Cardioplegia delivery can be affected by the coronary artery anatomy, aortic atresia or insufficiency, the presence of a left superior vena cava, or sinusoids in the right ventricle which produce a right ventricle-dependent coronary circulation (RVDCC). In all these situations, cardioplegia delivery must be modified to adequately protect the ventricles during cardioplegic arrest.

Deep Hypothermia Circulatory Arrest and Regional Cerebral Perfusion

With the availability of prostaglandin in the late 1970s, the ductus arteriosus could be maintained patent in neonates to increase their oxygen levels. This allowed for improved early survival in neonates with critical congenital heart disease. Since the early 1980s, deep hypothermia circulatory arrest (DHCA) was the primary technique used for correcting complex defects. Cooling the patient to between 18 and 20°C allowed for a period of circulatory arrest, during which cannulas could be removed to permit surgical visibility.

However, circulatory arrest was not without some long-term concerns including lower IQ, and behavioral and physical impairments. Since the early 2000s, regional cerebral perfusion has been used as an adjunct to deep hypothermia. Regional cerebral perfusion provides blood flow to the brain through the innominate artery which supplies blood to the left side of the brain through the circle of Willis and collateral vessels. Recent evidence demonstrates that an average of 35 minutes of DHCA with regional cerebral perfusion is well tolerated; there have been reports of DHCA times in excess of 120 minutes followed by good cardiac and neurological recovery. Monitoring of the cerebral circulation using cerebral oximetry has provided a real-time estimate of cerebral oxygen delivery. Both of these techniques, regional cerebral perfusion and cerebral oxygenation monitoring, are widely used in clinical practice and help improve outcomes.

Conduct of Cardiopulmonary Bypass

Cannulation

The aim of cannulation is to provide adequate blood flow with unobstructed venous drainage and an unobstructed operating field. This presents challenges in the pediatric patient. Both arterial and venous cannulas require careful selection based on maximum blood flow rate. The aim is to use the largest possible cannula, but this is often limited by the size of the vessels.

The site of arterial cannulation is determined by pathology and planned operation. Similar to adult surgery, the ascending aorta is the preferred site. However, access to the aortic arch in a neonate may be best achieved via cannulation of a small Gortex tube anastomosed to the innominate artery, which can also be used for regional cerebral perfusion. This technique may be used in patients with either an atretic aorta or interrupted aortic arch. Another strategy in such patients is cannulation through the pulmonary artery into the patent ductus arteriosus. Patients with an interrupted aortic arch may require cannulation in both the ascending and descending aorta.

Bicaval cannulation for venous drainage is the most frequently used technique in pediatrics because it allows access to the right atrium and right ventricle while providing complete venous return with little risk of air entrainment. A single venous cannula may be used when deep hypothermia circulatory arrest (DHCA) is going to be used to complete right-sided repairs or when surgery does not require opening the heart. During periods of DHCA the aortic cannula and/or venous cannula maybe moved to improve access and visibility to complete the repair.

In complex redo operations the femoral artery and vein may be cannulated in older children or the carotid artery and internal jugular vein in smaller children to enable safe sternal entry or if there is uncontrollable bleeding during re-sternotomy.

In patients with cyanosis or extensive collateral vessels or shunts that cannot be controlled, excessive venous return to the left atrium may cause left ventricular distension and myocardial damage. This can be managed by placing a vent in the left atrium, pulmonary vein or left ventricle.

Anticoagulation Management

Heparin is the primary anticoagulant used for CPB. Because of the larger pump prime volume in relation to the pediatric patient blood volume, it is important to maintain adequate circulating heparin levels by estimating circulating heparin level on CPB. For example, the 3 kg neonate will have a blood volume of approximately 85 ml/kg $\times$ 3 kg = 255 ml. A heparin loading dose of 400 units/kg = 1200 units. This will equal a concentration of 1200/255 = 4.7 units/kg. If the pump prime is 250 ml, then to maintain the same heparin concentration, 1175 units of heparin need to be added to the prime. The target ACT is similar to that in adult CPB, with equally big variation between centers.

Flow Rates and Oxygen Delivery

Oxygen delivery is dependent on three factors: blood flow rate, hemoglobin and pO_2. The blood flow rate is calculated based on the body surface area or weight and is usually 2.6 L per minute/meter square; blood flow rate based on kilogram weight ranges from 200 ml/kg/min for neonates to 125 ml/kg/min for larger pediatric patients. After much debate, the current consensus is to maintain hematocrit in excess of 24% during CPB in single ventricle patients; in those with a mixed circulation it is usually maintained at a level above 30% during the termination of bypass because of their low arterial oxygen saturation.

Monitoring

Monitoring during CPB includes arterial blood pressure, nasopharyngeal, esophageal and rectal temperatures, venous oxygen saturation and cerebral oximetry. Some centers also monitor central venous pressure. During CPB, continuous monitoring of the arterial blood flow with an ultrasonic flow meter is critical to maintain adequate blood flow to the patient when shunts are incorporated into the perfusion circuit. Before the termination of bypass, pressure lines are placed in the right and left atrium to evaluate right and left heart function during the weaning process and to assist with postoperative hemodynamic management.

Blood Gas Management

Blood gas management during bypass can either be one of two strategies, alpha stat or pH stat. Both strategies are explained in detail in Chapter 9.

Oxygen management is also critical in children with cyanosis. Because of their low pO2, they are susceptible to oxidative stress which releases oxygen free radicals when exposed to high pO2. In these patients it is important to start CPB at a low normal level of oxygen and then gradually increase over time on CPB.

Termination of CPB

As with adults, termination of CPB is a very critical time and follows similar principles to those discussed in Chapter 12. Monitoring of filling pressures is extremely important to avoid distension of the ventricles. Pediatric patients often have increased pulmonary vascular resistance and may require ventilation with nitrous oxide. During this period the anesthesiologist is carefully titrating inotropes to maximize the cardiac function. Good communication between the surgeon, perfusionist and anesthesiologist is critical during this time. Reversal of heparin with protamine is achieved in the same way as in adults.

Pathophysiology of Cardiopulmonary Bypass

The effects of CPB in pediatric patients were first identified by Kirklin's group in 1982 in his publication on whole body systemic inflammatory response.

Table 15.1. Blood volume estimation based on weight

Weight (kg)	Blood Volume (ml)
0–10 kg	85 ml/kg
10–25 kg	80 ml/kg
25–45 kg	70 ml/kg
≥45 kg	65 ml/kg

The inflammatory response is not dissimilar to that in adults but is exacerbated in infants due to the large surface area of the bypass circuit relative to the patients' size, cardiotomy suction and certain foreign materials which stimulate the immune system. The inflammatory response to CPB is discussed in detail in Chapter 17.

Hemodilution and Low Prime Circuits

As the pediatric patients presenting for surgery became younger and smaller, it became necessary to reduce the size of the perfusion circuit to reduce hemodilution and surface contact.

Patient blood volume is estimated according to Table 15.1. Even today, with perfusion circuits requiring prime volumes as low as 200 mL, this represents almost a 100% dilution of some patients' blood volume. This is in stark contrast to adult bypass circuits, where a standard prime volume of about 1000ml represents a 20–30% dilution, meaning that a neonate circuit needs to be thought of as equivalent to a 5 L pump prime volume in an adult patient. The severe hemodilution of clotting factors and platelets contributes to an increased risk of postoperative bleeding. In addition to reducing the size of the circuit as much as technically possible, it is often necessary to add blood to the prime to maintain adequate oxygen delivery and oncotic pressure. The use of fresh frozen plasma in the pump prime has advantages in preserving coagulation in neonates. Following protamine administration, platelet transfusion is often necessary to increase the platelet count. Some centers have whole blood available, which reduces the total number of donor blood exposures.

Neonatal oxygenators now have reduced priming volumes around 40 ml. With the use of 1/8" tubing, circuit prime volumes as low as 100 ml have been reported. However, there is some variation in the way

153

$$Required\ PRC = \frac{(Patient\ BV + CPB\ PV)\ x\ target\ Hct}{PRC\ Hct}$$

PRC = Packed Red Cells, BV = blood volume, PV = Prime volume, Hct = Hematocrit

Figure 15.1

that prime volume is measured. Calculation of the circuit priming volume should include venous reservoir volume at the minimum operating level and all primed tubing lines. Figure 15.1 shows the formula for calculating the packed red cell volume needed to maintain a target hematocrit.

It is essential that in the effort to reduce priming volume, no compromise is made in arterial line pressure and venous resistance. Institutional guidelines about choice of oxygenator and tubing, as well as cannula selection, should be carefully followed for each individual pediatric patient. Arterial and venous cannula pressure drop should not exceed 100 mmHg and 40 mmHg respectively at the maximum calculated blood flow rate for the individual patient.

Retrograde Autologous Prime

Retrograde autologous prime (RAP) is a method used to reduce the priming volume by displacing crystalloid solution with the patient's own blood immediately before going on bypass. Once heparinized and fully cannulated, blood from the patient is slowly withdrawn from both the arterial and venous lines into a collection bag. The anesthesiologist is responsible for giving the patient a vasoconstrictor to maintain the patient's blood pressure in a safe range (usually >80 mmHg systolic). Any major change in arterial pressure, EKG or arterial oxygen saturation is reason to discontinue RAP. Usually about 50% of the prime volume can be removed during RAP. This results in an increased hematocrit during bypass while reducing the need for blood products.

Conventional and Modified Ultrafiltration

Ultrafiltration is a method of hemoconcentration that is used both during and after CPB to increase hematocrit, plasma proteins including clotting factors and platelets. As the pump volume is diluted with cardioplegia solution, it is important to have a method to remove excess crystalloid fluid in order to maintain adequate hemoglobin levels. Ultrafiltration reduces the levels of inflammatory mediators IL-6 and IL-8, although the clinical utility is still subject to debate.

Zero balance ultrafiltration refers to replacing the filtered off fluid with an equal amount of crystalloid solution.

Modified ultrafiltration (MUF) is a method to filter the blood after CPB. MUF has changed over the years since the early 1990s when it was first introduced by Great Ormond Street Hospital in London. It is important that protamine administration is withheld until the end of MUF since blood is still circulating through the bypass circuit.

The original method was relatively simple. After coming off bypass, a circuit with a hemoconcentrator was connected to the arterial cannula. The tubing proximal to the hemoconcentrator was placed in a roller pump and the outlet tubing was connected to a venous cannula in the right atrium. Blood was slowly withdrawn retrograde from the aorta and pumped through the hemoconcentrator back into the right atrium. Numerous modifications of MUF circuitry and technology have been proposed since, all of which still involve using the existing cannulation and pose a risk of high negative pressure in the arterial line with the risk of cavitation or pulling air across the microporous membrane oxygenator.

Recently, there has been some suggestion that MUF is no longer necessary because the perfusion circuits have been reduced in size, requiring smaller priming volumes. Since it has the risk of air embolism, eliminating MUF avoids this potential complication.

There are major challenges to accomplishing successful cardiac surgery in pediatric patients. In part due to much improved extracorporeal technology, surgical outcomes have significantly improved over the years. Today, with the assistance of postoperative ECMO support, even more patients are surviving.

Suggested Further Reading

1. Harvey B, Shann KG, Fitzgerald D et al. (2012). International pediatric perfusion practice: 2011 survey results. *J Extra Corpor Technol*, 44(4), 186–193.

2. Sistino JJ, Bonilha HS. (2012). Improvements in survival and neurodevelopmental outcomes in surgical treatment of hypoplastic

left heart syndrome: a meta-analytic review. *J Extra Corpor Technol*, 44(4), 216–223.

3. Benziger CP, Stout K, Zaragoza-Macias, E et al. (2015). Projected growth of the adult congenital heart disease population in the United States to 2050: an integrative systems modeling approach. *Popul Health Metr*, 13, 29. doi:10.1186/s12963-015-0063-z

4. Kirklin/Barratt-Boyes Cardiac Surgery 4th edition, by Nicholas T. Kouchoukos, Eugene H. Blackstone, Frank L. Hanley, and James K. Kirklin Chapter 2: Hypothermia, Circulatory Arrest, and Cardiopulmonary Bypass.

5. Allen BS, Barth MJ, Ilbawi MN. (2001). Pediatric myocardial protection: an overview. *Semin Thorac Cardiovasc Surg*, 13(1), 56–72. doi:10.1053/stcs.2001.22738

6. Sistino JJ, Atz AM, Ellis C Jr. et al. (2015). Association between method of cerebral protection during neonatal aortic arch surgery and attention deficit/hyperactivity disorder. *Ann Thorac Surg*, 100(2), 663–670. doi:10.1016/j.athoracsur.2015.04.119

7. Wypij D, Jonas RA, Bellinger DC et al. (2008). The effect of hematocrit during hypothermic cardiopulmonary bypass in infant heart surgery: results from the combined Boston hematocrit trials. *J Thorac Cardiovasc Surg*, 135(2), 355–360. doi:10.1016/j.jtcvs.2007.03.067

8. McCall MM, Blackwel, MM, Smyre JT et al. (2004). Fresh frozen plasma in the pediatric pump prime: a prospective, randomized trial. *Ann Thorac Surg*, 77(3), 983–987; discussion 987. doi:10.1016/j.athoracsur.2003.09.030

9. Naik SK, Knight A, Elliott M. (1991). A prospective randomized study of a modified technique of ultrafiltration during pediatric open-heart surgery. *Circulation*, 84(5 Suppl), III422–431.

10. McRobb CM, Ing RJ, Lawson DS et al (2017). Retrospective analysis of eliminating modified ultrafiltration after pediatric cardiopulmonary bypass. *Perfusion*, 32(2), 97–109. doi:10.1177/0267659116669587

Coagulopathy and Hematological Disorders Associated with Cardiopulmonary Bypass

Bruce D Spiess and Erik Ortmann

Pathophysiology of Coagulopathy After Cardiopulmonary Bypass

CPB as well as surgical trauma have a significant impact on the usually well-balanced coagulation system. This often leads to bleeding complications, and interventions to restore this balance are frequently attempted perioperatively. The coagulation and inflammatory systems are so complex that restoration of homeostatic balance cannot be achieved by giving blood products alone.

Major known causes of CPB-associated coagulopathy are dilution, complex and variable platelet dysfunction, fibrinolysis, the effects of heparin and protamine, hypocalcemia, hypothermia, as well as activation of the coagulation system after contact with artificial surfaces and from tissue factor release from the endothelium in response to ischemia and reperfusion.

The priming volume of a standard adult CPB circuit leads to 20–30% hemodilution, while loss of activity for isolated clotting factors becomes clinically significant at 30–50% of normal activity. The importance of minimizing hemodilution can therefore not be overstated. Today, many centers make efforts to reduce hemodilution by using smaller CPB circuits and by retrograde autologous priming. Chapters 2, 7 and 8 discuss circuit design and other strategies to decrease priming volume.

Historically, artificial surfaces were considered the primary activators of coagulation. Today we know that ischemia reperfusion injury, endothelial release of thrombin and the presence of tissue factor may outweigh extrinsic activation:

- Endothelial cells at rest are highly anti-inflammatory and anti-thrombotic; when stressed, however, they become active exporters of thrombin.
- Arteriolar microemboli may lead to localized ischemia and reperfusion, which is a potent stimulus of thrombin formation. In these conditions endothelial cells rapidly shift from being anti-thrombotic to being prothrombotic.
- Cardiotomy suction blood carries cell debris and tissue factor directly into the circulating blood, causing thrombin and fibrin generation via the extrinsic pathway.

The platelet count decreases during CPB through hemodilution and mechanical destruction. A degree of platelet dysfunction is caused by hypothermia, but this is partially reversible with rewarming. They undergo reversible aggregation during CPB, show more and more changes in morphology with increasing length of bypass and degranulate partially.

Even high doses of heparin do not "paralyze" the hemostatic system. Thrombin generation is ever present during CPB and heparin combined with anti-thrombin merely blocks the formation of fibrin. Thrombin triggers fibrinolysis, which in turn can lead to the breakdown of clots; the resulting fibrin degradation products (particularly D-dimers) further impair fibrin polymerization.

Residual heparin can cause bleeding after cardiopulmonary bypass and needs to be reversed with protamine. Non-heparin-bound protamine has anticoagulant effects, and high protamine-heparin ratios should be avoided as much as incomplete reversal of heparin. Heparin rebound might occur by redistribution from tissue or cell surfaces even hours after initial reversal.

Role of Preoperative Medication in Coagulopathy

Cardiac patients are prescribed a wide range of medications for a variety of underlying conditions. Many of these drugs have effects on platelets, vascular reactivity, hepatic or renal function and may be linked to bleeding or thrombosis risk. Some commonly prescribed drugs, such as cephalosporin antibiotics, can have anti-platelet effects. What makes a patient bleed is likely to be a complex combination of drugs, effects of acute and chronic inflammation, oxidative stress, inflammation on CPB and the patient's own genetic makeup.

Genetic Factors

Genetic predilection for disease is complex as is the response to drugs. Examples are that:

- patients with angina are more hypercoagulable than the general population
- blood group O patients have more bleeding, transfusion and postoperative chest tube output than those with groups A, B or AB
- anti-platelet (P_2Y_{12}) agents and aspirin have a significant proportion of non-responders.

Anti-platelet Agents

- Glycoprotein IIb/IIIa inhibitors and monoclonal antibodies – the success of cardiology interventions has relied for years on acutely blocking the fibrinogen receptor on the platelet surface with short acting drugs, such as eptifibatide and tirofiban, or longer acting monoclonal antibodies, such as abciximab, and other IIb/IIIa inhibitors. Abciximab has a 10–30 minute redistribution half-life, but its terminal half-life and effects on platelets may last up to 15 days.
- Aspirin – functions by acetylating cyclooxygenase enzymes in platelets. Cyclooxygenase-1 (COX-1) is involved in the formation of thromboxane, a prostaglandin signaler for platelets to partially activate. Following even low dose aspirin administration, COX-1 is irreversibly inhibited within megakaryocytes and as such will "poison" growing platelets for their life span of 7–10 days. It takes 3–7 days after aspirin discontinuation to increase non-aspirin tainted platelets. Aspirin does not appear to lead to a higher incidence of bleeding complications after CAGB and the current recommendation is not to stop it prior to surgery.
- P_2Y_{12}-blockers – these drugs affect platelet activation via the ADP receptor and include the thienopyridines (clopidogrel, prasugrel and ticlopidine) and ticagrelor. Clopidogrel acts for the life of the platelet, i.e. 7–10 days. Ticagrelor

and its major metabolite are active. Although the half-life is 7–9 hours, restoration of platelet activity takes significantly longer.

There is very strong evidence that discontinuation of clopidogrel prior to elective cardiac surgery is not just preferable but is a must. A European Society of Cardiology meta-analysis, including 54 separate studies and over 50,000 patients, showed that preoperative dual anti-platelet therapy with clopidogrel and aspirin significantly increased major bleeding and transfusion as well as increasing the risk of re-exploration for bleeding 2.5-fold, while not conferring an advantage by decreasing the incidence of perioperative myocardial infarction when compared to patients whose clotting had been allowed to return to baseline. Another meta-analysis comprising of 30 studies showed that mortality increased 47% if dual anti-platelet therapy was continued to surgery. It is conjectured that much of the increased risk of death was due to bleeding and excessive use of allogeneic blood products.

The use of single, dual or even triple anti-platelet therapy creates a therapeutic dilemma in patients with recently fitted coronary stents. Dual anti-platelet therapy is recommended up to six months immediately after stent placement and for up to 12 months in patients who have had an acute coronary event. As seen above, it is recommended to stop dual therapy for 5–7 days prior to elective surgery. Unfortunately, there are reports of acute coronary events soon after stopping these drugs and there is some evidence that acute hypercoagulable state occurs after withdrawing the therapy. In cases where an operation becomes urgently necessary after a percutaneous intervention the anti-platelet effects can be overcome by transfusing platelet concentrates, so that the platelet number overwhelms any residual drug.

Table 16.1 summarizes the characteristics of commonly encountered anti-platelet drugs.

Vitamin K Antagonists

Vitamin K coagulation proteins are involved with the extrinsic cascade (Factor VII) and the final common pathway (II, IX and X). Carefully titrated and monitored, warfarin therapy provides a 30–50% reduction in the risk of pulmonary embolism and/or stroke in atrial fibrillation. However, it comes with a 3–5% risk of major bleeding per year.

Table 16.1. Summary of commonly encountered anti-platelet drugs

	Plasma half-life	Time to effect offset	Reversal agent available
Aspirin	15–30 minutes	7–10 days	no
Clopidogrel	8 hours	7–10 days	no
Prasugrel	7 hours	7–10 days	no
Ticagrelor	7 hours	5 days	yes (PB2452, in clinical stage trials)
Abciximab	10–15 minutes	12 hours	no
Eptifibatide	2.5 hours	2–4 hours	no
Tirofiban	2 hours	2.5 hours	no

The therapeutic window of warfarin is 2–3 times international normalized ratio (INR). Cardiac patients are at risk of sudden and rapid increases in INR without altering the dose. This is especially true for those:

- with right sided heart failure, tricuspid insufficiency and vena cava congestion where liver protein synthesis is reduced and
- with acute or chronic heart failure where gut absorption of vitamins as well as the microbiome are changed.

With INR levels above 1.2 associated with excess bleeding most practices agree there is no "safe" INR elevation for bleeding risk in the operating room. Accordingly, most surgical teams aim to correct the INR close to 1.0.

The most appropriate way to acutely reverse warfarin is to administer 4 factor prothrombin complex concentrate (4FPCC). The use of PCC has been found to be superior to fresh frozen plasma (FFP) in restoring a normal INR as well as maintaining it for 24–48 hours. Most institutions will co-administer Vitamin K to use this 24–48 hour window to support the hepatic synthesis of Vitamin K dependent coagulation factors. There is no clear guidance about the timing of intraoperative 4FPCC administration. Some teams opt to give a 50% dose after anesthetic induction and fully correct after CPB while others do not give any reversal until the patient has been weaned.

Novel Oral Anticoagulants

This group of new and evolving pharmaceutical agents block either factor Xa or factor II (thrombin). Novel oral anticoagulants (NOACs) or direct acting oral anticoagulants (DOACs) are utilized today for treatment of hypercoagulable states such as venous thromboembolism and for prevention of clot with atrial fibrillation. NOACs/DOACs have a similar effectiveness at reducing the incidence of VTE as warfarin but come with an enhanced safety profile. Most NOACs have a half-life of 7–14 hours, minimizing the risk of bleeding once patients have been off the drug for 24–48 hours. There does not seem to be a rebound hypercoagulability with NOACS.

The management of patients coming to the operating room without having stopped their NOAC or DOAC is controversial. These agents block the final common coagulation pathway and FFP seems the logical treatment. Unfortunately, FFP has, at best, the same level of proteins as normal plasma and a huge volume would be required to overcome the effects of these drugs. Several direct binding agents are approved for NOAC reversal in acute bleeding:

- Andexanet-α will within 30 minutes fully reverse the effects of Rivaroxaban and Apixaban and
- the monoclonal antibody idarucizumab can reverse the effect of dabigatran.

These two direct reversal agents are very expensive. 4FPCC appears to at least partially reverse NOACs and could present an alternative in cases where no specific reversal agent is available. It must be noted, though, that it does not have a specific indication for that use.

Assessment of Coagulopathy

Coagulopathy after cardiopulmonary bypass should ideally be treated in a goal-oriented manner. The ideal bleeding/coagulation assessment tool is currently elusive but should have the features summarized in Table 16.2. Timely test results are critical to effective treatment success as coagulopathy is a dynamic process, made worse by ongoing blood loss.

Standard laboratory tests (SLT), such as platelet count, fibrinogen levels, aPTT or PT, usually have a turnaround time of 30–90 minutes. In addition, SLTs

Table 16.2. The ideal coagulation test

Features	Areas of Assessment
Point-of-care test	Plasmatic coagulation
Fast results	Platelet function
Easy to use by non-laboratory staff	Fibrinogen activity
Unprocessed whole blood	Clot stabilization
Able to neutralize heparin effect	Fibrinolysis
Able to correct for hypothermia	Drug effects

are poor discriminators – an abnormal aPTT or ACT does not differentiate between factor deficiency and residual heparin effect. Having to wait for blood results for an hour after giving protamine often leads to initial blind, empiric treatment of any bleeding after CPB.

The alternative approach is to assess whole blood coagulation with viscoelastic tests (VET), such as thromboelastography/elastometry (e.g. ROTEM™, TEG™, ClotPro™) or resonance technology (e.g. TEG6s™, Quantra™). These point-of-care devices (POC) utilize whole blood samples with draw-to-result times of around 20 minutes. They offer assays sensitive and insensitive to heparin, which allow early testing while still on bypass and fully heparinized, as well as detection of residual heparin when testing after protamine. Results include clotting time (integrity of clotting factors), total clot firmness with fibrinogen and platelet contribution and fibrinolysis (lysis index). Figure 16.1 gives an overview of the information that can be gained from VET. Recent practice guidelines strongly recommend VET over SLT in the management of excess bleeding after cardiac surgery.

VET should be used in conjunction with an institutionally agreed algorithm for the treatment of post-CPB bleeding (see Figure 16.2). There is increasing evidence that the judicious use of VET and bleeding algorithms reduce transfusion requirements, particularly when clinicians accept that an abnormal test result by itself should not prompt treatment if there is no clinical evidence of coagulopathic bleeding.

Therapeutic Interventions and Management of Bleeding Patients

There are no simple answers and there is no magic bullet when it comes to treatment of bleeding in heart surgery. Blood coagulation is a cellular event taking place at a specific site of endothelial cell dysfunction, i.e. the site of surgical disruption of capillaries and small vessels.

Temperature: Besides using coagulation tests, temperature control is of utmost importance as blood does not coagulate below 30–32°C. It is not the central core temperature that matters but wound temperature. Measuring the temperature at a patient's sternal edge in a cold operating room can yield surprising results. This might explain why more often than not the bleeding markedly slows down once the chest is closed and the wound is no longer exposed to a 20°C environment.

Platelets: Platelet transfusions are obtained from pooled donors or from apheresis (single donor). They are the scarcest of blood products and in very high demand.

Platelets are the part of the coagulation system that is most affected by CPB and by inflammation. VETs are poor at picking up platelet dysfunction and the post-CPB platelet count currently provides the best guidance for transfusion. Institutional thresholds vary but generally are between 50.000 and 100.000/l.

Unfortunately, a large proportion of packed platelets are dysfunctional, dying or apoptotic and can act as prothrombotic microparticles. Platelet transfusions carry large concentrations of cytokines and can be a major risk for septic/bacterial transfusions with an incidence of approximately 1/2000 transfusions.

FFP and Cryoprecipitate: FFP contains all the protein coagulants found in circulating plasma at normal levels unless it has been processed at 1–6°C to produce cryoprecipitate. Cryoprecipitate is rich in Factor VIII, von Willebrand Factor and fibrinogen. At first glance it appears logical to use FFP to replenish proteins consumed by coagulopathy during bypass. When taking the dilution in the patient's circulation into account, at least 15 ml/kg body weight of FFP are necessary to achieve a meaningful rise toward normal levels of coagulation factors. Transfusing such a large amount of volume will lead to a significantly decreased platelet and red cell count, and further transfusion with associated risks and significant volume overload.

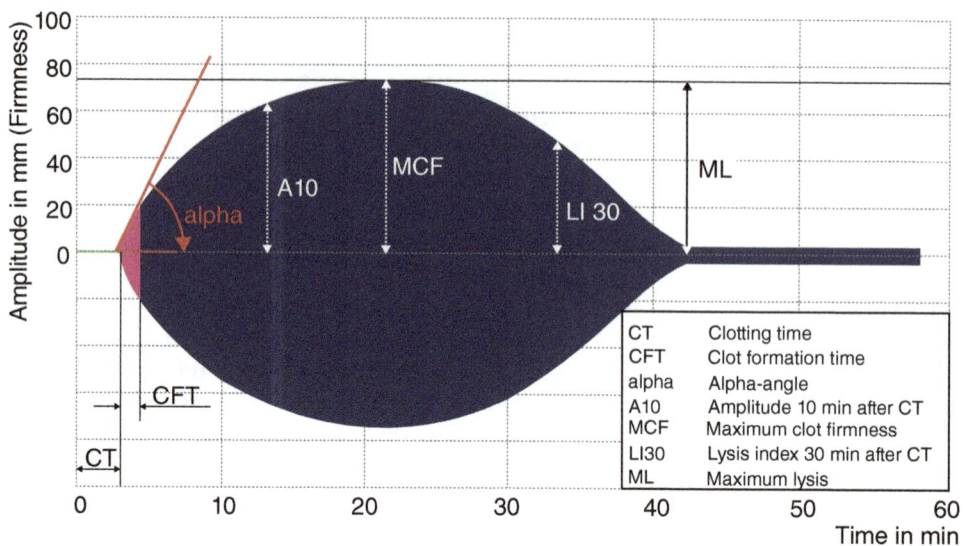

Figure 16.1 Picture of typical Temogram.

CT (s) – The CT parameter facilitates the decision to substitute clotting factors or to reverse anticoagulation.

CFT (s) – The CFT parameter facilitates the decision to substitute with platelets, fibrinogen or both. A shortened CFT is indicative for hypercoagulation (as well as increased MCF parameter)..

MCF (mm) – A low MCF indicates a low clot firmness. The MCF value is used to facilitate the decision for substitution therapy with platelets or fibrinogen. A high MCF value may indicate a hypercoagulable state.

A (x)-values represent the clot firmness. An A(x)-value is the amplitude after a certain time x after CT (e.g. A10 after 10 min)..

LOT (s) - The time span from CT to the start of significant lysis in s. Significant lysis is defined as a decrease of the amplitude of 15% as compared to MCF.

ML (%) – The parameter of maximum lysis (ML) describes the degree of fibrinolysis relative to maximum clot firmness (MCF) achieved during the measurement (% clot firmness lost). Image provided courtesy of Werfen.

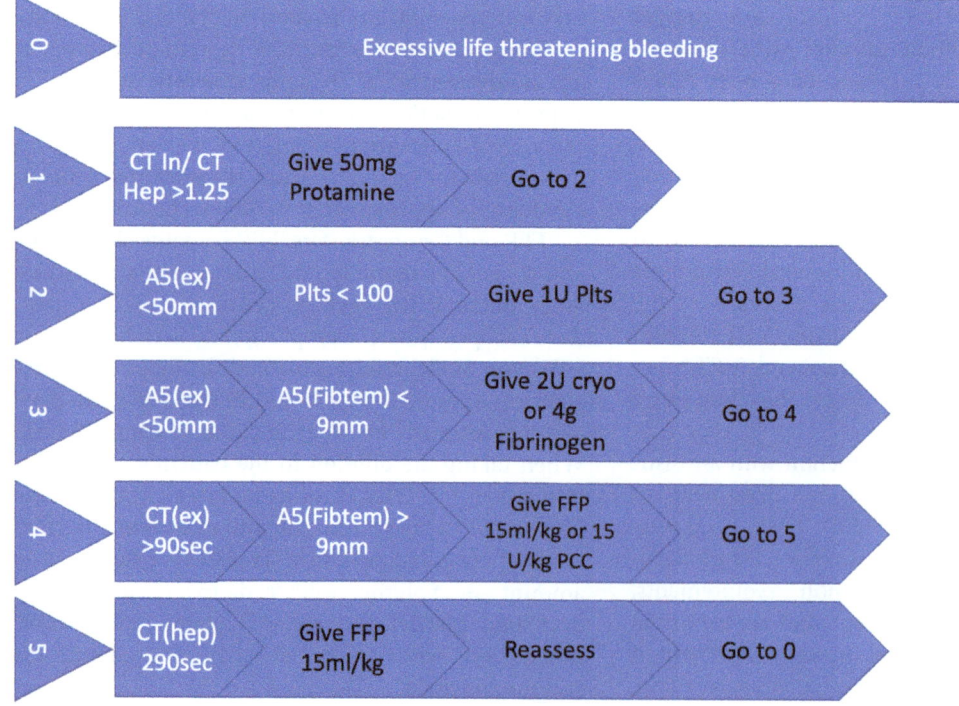

Figure 16.2 Typical ROTEM based algorithm for managing post-CPB bleeding with POC tests.

Unfortunately, the use of coagulation products from the blood bank is over-utilized in many clinical practices. Unguided transfusion does not decrease bleeding and increases adverse events, including length of hospital stay, pneumonia, renal failure and mortality. The data from combat casualty and major trauma, promoting 1:1:1 transfusion of red cell to FFP to platelet after a full blood volume loss, cannot be extrapolated to cardiac surgery and CPB coagulopathy.

Factor concentrates: Today both cryoprecipitate and FFP can be replaced with prothrombin complex concentrate (PCC) and fibrinogen concentrate.

Factor concentrates are available as single factors (Factor VIIa, VIII, IX and others) or as a combination of three or four factors. The latest iteration are the 4FPCCs, which do not just contain pro-coagulant factors but also Protein C, S, Anti-Thrombin III and a very small amount of heparin. Modern 4FPCCs contain the 25-fold concentration of pro-coagulant proteins compared to FFP.

PCC and fibrinogen concentrate figure prominently in difficult bleeding after CPB, particularly in algorithms based on viscoelastic testing. Concentrates, however, should not be given prophylactically. There are several reports of catastrophic thromboembolic complications following aggressive treatment of post-CPB bleeding with PCC, especially with older 3-Factor PCCs.

1-desamino-8-D-arginine-vasopressin (DDAVP): DDAVP is a synthetic analogue of vasopressin, which has no or little vascular contractility effect. DDAVP can enhance platelet function through the release of vWF and multimeric building blocks of vWF. The use of DDAVP after CPB in patients with renal failure and uremia has gained some attraction but data are scarce.

Practical management: Coagulation testing with VET within a structured algorithm is recommended as best practice (Figure 16.2). Assessment should start prior to coming off CPB using tests that neutralize heparin in vitro. They should be done with enough time to arrange for the necessary coagulation products to arrive in the operating room should coagulopathic bleeding develop following protamine administration.

In case of deranged VET results, coagulation factors should be substituted using 4FPCC. Keeping in mind the potential for thromboembolic events, starting with a low dose approach is recommended. Fibrinogen concentrate and platelets should be transfused in accordance with a bleeding algorithm. The effect of residual heparin should be excluded by comparing intrinsically activated coagulation times on VET with heparin insensitive assays and treated with additional protamine if necessary.

If coagulopathic bleeding persists after the "first round" of tests and products, the above cycle starting with viscoelastic testing should be repeated until safe transfer to the ICU is possible.

Blood Conservation Techniques

Anemia as well as red blood cell transfusion have both been linked to unfavorable outcomes after cardiac surgery. Perioperative blood and coagulation management needs to strike the right balance between avoiding low hemoglobin concentrations and avoiding unnecessary transfusion.

Antifibrinolytic Agents

Fibrinolysis is triggered by thrombin activation and physiologically occurs in parallel to clotting and leads to balanced hemostasis. This process is governed by physiological activators (tissue and urinary plasminogen activator) and inhibitors (plasminogen activator inhibitor-1 and -2 and alpha-2-antiplasmin).

Despite the presence of high dose heparin, thrombin and fibrin are constantly formed within the CPB circuit. Unsurprisingly, this is accompanied by activation of fibrinolysis, as demonstrated by elevated levels of tissue plasminogen activator during CPB, using up fibrinogen and potentially impairing clot formation after reversal of heparin. Blocking antifibrinolytic activity has been shown to reduce postoperative blood loss in cardiac surgical patients. The prophylactic administration of antifibrinolytic agents has become a standard practice and is recommended in current guidelines.

The synthetic lysine-analogues tranexamic acid (TXA) and epsilon-aminocaproic acid (EACA) are the most commonly used antifibrinolytics in cardiac surgery. They prevent the activation of plasminogen to plasmin by reversibly blocking its lysine-binding-site. There does not seem to be an increased risk of prothrombotic events with both substances but high doses of TXA have been linked to an increased incidence of seizures. Lower dose regimens, with either:

- a single bolus of up to 25 mg/kg or
- a bolus of up to 10 mg/kg followed by an infusion of typically 1 mg/kg/h for the duration of the operation

161

are currently recommended. Higher dose regimens have not shown further decreases in blood usage.

Until 2008 the non-specific serine protease inhibitor aprotinin was the antifibrinolytic of choice in cardiac surgery. It has been shown to significantly reduce blood loss in numerous studies. Following a series of controversial studies raising concerns of higher rates of renal and cardiovascular complications with aprotinin, it was withdrawn from the United States market. In recent years there has been a resurgence in interest in aprotinin. Its marketing license has been reinstated by Health Canada and by the European Medicines Agency and registry data re-evaluating its safety are eagerly awaited.

Avoiding Hemodilution

Surgical misadventure aside, one of the main threats to hemoglobin concentration is hemodilution. Excessive iv fluids and, more importantly, the CPB priming solution can cause significant dilution. Strategies such as optimizing the circuit, using minimal invasive extracorporeal circulation (MiECC), or retrograde autologous priming are discussed in Chapter 8.

Acute normovolemic hemodilution (ANH), where whole blood is removed into a blood storage bag before heparinizing and replacing it with the same amount of crystalloid or colloid fluid, has fallen out of favor in recent years. ANH has theoretical advantage that not only red cells but also coagulation factors and platelets are spared the exposure to bypass and are available to support coagulation at the end of surgery. While ANH has been shown to reduce the risk of bleeding and transfusion, it is most effective when larger volumes of up to 800 ml of blood are removed. Only a very limited number of patients will have a high enough Hb (>150 g/l) to tolerate ANH without the risk of significant hemodynamic instability.

Cardiotomy suction reduces the actual blood loss as shed blood is returned from the surgical field to the CPB reservoir. This blood is filtered to remove cell debris but remains potentially highly activated with inflammatory mediators and coagulation products, potentially accelerating the cycle of clotting and fibrinolysis.

Ultrafiltration during CPB helps to increase hematocrit, concentration of clotting factors and platelets indirectly by removing extracellular water from the blood. This requires the venous reservoir to be well filled to still be able to run bypass safely without triggering a level alarm. Patients most likely to benefit from ultrafiltration are those with decompensated heart failure or renal failure and volume overload. It can also be useful where high volume crystalloid cardioplegia techniques with Custodiol or Brettschneider are employed. Residual volume in the pump after separating the patient from bypass can be concentrated using an ultrafilter. Cell salvage systems ("cell saver") can be used to minimize the loss of red blood cells before, during and after CPB. These automated systems heparinize blood during collection into a reservoir, filter it and process it by centrifuging and washing it to produce a red cell concentrate. Fluid, plasma with clotting factors, platelets and the anticoagulant heparin are largely removed during the washing process. Cell saved blood helps to maintain a sufficient hematocrit, but additional replacement of coagulation factors and platelets is likely to be necessary to treat coagulopathy.

Special Conditions

Although the conditions discussed below are infrequently encountered in normal practice, they can create problems for clinicians who are unaware of them. It is worth having a working knowledge of them and developing locally agreed protocols on how to deal with them.

Jehovah's Witnesses

There are more than 7 million followers of the Jehovah's Witness (JW) faith worldwide. Since 1945 the majority of members of this community refuse allogeneic blood transfusion, even in life-threatening situations.

JW patients do not accept whole blood, red blood cell, platelet or plasma transfusion. Some other treatments are left to the individual's decision and may be accepted:

- derivatives of blood: albumin, coagulation factors, immunoglobulins, interferons, hemoglobin, cryoprecipitate
- recombinant factors: erythropoietin, rFVIIa
- procedures: cardiopulmonary bypass, cell salvage, normovolemic hemodilution, hemofiltration or dialysis, provided continuity with the patient's circulation is maintained at all times.

It is essential to have an informed discussion with the patient to determine their wishes, which are generally detailed in an advance directive document, prior to surgery and to meticulously document the consent process. The question whether the refusal of transfusion extends to life-threatening situations should be asked explicitly and the answer needs to be documented.

If Jehovah's Witnesses present for cardiac surgery their acceptance of extracorporeal circulation is usually tied to there being continuity at all times between the bypass circuit and the patient's own circulation. The same principle applies to cell salvage.

It is paramount to the successful management of JW patients to avoid situations of anemia and coagulopathy. All accepted measures of modern patient blood management should be part of a multidisciplinary institutional treatment protocol for JW patients undergoing cardiac surgery.

- Preoperative optimization – Treatment with (intravenous) iron and erythropoietin is essential to aim for a high-normal hemoglobin level of at least 140–150 g/dL. Cardiac catheterization should happen weeks before surgery, if possible, to avoid an inadvertent loss of Hb too close to surgery. All medication potentially impairing coagulation (platelet inhibitors, warfarin, DOAC, etc.) should be stopped early, and bridged where necessary.

- Tolerance of anemia – Oxygen delivery (DO_2) can be improved during CPB by maintaining normovolemia, increasing the cardiac output (i.e. pump flow), fully oxygenate the available hemoglobin and potentially utilize dissolved oxygen transport with high partial pressures of oxygen (0.3 ml O_2/100 mmHg). Oxygen consumption (VO_2) can be reduced by sufficiently deep anesthesia, including muscle relaxation, and hypothermia.

- Intraoperative management of cardiopulmonary bypass may include acute ANH, RAP, the use of vasopressors over volume to maintain blood pressure, hypothermic bypass (32–34°C), cell salvage and ultrafiltration. Residual pump blood should be reinfused via the aortic cannula to keep a closed circulation. Meticulous surgical hemostasis is of the essence including the use of topical hemostatic agents. Antifibrinolytic agents are a standard of care and in case of coagulopathic bleeding the early use of accepted hemostatic agents should be considered.

Cardiac surgery can be performed in JW patients with outcomes comparable to those of routine cases, despite the limited therapeutic options with blood transfusion and treating coagulopathy. This has not only been shown for patients undergoing CABG surgery, but also for more complex procedures including LVAD implantation and heart transplantation, especially where a preoptimization protocol was used. This demonstrates the effectiveness of blood conservation techniques as a holistic concept to decrease blood usage in cardiac surgery without increasing risk.

Sickle Cell Anemia

Sickle cell anemia is an autosomal genetic hemoglobinopathy with mutations of the β-globin gene, which results in abnormal β-chains, leading to abnormal hemoglobin S (HbS) rather than the normal HbA. Due to a relative resistance of HbS to malaria, prevalence of the sickle cell gene is highest in African and Middle Eastern populations. Depending on the genotype, there is the heterozygous (HbAS) *sickle cell trait* with around 40% HbS and the homozygous (HbSS) *sickle cell disease* with only abnormal HbS. Combination with other haemoglobinopathies is also possible (e.g. HbSC, β-thalassemia). Diagnosis includes HbS-screening test, full blood count for assessing anemia, and hemoglobin electrophoresis to confirm and quantify the HbS fraction in *sickle cell trait* patients.

Deoxygenated HbS is decreased in solubility and forms polymers, creating the typical sickle-shaped erythrocytes. As a consequence, blood viscosity increases and capillaries are blocked, often leading to embolic-like organ infarction. Typical clinical features are anemia, acute and chronic pain, bone pain and necrosis, splenic sequestration, pulmonary hypertension, stroke and vaso-occlusive or aplastic crises. Sickle cell crises can be triggered by hypoxemia, hypothermia and acidosis, which are all conditions frequently encountered during cardiopulmonary bypass. HbS polymerizes at around PaO_2 of 40–50 mmHg, which means sickling can occur under physiological conditions in HbSS patients. Characterization of the genotype and knowing the percentage of HbS are crucial for choosing the management plan for operations involving CPB.

General principles for management of patients with sickle cell disorders are:

- Avoiding hypothermia (use of warm cardioplegia where necessary), dehydration, acidosis and most importantly hypoxemia
- Blood transfusion with HbS-negative blood while avoiding cell salvage and retransfusion of residual pump blood
- If hypothermia is unavoidable (in operations such as pulmonary thrombendarterectomy, see Chapter 9) exchange transfusion aiming for an HbS of less than 30%, ideally three to five days prior to surgery, is necessary.

Accepting a lower hematocrit might improve blood viscosity and perfusion during CPB in these patients.

Cold Agglutinins

Cold agglutinins (CA) are mostly IgM-antibodies against surface antigens of red blood cells. Antibody-antigen interaction only becomes relevant below a certain threshold temperature, the so-called CA antibody specific thermal amplitude. Because of the pentameric structure of IgM, CA antibodies can bind to multiple erythrocytes causing hemagglutination below their thermal amplitude, potentially leading to occlusion of small blood vessels and tissue damage. Even though the agglutination resolves when temperature rises again, the antibody-antigen interaction triggers a non-reversible complement activation, which leads to hemolysis.

The incidence of cold agglutinin disease is low. A study screening nearly 15,000 cardiac surgical patients found true antibodies in only 0.13%. Two forms of cold agglutinin disease have been described:

- a primary form, which is associated with lymphoproliverative disorders and
- a secondary form, which is part of an immune response to various viral and bacterial infections (e.g. mycoplasma pneumonia, EBV, CMV, influenza, HIV, chlamydia) or a neoplastic process (e.g. adenocarcinoma) and is usually less severe and self-limiting.

In preparation for cardiac surgery, patients with CA need to have their titer and the thermal amplitude evaluated. A titer below 1:32 and an amplitude below 20°C is considered low risk for cardiac surgery. A significant titer is thought to be over 1:64 and a thermal amplitude of above 30°C seems relevant in patients undergoing cardiopulmonary bypass.

The patient temperature needs to be kept above the threshold temperature, CPB should be conducted with normothermic perfusion and warm cardioplegia should be used. If cold crystalloid cardioplegia is used, the coronary system should be flushed out with a warm crystalloid solution to remove red blood cells prior to administering the cold solution. In preparation for procedures where hypothermia cannot be avoided (e.g. aortic arch surgery), preoperative treatment with plasmapheresis or monoclonal antibodies (rituximab) can reduce the antibody titer.

The perfusionist is often the first person to spot cold agglutination in patients that have not been diagnosed. Agglutination generally occurs first in the cardioplegia circuit when cold cardioplegia is mixed with the patient's own blood.

Suggested Further Reading

1. Besser MW, Klein AA. The coagulopathy of cardiopulmonary bypass. *Crit Rev Clin Lab Sci.* 2010; 47: 197–212.

2. Hofer J, Fries D, Solomon C et al. A snapshot of coagulopathy after cardiopulmonary bypass. *Clin Appl Thromb Hemost.* 2016; 22: 505–511.

3. Task Force on Patient Blood Management for Adult Cardiac Surgery of the European Association for Cardio-Thoracic S, the European Association of Cardiothoracic A, Boer C et al. 2017 EACTS/EACTA Guidelines on patient blood management for adult cardiac surgery. *J Cardiothorac Vasc Anesth.* 2018; 32: 88–120.

4. Ortmann E, Besser MW, Klein AA. Antifibrinolytic agents in current anaesthetic practice. *Br J Anaesth.* 2013; 111: 549–563.

5. RCoS. Caring for patients who refuse blood – a guide to good practice. 2016.

6. Jassar AS, Ford PA, Haber HL et al. Cardiac surgery in Jehovah's Witness patients: ten-year experience. *Ann Thorac Surg.* 2012; 93: 19–25.

7. Tanaka A, Ota T, Uriel N et al. Cardiovascular surgery in Jehovah's Witness patients: The role of preoperative optimization. *J Thorac Cardiovasc Surg.* 2015; 150: 976-83.e1–3.

8. Vaislic CD, Dalibon N, Ponzio O et al. Outcomes in cardiac surgery in 500 consecutive Jehovah's Witness patients: 21 year experience. *J Cardiothorac Surg.* 2012; 7: 95.

9. Patel PA, Ghadimi K, Coetzee E et al. Incidental cold agglutinins in cardiac surgery: Intraoperative surprises and team-based problem-solving strategies during cardiopulmonary bypass.

J Cardiothorac Vasc Anesth. 2017; 31: 1109–1118.

10. Jain MD, Cabrerizo-Sanchez R, Karkouti K et al. Seek and you shall find – but then what do you do? Cold agglutinins in cardiopulmonary bypass and a single-center experience with cold agglutinin screening before cardiac surgery. *Transfus Med Rev.* 2013; 27: 65–73.

Inflammation and Organ Damage during Cardiopulmonary Bypass

R Clive Landis and Sherif Assaad

The transition from physiological circulation to cardiopulmonary bypass (CPB) represents a major change to the homeostasis of the body including alterations in the distribution of blood flow and oxygen delivery to organs (see Figure 17.1a). Tissue oxygen delivery is influenced to a large extent by CPB flow rate (see Figure 17.1b). During CPB cerebral and systemic oxygen saturation are significantly reduced by lower blood flow regardless of systemic arterial pressure. Moreover, vasopressors, frequently administered to restore blood pressure, are associated with a further decrease in cerebral and systemic oxygen saturation. Organ dysfunction on CPB may thus be in part attributed to changes in the regional distribution of blood flow and the dependence of oxygen delivery on the maintenance of adequate CPB flow rates.

Layered on top of disturbances in oxygen delivery to the tissues is a systemic inflammatory response triggered by contact of leukocytes and other blood components with the artificial surfaces of the extracorporeal circuit. This results in a storm of cytokine and protease release from leukocytes in addition to activation of complement, kallikrein, coagulation and fibrinolytic pathways. While most of these host responses are appropriate and desirable in the context of a localized injury or infection, they are not desirable systemically and contribute to the morbidity and mortality associated with cardiopulmonary bypass.

Systemic Inflammatory Response

There is some controversy over the definition of the systemic inflammatory response, which has evolved as an amalgam of formal and informal definitions. The only formal definition is borrowed from critical care and the 1992 diagnostic criteria of the Systemic Inflammatory Response Syndrome (SIRS) in sepsis. Unfortunately, the SIRS criteria are widely regarded as too non-specific to add any discriminant value to the systemic inflammatory response, with moderate tachycardia and pyrexia >38°C qualifying a patient with the syndrome. SIRS has *de facto* been abandoned in the field of cardiopulmonary bypass, with a small minority of papers (<14%) on this topic even mentioning SIRS and even fewer reporting on the four criteria necessary to define SIRS.

Despite the lack of a practical definition, there is acceptance that an iatrogenic inflammatory response is most likely triggered to a greater or lesser extent in *all* patients undergoing cardiac surgery with CPB and that this contributes to the perioperative complications summarized in Table 17.1. This chapter focuses on CPB-associated gastrointestinal, pulmonary and myocardial dysfunction. Renal and cerebral complications are discussed in further detail in Chapters 18 and 19.

Table 17.1. Complications after cardiac surgery

Renal failure	3.1 %
Stroke or coma	2.8 %
Gastrointestinal complications	2.5 %
Re-op for bleeding	2.3 %
Sternal infections	1.4 %
Periop myocardial infarction	1.1 %
Acute respiratory distress syndrome	0.9 %
Dialysis	0.9 %
Multisystem failure	0.6 %

Patients after first time coronary artery bypass in the USA (Society of Thoracic Surgeons, 1997 Database; 161,018 patients). Adopted from Hessel; Seminars in Cardiothoracic and Vascular Anesthesia 2004.

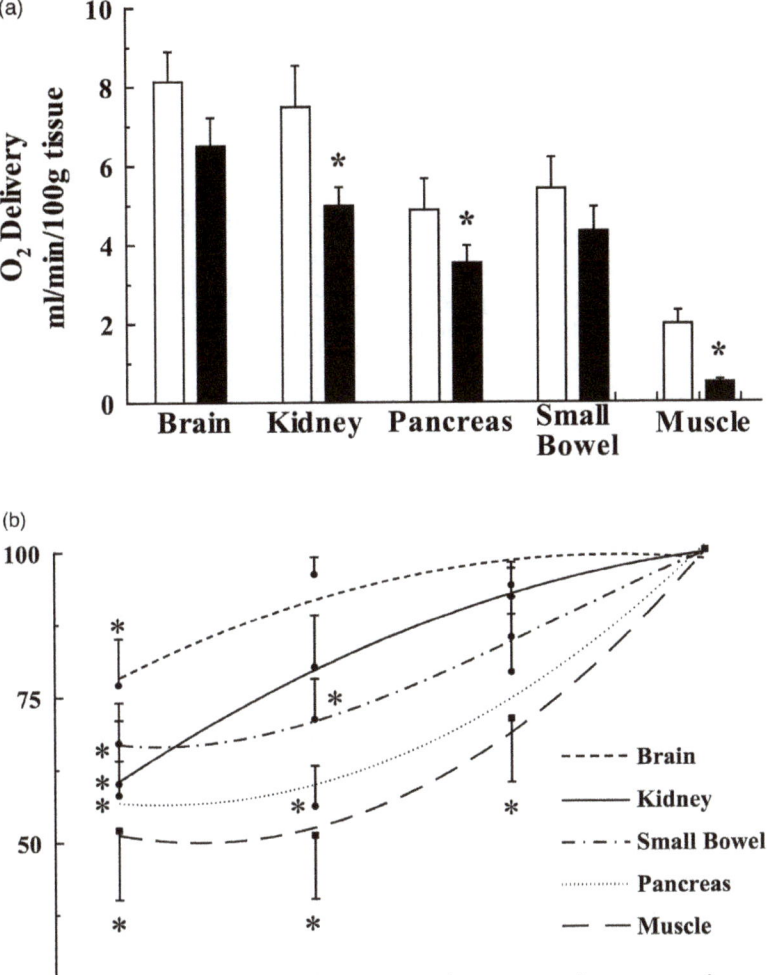

Figure 17.1 (a) Regional O_2 delivery with onset cardiopulmonary bypass, (b) Change in organ DO_2 with changes in CPB flow rate. (Adapted from Boston US, Slater JM, Orszulak TA, Cook DJ. Hierarchy of regional oxygen delivery during cardiopulmonary bypass. *Ann Thorac Surg.* 2001 Jan;71(1):260–264.)

From Teflon to Velcro: How Endothelial Lining Links the Systemic Inflammatory Response to Organ Injury

Endothelial cells have been recognized as gatekeepers, separating the activated milieu in the circulation from the tissues (Figure 17.2a). Even modest hypoxia can activate endothelial cells, thereby forming a nexus for prothrombotic events and exudation of inflammatory mediators and leukocytes into the tissues. Several studies have shown that the endothelium lining microvascular beds (e.g. in the brain and kidneys) can become activated by periods of ischemia/reperfusion. Such activated endothelium becomes prothrombotic, is open to solute exchange and supports the transport of activated leukocytes into organs (Figure 17.2b). This mode of organ injury occurs in addition to more direct hypoxic injury to tissues, such as to the sensitive medullar region of the kidney. Maintaining optimal and continuous tissue perfusion

167

therefore takes on further importance from the perspective of the systemic inflammatory response.

Dysfunction of Specific Organ Systems

Gastrointestinal Dysfunction

Gastrointestinal (GI) complications post cardiac surgery are relatively uncommon with an incidence of 2–4 %, but a mortality rate of 15–60%. This represents about 11 times (range 4–32 times) the mortality in patients not experiencing GI complications. The median time for presentation of GI complications is eight days.

Despite improvements in surgical techniques and perfusion strategies, the incidence and the mortality rate have not changed in the last two decades. The clinical assessment of patients with GI complications is often delayed because patients might be sedated, partially unresponsive, mechanically ventilated or the classical symptoms and signs are masked by other cardiac and pulmonary complications. Table 17.2 summarizes the most common GI complications.

In a study of 4,883 patients who underwent cardiac surgery, several risk factors were identified as predisposing for GI complications, including prolonged skin-to-skin time (>240 minutes) and prolonged cardiopulmonary bypass time (>121 minutes). Acute kidney failure and pneumonia were identified as postoperative risk factors. Interestingly, the type of surgery and new onset postoperative atrial fibrillations were not found to be risk factors.

Pathogenesis of GI Complications

Depressed systemic hemodynamics: CPB causes profound reductions in blood flow in the splanchnic circulation intraoperatively and for up to several hours postoperatively. Severe intestinal ischemia may occur during CPB even when the indices of global body perfusion remain normal. This may be due to the release of a variety of endogenous vasoactive factors, such as vasopressin, catecholamines and thromboxanes, and to the administration of vasopressors to maintain perfusion pressure. Both of these lead to a redistribution of regional blood flow away from the mucosa of the GI tract.

SIRS: The combination of reduced splanchnic blood flow and the CPB-induced SIRS reduce the efficacy of both the absorptive and barrier functions of the GI tract. The increase in gastrointestinal mucosal permeability results in the translocation of bacterial

(a)

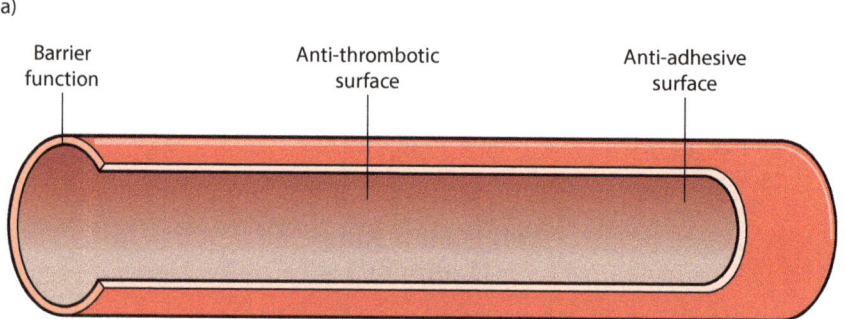

Barrier function   Anti-thrombotic surface   Anti-adhesive surface

NO (nitric oxide) mediates endothelial dependant relaxation

AT-III inhibits thrombin
tPA promotes fibrinolysis
PGI₂ inhibits platelet activation

Absence of inducible selectin and intercellular adhesion molecules required for leukocyte recruitment

Figure 17.2 Contrasting properties of resting versus activated or denuded endothelium. Diagram depicts a cut away section of a blood vessel lined with (**a**) resting intact endothelium or (**b**) activated or denuded endothelium. Resting, intact endothelium provides barrier function, an anti-thrombotic surface, an anti-adhesive surface and nitric oxide mediated vasorelaxation. Vascular beds or grafted vessels that have been activated by inflammatory mediators, transient ischemia, anaerobic metabolism or endothelial denudation lose their homeostatic barrier properties and promote thrombosis, solute exchange, adhesion and extravasation of cytodestructive neutrophils, and loss of nitric oxide mediated vasodilation.

Key: **NO** = nitric oxide; **At-III** = antithrombin-III; **tPA** = tissue plasminogen activator; **PI2** = prostaglandin I2; **PAI-1** = plasminogen activator inhibitor-1; **ICAM-1** = intercellular adhesion molecule-1.

endotoxins from the GI tract into the bloodstream, amplifying SIRS and subsequent organ damage.

Prolonged mechanical ventilation > 24 hours: Mechanical ventilation using large tidal volumes with high airway pressures may lead to release of proinflammatory cytokines. In conjunction with stimulation of the sympathetic nervous system and decreased

Table 17.2. Visceral complications after cardiac surgery

	Incidence (%)	Mortality (%)
Gastrointestinal bleeding	30.7	26.9
Ischemic bowel	17.7	71.3
Pancreatitis	11.2	27.5
Cholecystitis	10.9	26.9
Paralytic ileus	4.5	10.8
Perforated peptic ulcer	4.2	43.8
Hepatic failure	3.5	74.4
Diverticulitis	2.6	17.1
Small bowel obstruction	2.0	18.5
Pseudo-obstruction of colon	1.9	21.4

Adapted with modifications from: **Hessel;** Seminars in Cardiothoracic and Vascular Anesthesia 2004

cardiac output, which are also often associated with mechanical ventilation, this may result in splanchnic hypoperfusion and mucosal injury.

Table 17.3 gives an overview of the risk factors for GI complications.

Specific GI Complications

- GI bleeding – bleeding from the upper GI tract is far more common than bleeding from the lower GI tract. Lower GI tract bleeding is usually associated with bowel ischemia or preexisting large bowel disease.
- Bowel ischemia or perforation – bowel ischemia after cardiac surgery is one of the most serious complications in the postoperative period. It accounts for 18 % of all GI complications and is associated with a mortality rate of >70%. It is more common in advanced age, females, emergency surgery, complex surgery, end stage renal disease, prolonged bypass and perioperative use of IABP and vasopressors. The earliest presenting signs are progressive metabolic acidosis, leukocytosis and ileus. Early diagnosis and intervention, for example CT scan or laparotomy, may be lifesaving.
- Hepatic dysfunction – as a result of reduced splanchnic perfusion, hepatic metabolism is reduced during CPB. Hepatic blood flow has been reported to decrease by 19% after CPB is

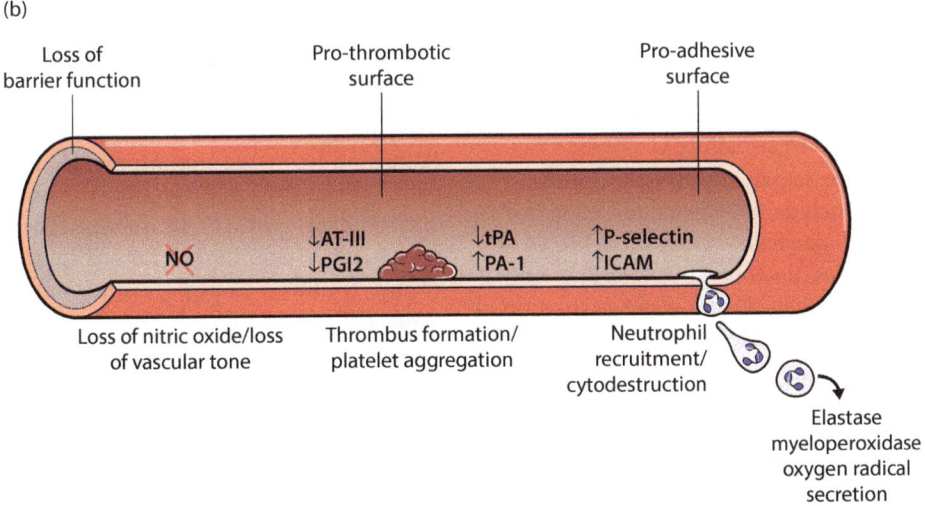

(b)

Loss of barrier function   Pro-thrombotic surface   Pro-adhesive surface

NO

↓AT-III   ↓tPA   ↑P-selectin
↓PGI2   ↑PA-1   ↑ICAM

Loss of nitric oxide/loss of vascular tone   Thrombus formation/platelet aggregation   Neutrophil recruitment/cytodestruction

Elastase myeloperoxidase oxygen radical secretion

Figure 17.2 *(cont.)*

Table 17.3. Risk factors associated with GI complications post cardiac surgery

Preoperative	Age > 75 years
	History of congestive heart failure or ejection fraction < 40%
	Renal insufficiency
	Increased preoperative total bilirubin >1.2 mg/dl
	Preoperative partial thromboplastin time (PTT) >37 seconds
	Type of cardiac surgery
	• Emergency
	• Reoperation
	• Valve or combined procedure
	• Cardiac transplantation
Intraoperative	Intraoperative circulatory failure
	CPB duration > 100 minutes
	Aortic cross-clamp duration > 55 minutes
	Transfusion of packed red blood cells
Postoperative	Low cardiac output
	Use of inotropes or vasopressors or intra-aortic balloon pump (IABP)
	Reoperation for bleeding
	Loss of normal sinus rhythm
	Ventilation > 24 hours
	Intensive care unit stay > 1 day

commenced. There may be a transient rise in the levels of hepatic enzymes, which usually peaks early in the postoperative period. Only a small number of patients show clinically evident jaundice, although bilirubin levels can rise in about 20% of cases. Moderate or severe degrees of hepatic dysfunction are rare and usually occur in concert with multi-organ failure.

Risk factors for hepatic dysfunction post cardiac surgery include female gender, congestive heart failure, valvular heart surgery, combined surgical procedures, postoperative bleeding and transfusion. Consequences of hepatic dysfunction relevant to CPB specifically include:

○ Impaired drug metabolism
○ Reduced plasma protein concentrations leading to reduced plasma oncotic pressure and alteration in the volume of distribution of drugs
○ Impaired coagulation due to reduction in production of clotting factors

○ Impaired ability to generate heat and regulate temperature
○ Impaired glucose metabolism.

• Pancreatitis – overt pancreatitis, characterized by a rise in serum amylase to over 1000 IU/l, occurs in 0.1–1% of cases following cardiac surgery and accounts for 11% of GI complications. Uncomplicated pancreatitis carries a mortality of 5–10%, but cases progressing to necrotizing pancreatitis or to the development of a pancreatic abscess or a pseudocyst usually result in death. Lesser degrees of pancreatic cellular injury with mild elevations in serum amylase concentrations are common. The etiology is probably related to perioperative reduction in splanchnic blood flow causing pancreatic ischemia. Calcium, frequently used to treat intraoperative hypotension, has not been identified clearly as an independent risk factor.

Pulmonary Dysfunction

Pulmonary complications remain a leading cause of morbidity after cardiac surgery. The incidence is 7.5% and the mortality rate is 21%. The spectrum of pulmonary complications ranges from atelectasis to acute respiratory distress syndrome (ARDS). The incidence of post-CPB ARDS is <2%. The mortality rate associated with post-CPB ARDS, however, is >50%.

Median sternotomy results in more than a 50% postoperative reduction in vital capacity (VC) and forced expiration (FEV1) from preoperative values. These changes last for about four months postoperatively and are caused by poor coordination of rib cage expansion following sternotomy, pleural effusion and pain. The use of the internal mammary artery for grafting exacerbates these changes. There is no difference between on-pump versus off-pump surgery with regard to these changes except that CPB may be associated with the release of bronchoconstricting mediators causing an increase in expiratory resistance.

Table 17.4 provides an overview over the most common causes of respiratory failure after cardiac surgery.

Although some of the factors listed relate to cardiac surgery in general and are not specific to CPB, the combined effect is the development of

Table 17.4. Common causes of postoperative respiratory failure

Atelectasis

Increase in lung water content as a result of increased capillary permeability caused by SIRS

Impaired hemodynamics in the immediate postoperative period

Additional fluid load during CPB

Altered production of surfactant
- lung collapse during CPB
- SIRS causing decreased static and dynamic lung compliance

Transfusion-related acute lung injury (TRALI)

Altered chest wall mechanics resulting from sternotomy

Pneumothorax or hemothorax

Phrenic nerve injury impairing diaphragmatic function

intrapulmonary shunts that cause a mismatch between ventilation and perfusion. This manifests as a higher inspired oxygen concentration requirement to maintain an acceptable level of blood oxygenation. This mismatch tends to resolve gradually postoperatively, but patients may require supportive measures such as positive endexpiratory pressure (PEEP) during mechanical ventilation or continuous positive airway pressure (CPAP) when spontaneously breathing until resolution occurs. In mechanically ventilated patients, tidal volumes in excess of 10 ml/kg were found to be a risk factor for organ failure and prolonged intensive care unit stay. Diuretics, as an adjunct to careful fluid balancing, may help to reduce interstitial lung water. In hemodynamically stable patients, with adequate gas exchange and no evidence of neurologic insults or bleeding, adequate pain control and early extubation allow early ambulation and the ability to cough and clear pulmonary secretions, which reduces the incidence of pulmonary complications.

Myocardial Dysfunction

The period of CPB during cardiac surgery can be divided into three phases:
- Onset of CPB until application of the cross-clamp
- The period of cross-clamping and cardioplegic or fibrillatory arrest
- The reperfusion period following removal of the cross-clamp and ultimately separation from CPB.

During these periods the heart is subjected to insults from microemboli, SIRS, regional hypoperfusion, complete ischemia and reperfusion injury. The injurious effects incurred from these insults, together with the potential for inadequate myocardial protection and distension of the flaccid heart during the period of cross-clamping, result in myocardial edema and reduced ventricular contractility, which may persist into the postoperative period. Furthermore, if the heart is subject to excessive preload or high afterload during weaning from CPB, left ventricular end-diastolic volume, myocardial wall stress and oxygen consumption are all increased, further contributing to deterioration in cardiac function.

Therapeutic Strategies for Attenuating the Systemic Inflammatory Response

How to Measure Anti-inflammatory Interventions?

There is no practical working definition of the systemic inflammatory response. The only formal definition of SIRS does not provide discriminant value, with moderate tachycardia and pyrexia >38°C qualifying for the syndrome. In the absence of a workable definition, different scoring systems, such as ODIN (Organ Dysfunctions and/or Infection) or APACHE (Acute Physiology and Chronic Health Evaluation), have been adopted by different groups to link the CPB-associated systemic inflammatory response to clinical endpoints, providing better discriminant value.

An alternative approach put forth by the "Outcomes" Consensus Panel in 2010 is to measure "softer" outcomes, such as time to extubation, renal and cardiac injury biomarkers, length of ICU stay and neurocognitive deficits tailored to heart surgery, as surrogate but still clinically meaningful endpoints.

Anti-inflammatory Interventions

Using the "Outcomes" Consensus Panel's surrogate endpoints, a multidisciplinary consortium of surgeons, anesthetists, perfusionists and basic scientists synthesized the evidence covering the complete spectrum of anti-inflammatory interventions deployed in the setting of cardiopulmonary bypass. This included pharmacological, perfusion-related and surgical/perioperative management interventions. Ninety-eight anti-inflammatory interventions including off-pump surgery, minimized circuits, biocompatible circuit coatings, leukocyte filtration, complement C5 inhibition, preoperative aspirin and corticosteroid prophylaxis were part of the analysis. Unfortunately no single intervention was supported by strong level A evidence (multiple randomized controlled trials [RCTs] or meta-analysis) of clinical benefit. The somewhat gloomy conclusions from the review were consistent with the fact that there are few statistically well powered studies and meta-analyses examining hard endpoints. A Cochrane review concluded that corticosteroids had no effect on mortality, cardiac or pulmonary complications in cardiopulmonary bypass patients, while meta-analyses investigating leukocyte filtration and ultrafiltration strategies found that these were sometimes associated with heightened leukocyte activation.

A secondary analysis of the "Outcomes" criteria revealed that suppression of a single inflammatory biomarker was insufficient to confer clinical benefit. This is consistent with a "multiple hit" hypothesis, in which clinically effective suppression of the systemic inflammatory response will require combinations of treatments and interventions to hit multiple targets in the multiple pathways activated. The evidence therefore points toward the fact that narrowly targeted interventions fail to demonstrate clinical benefit when used on their own. This is hardly surprising if we take into account the broad array of host defense pathways – complement, coagulation, kinins, fibrinolysis, leukocytes, platelets, hemolysis, and inflammatory mediators – activated across the surgical population.

The mechanisms of the currently most plausible interventions are summarized below.

Pharmacological Strategies

- *Steroids* – administrating pre-CPB corticosteroids may attenuate the inflammatory response by inhibiting the release of the inflammatory cytokines IL-6, IL-8 and enhancing the release of the anti-inflammatory cytokine IL-10. In one study this was associated with a decrease in ICU and hospital stay and in the incidence of postoperative atrial fibrillation. This did not translate into survival benefits or a reduction in the cardiac or pulmonary complications. On the contrary, there was an increase in the incidence of

gastrointestinal bleeding and hyperglycemia requiring insulin infusion. The routine administration of prophylactic corticosteroids is thus not recommended.

- *Statins* – are primarily used in the treatment of hypercholesterolemia. They also have anti-inflammatory effects with a reduction in post-CPB renal and cerebrovascular complications. Statins may have a potential benefit on graft patency and reduction in mortality and equivocal benefit on reduction of postoperative atrial fibrillation. For these reasons, continuation of perioperative statins may be recommended pending more definitive evidence of efficacy.

- *Angiotensin converting enzyme inhibitors (ACE-I)* – ACE-I are antihypertensive agents that are used as an adjunct in the treatment of heart failure with beneficial effects on cardiac remodeling. They have anti-inflammatory effects as shown by attenuation of the IL-6 rise in the postoperative period and antifibrinolytic effects that might decrease the incidence of graft thrombosis. Long-term survival benefits and reduction in cardiac adverse events are still controversial, particularly in patients with normal ejection fraction.

Perfusion Strategies

- *Heparin-bonded circuitry* – proponents of bonded circuits used them with the intention of reducing the degree of complement activation. Despite high initial hopes they have not been proven to be effective in attenuating coagulation disorders or fibrinolysis.

- *Hemofiltration/ultrafiltration* – convection and osmosis under hydrostatic pressure have been incorporated into CPB circuits to remove low-molecular-weight substances from plasma with the aim of reducing the circulating levels of proinflammatory mediators. Current techniques are more effective in the pediatric than the adult population.

- *Leukocyte depletion* – such filters are often incorporated into the CPB circuit to reduce the number of circulating activated white cells. Their value is presently unclear, but leukocyte depletion may have a protective effect in reducing the severity of lung, renal and myocardial injury after

CPB. The most consistent benefit is found in higher risk patients with preexisting lung disease and ventricular dysfunction as well as patients undergoing transplantation or procedures with prolonged CPB duration. Leukocytes in allogenic blood transfusions have important immunomodulatory effects in the recipient. The use of leukocyte depleted stored blood has been shown to decrease mortality in some cardiac surgical patients. This is predominantly due to a decrease in non-cardiac causes of death, in particular multi-organ failure. However, a number of studies have shown that leukocyte adhesion to filters may cause their activation and subsequent release of inflammatory proteases and cytokines.

- *Maintaining ventilation and pulmonary artery perfusion* – keeping the lungs ventilated and, where possible, perfused during CPB decreases the incidence of postoperative atelectasis and lung ischemia-reperfusion injury and hence decreases the incidence of post-CPB pulmonary dysfunction. Although this strategy has been associated with lesser inflammatory and proteolytic response, its clinical benefit is still to be proven.

- *Minimal invasive extracorporeal circulation (MiECC)* – recently, there has been growing interest in the use of MiECC to replace conventional cardiopulmonary bypass circuits. The use of MiECC circuits has been shown to lead to less thrombin generation due to improved biocompatibility, elimination of the blood-air interaction in the reservoir and exclusion of unprocessed shed blood reinfusion. Despite some studies showing potential clinical advantages, such as lower incidence of postoperative AF and renal dysfunction and a reduction in blood transfusion, MiECC circuits have not gained wide clinical acceptance yet. See Chapter 8 for more detail.

- *Pulsatile flow* – most cardiac centers use non-pulsatile roller or centrifugal pumps to drive circulation during CPB. Though the exact mechanism is not fully understood, it is believed that non-pulsatile laminar flow, as opposed to physiological pulsatile flow, causes deterioration of microcirculatory perfusion and shedding of the endothelial glycocalix. Proponents of pulsatile flow argue that as a result of non-pulsatile, laminar flow there is an increase in endotoxins, endogenous vasoconstrictors and platelet activation leading to local cellular damage. On the other hand, pulsatile flow has the theoretical advantage of delivering more surplus hemodynamic energy (SHE) to the microcirculation. This should result in preservation of the microcirculation, improved blood flow to vital organs and attenuation of the systemic inflammatory response. Despite these potential advantages, the use of pulsatile flow on CPB is controversial because of the absence of data showing clinically significant benefits.

- *Avoiding CPB* – off-pump CABG (OPCABG) is an alternative technique for coronary revascularization, which is still controversial and highly dependent on institutional experience and preference. Clinical reports have shown that oxidative stress and markers of inflammation (particularly IL-8, IL-6, TNF and E-selectin) are significantly reduced during OPCABG when compared to CABG performed on CPB. OPCABG has also been shown to be associated with a reduction in blood transfusion. Full heparinization may not be necessary and this, together with the avoidance of hemodilution through the CPB priming volume, may be more important in reducing transfusion requirements than any advantageous effects from ameliorating the systemic inflammatory response. Despite these potential advantages, large-scale studies failed to show benefits in long-term survival or neuropsychological outcomes after OPCABG compared to on-pump CABG. On the contrary, OPCABG patients have poorer graft patency at one year.

Disturbances in blood flow and its distribution, along with systemic inflammatory responses, are characteristics of CPB which put vital organs at risk. While the specific injury patterns of various organs have become better elucidated, methods to mitigate damage for many of these remain elusive. It is likely that clinically effective suppression of the systemic inflammatory response will require combinations of treatments and interventions to hit the multiple pathways activated.

Suggested Further Reading

1. Prondzinsky R, Knupfer A, Loppnow H et al. Surgical trauma affects the proinflammatory status after cardiac surgery to a higher degree than cardiopulmonary bypass. *J Thorac Cardiovasc Surg* 2005 April;129(4):760–766.

2. Dieleman JM, van Passen J, van Dijk D et al. Prophylactic corticosteroids for cardiopulmonary bypass in adults. *Cochrane Database Syst Rev* 2011;(5):CD005566.

3. Warren O, Alexiou C, Massey R et al. The effects of various leukocyte filtration strategies in cardiac surgery. *Eur J Cardiothorac Surg* 2007 April;31(4):665–676.

4. Zhu X, Ji B, Wang G et al. The effects of zero-balance ultrafiltration on postoperative recovery after cardiopulmonary bypass: a meta-analysis of randomized controlled trials. *Perfusion* 2012 September;27(5):386–392.

5. Ranucci M, Balduini A, Ditta A et al. A systematic review of biocompatible cardiopulmonary bypass circuits and clinical outcome. *Ann Thorac Surg* 2009 April;87(4):13111319.

6. De Backer D, Dubois MJ, Schmartz D et al. Microcirculatory alterations in cardiac surgery: effects of cardiopulmonary bypass and anesthesia. *Ann Thorac Surg* 2009 November;88(5):13961403.

7. Litmathe J, Boeken U, Bohlen G et al. Systemic inflammatory response syndrome after extracorporeal circulation: a predictive algorithm for the patient at risk. *Hellenic J Cardiol* 2011 November;52(6):493–500.

8. Hessel, EA 2nd. Abdominal organ injury after cardiac surgery. *Semin Cardiothorac Vasc Anesth*, 2004. 8(3):243–263.

9. Weissman, C. Pulmonary complications after cardiac surgery. *Semin Cardiothorac Vasc Anesth* 2004. 8(3):185–211.

10. Buggeskov KB, Grønlykke L, Risom EC et al. Pulmonary artery perfusion versus no perfusion during cardiopulmonary bypass for open heart surgery in adults. *Cochrane Database Syst Rev* 2018 February 8;2:CD011098.

11. Ng CS, Wan S. Limiting inflammatory response to cardiopulmonary bypass: pharmaceutical strategies. *Curr Opin Pharmacol* 2012. 12(2):155–159.

12. Dvirnik N, Belley-Cote E, Hanif H et al. Steroids in cardiac surgery: a systematic review and meta-analysis. *Br J Anesth* 2018 120 (4):657–667.

13. Butler J, Rocker GM, Westaby S. Inflammatory response to cardiopulmonary bypass. *Ann Thorac Surg* 1993 February;55(2):552–9.

14. Landis RC, Arrowsmith JE, Baker RA, et al. Consensus Statement: minimal criteria for reporting the systemic inflammatory response to cardiopulmonary bypass. *Heart Surg Forum* 2010 April;13(2) E116–123.

15. Shann KG, Likosky DS, Murkin JM, et al. An evidence-based review of the practice of cardiopulmonary bypass in adults: a focus on neurologic injury, glycemic control, hemodilution, and the inflammatory response. *J Thorac Cardiovasc Surg* 2006 August;132(2):283–90.

16. Landis RC, Brown JR, Fitzgerald D, et al. Attenuating the Systemic Inflammatory Response to Adult Cardiopulmonary Bypass: A critical Review of the Evidence Base. *J Extra Corpor Technol* 2014 September;46(3):197–211.

17. Myers GJ, Wegner J. Endothelial Glycocalyx and Cardiopulmonary Bypass. *J Extra Corpor Technol* 2017 September;49(3):174–181.

18. Landis RC, Durandy Y "Dear SIRS … unfaithfully yours". *Anaesth Intensive Care* 2017 March;45(2):274–275.

Neuromonitoring and Cerebral Morbidity Associated with Cardiopulmonary Bypass

Etienne J Couture, Stéphanie Jarry and André Y Denault

Neurological complications after a cardiac surgery are common and have a large impact on patient outcomes. They are the result of a combination of numerous factors, many of them associated with cardiopulmonary bypass (CPB). Blood pressure control is essential to reduce the incidence of cerebral hypoperfusion and ischemic stroke during and after cardiac surgery. Cerebral oxygen saturation can be tracked using near-infrared spectroscopy to assess cerebral perfusion and oxygenation. Careful temperature management plays a key role in preventing cerebral morbidity. Despite multiple attempts to find pharmacologic strategies to prevent neurologic injury, no such solution has been found to reduce the burden of neurologic complications associated with cardiac surgery.

Risk Factors

The incidence of stroke after cardiac sugery has been reported to be as high as 6%. Unfortunately, postoperative neurocognitive dysfunction is even more common with a rate of up to 60%. Numerous studies have identified independent predictors of perioperative stroke, the most commonly named variables are summarized in Table 18.1.

Different surgical procedures come with different risks of stroke. Figure 18.1 shows the results of a retrospective review of 16,184 patients undergoing various cardiac procedures. It is interesting to note that the operations done without CPB, i.e. off-pump coronary artery bypass grafting (OPCABG) and minimal invasive direct coronary artery bypass grafting, show the lowest incidence of stroke. This gives credence to the theory that the majority of cerebral infarcts are embolic in nature. In the majority of studies, the lesions identified by computed tomography (CT) were indicative of a macroembolic etiology with the culprit lesion most commonly located in the distribution of the major cerebral arteries, mainly the middle cerebral artery. Aortic cross-clamping and cannulation are likely to play a huge role in the shedding of atheromatous emboli from the ascending aorta.

Blood Pressure Control

Blood pressure control during CPB is important to ensure appropriate perfusion of end-organ tissues such as the brain, the kidneys and the gastrointestinal tract. Organ perfusion pressure, defined as arterial minus venous pressure, is a key factor to assuring adequate blood flow, oxygenation and metabolic function. The "tools" built into the CPB machine provide control of multiple parameters, such as blood temperature, flow and carbon dioxide, all of which can be used to optimize cerebral blood flow (CBF).

Hypotension during CPB can be the result of hemodilution or of vasodilatation due to pro-inflammatory processes, anesthetic drugs and preoperative use of angiotensin-converting enzyme inhibitors (ACEI) or calcium channel blockers. Hypotension may compromise the clearance of emboli and reduce cerebral perfusion, especially to the watershed areas of the brain.

Hypertension, on the other hand, can result from inadequate levels of anesthesia or analgesia, endogenous release of catecholamines or vasoconstriction due to hypothermia. Hypertension may lead to cerebral hyperperfusion and hyperemia.

Good blood pressure control is very important to ensure optimal neurologic outcomes as both hypotension and hypertension can be deleterious. The 2019 European guidelines on the conduct of CPB recommend adjusting mean arterial pressure (MAP) to within the range of 50–80 mmHg with the use of vasoconstrictors and vasodilators, after ensuring adequate depth of anesthesia and optimal pump flow. A MAP less than 50 mmHg is not recommended as this may fall below the lower limit of cerebral autoregulation, commonly estimated to be around that point despite the wide interindividual variety.

Blood Pressure Control and Stroke

Stroke with clinical symptoms occurs with an incidence of 1–2% after cardiac surgery; neurologic injury, however, occurs in up to 50% of patients and can be silent or only exhibit subtle symptoms such as mild postoperative neurocognitive dysfunction. The optimal MAP during CPB remains a focus of inquiry as multiple trials to find the optimal target MAP during CPB have yielded conflicting results. A retrospective study of 7,457 patients demonstrated the effects of a sustained MAP < 65 mmHg during CPB on postoperative stroke. Every 10-minute period of MAP between 55 and 64 mmHg was associated with a 13% increase in the odds of having a stroke; every 10-minute period of MAP < 55 mmHg was associated with a 16% increase. The study is not able to recommend an ideal MAP target but suggests that the MAP should be kept at least at 65 mmHg in order to reduce the incidence of postoperative neurological complications. A randomized controlled trial of 248 patients undergoing coronary artery bypass grafting (CABG) reported significantly higher rates of cardiac and neurological events with a low MAP strategy (50–60 mmHg) when compared with a high MAP strategy (80–100 mmHg) (12.9 versus 4.8%, p = 0.026). The incidence of permanent neurologic injury was also higher in the low MAP group (7.2 versus 2.4%). Conversely, another study targeting a high MAP (70–80 mmHg) and comparing it to a low MAP (40–50 mmHg) at similar pump flow did not show any difference between the two groups in the volume or number of new perioperative cerebral infarcts detected by magnetic resonance imaging (MRI) or the incidence of postoperative cognitive dysfunction. However, this study showed a trend

Table 18.1. Patient and operation factors associated with increased risk of perioperative stroke

History of cerebrovascular disease

Any grade of internal carotid artery stenosis

Peripheral vascular disease

Age > 70 years

Diabetes mellitus

Hypertension

Infective endocarditis

Emergency/urgent operation

Redo surgery

CPB time > 2 hours

High transfusion requirement

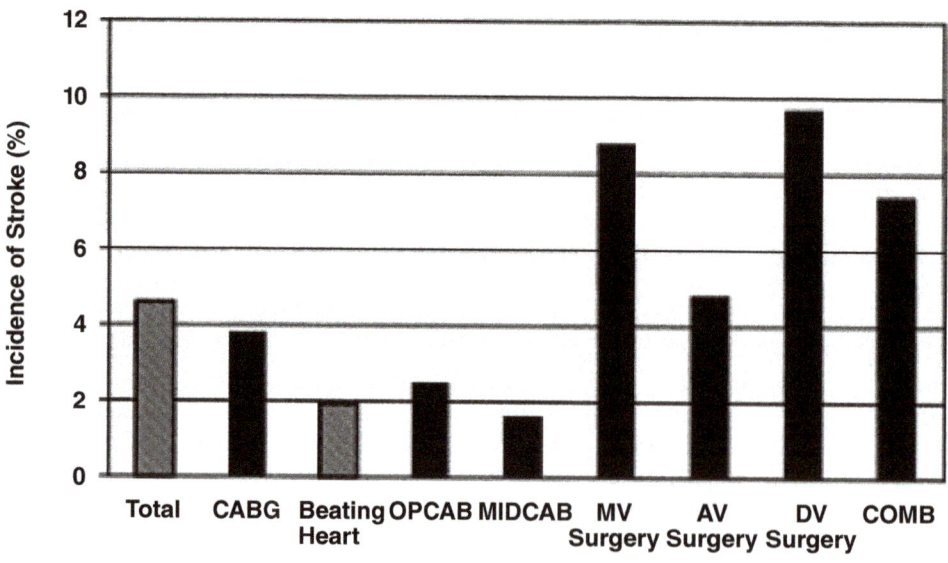

Figure 18.1 Incidence of stroke in relation to different surgical procedures. CABG = coronary artery bypass grafting, beating heart = OPCABG + MIDCABG, MV = mitral valve surgery, AV = aortic valve surgery, DV = double valve surgery, COMB = any other combined procedure. (From Bucerius J, Gummert JF, Borger MA et al. Stroke after cardiac surgery: a risk factor analysis of 16,184 consecutive adult patients. *Ann Thorac Surg.* 2003 Feb;75 (2):472–4788.)

toward a higher rate of stroke (7.0% versus 1.1%; p = 0.06) and death (4.1% versus 0%; p = 0.06) in the high MAP group. A different study comparing an on-pump MAP based on preoperative values versus a set MAP of 80 mmHg has shown the same rates of mortality, major neurological or cardiac complications, deterioration of cognitive function and decline in functional status.

The ultimate individual approach is to use continuous cerebral blood flow autoregulation assessment on the operating table to personalize blood pressure management during CPB. Despite the potential benefits, the current evidence does not support the hypothesis that basing the MAP during CPB on cerebral autoregulation monitoring reduces the frequency of stroke or delayed neurocognitive recovery after surgery compared with usual care. However, personalized MAP management using a cerebral autoregulation approach does reduce the incidence of delirium and alterations in memory after surgery.

Blood Pressure Control and Delirium

The impact of hypotension on the incidence of postoperative delirium and cognitive dysfunction remains subject to debate. In a randomized controlled trial of 92 patients undergoing CABG, those in the high MAP group (80–90 mmHg) had less delirium (0 versus 13%) and a smaller reduction in Mini-MentalStatus score (1.1±1.9 versus 3.9±6.5) when compared to a low MAP group (60–70 mmHg). On the other hand, a prospective cohort study based on 734 cardiac surgical patients did not find an association between intraoperative hypotension – defined by MAP lower than 50 mmHg, MAP decreased by more than 30% relative to the baseline or even a MAP decrease by more than 40% relative to the baseline – and postoperative delirium.

Cerebral Blood Flow

In recent years, CBF autoregulation has been proposed as a new parameter that can be personalized from patient to patient. Different tools have been used in order to find the best MAP during CPB. Among them are the mean velocity index (Mx) and the cerebral oximeter index (Ox). The lower and upper limit of autoregulation can be defined using a Pearson's correlation coefficient calculated from MAP and cerebral oximetry using near-infrared spectroscopy (NIRS) or mean CBF velocity using transcranial Doppler. The correlation coefficient approaches 1 when CBF falls outside the limits of autoregulation, meaning that any change in MAP will be associated with a linear change in CBF; when the correlation coefficient is 0, the autoregulation is preserved and there is no correlation between MAP and CBF. The lower limit of autoregulation is defined as the MAP where the correlation between cerebral oximetry and CBF mean velocity increases above a threshold of 0.4, meaning that any decrease in MAP is associated with a decrease in CBF. The upper limit of autoregulation is defined in a similar fashion.

Ultrasound-tagged NIRS to determine the limits of autoregulation showed no difference in the amount of blood pressure excursions above and below the optimal MAP during CPB and in the first three hours after ICU admission in patients with or without delirium at postoperative days one and three. However, there were more blood pressure excursions above the optimal MAP in patients with delirium and this was positively correlated with the severity of delirium on postoperative day two.

In a similar study using the concept of optimal blood pressure based on CBF autoregulation derived from cerebral oximetry, the same group found a significant difference in the rate of postoperative delirium in patients whose MAP exceeded the upper limit of autoregulation compared to patients whose MAP did not. The magnitude and duration of MAP above the upper threshold during CPB was associated with an increased risk of delirium, while MAP below the autoregulation threshold was not.

The Cerebral Autoregulation Study Group from Johns Hopkins University compared CPB patients with a local standard MAP target of 60 mmHg or higher with a group of patients with a target MAP above the lower limit of autoregulation based on systemic arterial and middle cerebral artery pressure. Despite an only marginally higher MAP in the autoregulation group (73.9 mmHg versus 71.3 mmHg, p = 0.01), the incidence of postoperative delirium was lower compared to the standard of care group (37.9% versus 52.7%, p = 0.04). These results highlight the importance of individualizing the MAP target during CPB in order to avoid hypoperfusion and hyperemia.

Cerebral Oxygen Saturation

The balance between cerebral oxygen consumption and supply can be assessed by cerebral oxygen saturation, which is measured using NIRS and is the result of the local change in the concentration of oxyhemoglobin over total hemoglobin. NIRS optodes are commonly applied to the forehead to measure the regional cerebral oxygen saturation (rSO_2) in the frontal cortex.

There are three different mechanisms of cerebral desaturation:

- altered cerebral metabolism
- decreased blood oxygen content and
- compromised cerebral blood supply.

Cerebral desaturation is generally defined as a decrease of 20% from baseline or an absolute value of less than 50%. These thresholds were defined during clamping for carotid endarterectomy, using transcranial Doppler, electroencephalography or somatosensory evoked potential as they are able to detect ipsilateral cerebral ischemia during carotid artery clamping with a sensitivity of 44–100% and a specificity of 44–82%.

The usefulness of cerebral oximetry during cardiac surgery has been evaluated in multiple trials. One multicenter study found that 61% of patients experience at least one episode of cerebral desaturation during CPB. 34% of these resolved with usual care, while 66% resolved in response to an intervention based on a management algorithm. Only 5% of cerebral desaturations remained unresolved. A multicenter Canadian study evaluated the use of cerebral saturation by randomizing patients into either an intervention group where the clinician was aware of the cerebral saturation and a control group where the cerebral saturation was recorded but blinded to the clinician. 63% of patients had at least one episode of cerebral desaturation, which was successfully reversed in 97% in the intervention group. These studies highlight that cerebral oxygen desaturation is common during cardiac surgery and these episodes can be appropriately reversed in more than 95% of the time using an intervention algorithm (see Figure 18.2). These studies, however, do not show any advantages in neurological outcome conferred by using NIRS.

There are several factors that contribute to the low sensitivity and specificity of NIRS for diagnosing cerebral ischemia. Its sensitivity is limited by the small sampling window over the frontal cortex, and its inability to monitor global cerebral oxygenation. Its specificity is limited by the fact that rSO_2 can be influenced by a variety of factors such as systemic and regional hemodynamics, blood oxygen transport and tissue metabolism. NIRS also lacks the ability to differentiate the causes of low rSO_2 (i.e. emboli versus hypoperfusion). Despite the absence of unequivocal evidence to suggest that its use reduces the incidence and severity of postoperative neurological complications, NIRS is widely used in deep hypothermic circulatory arrest (DHCA) to assess cerebral oxygenation during cooling, arrest and rewarming.

Measuring cerebral oxygen saturation during cardiac surgery is best utilized as one component of multimodal neurologic and hemodynamic monitoring and interpreted in the context of the patient's pathology and the operation. NIRS can only access a small area of the frontal cortical area. The use of this technology is not intended to detect or lower the incidence of stroke, which is more associated with embolic phenomena. Emboli detected using transcranial Doppler can often go undetected by cerebral oximetry (see Figure 18.3). Light transmission and absorption used for NIRS takes place in arteries, capillaries and veins and thus does not differentiate between arterial and venous blood. NIRS monitoring algorithms assume a fixed distribution of venous and arterial blood, between 70:30 and 75:25, depending on the manufacturer. The internal algorithms of these devices do not take into account any variation in blood flow or distribution caused by changes in CO_2 levels or temperature, as are commonly encountered during CPB.

Monitoring venous oxygen saturation at the jugular bulb ($S_{JV}O_2$) using a fibreoptic catheter provides a continuous measure of the global balance between cerebral oxygen supply and demand. Retrograde insertion of the $S_{JV}O_2$ catheter comes with the attendant risk of vascular injury and typically requires fluoroscopy to ensure correct placement. The normal range for $S_{JV}O_2$ is quoted to be 55–75% but may be as high as 85% in some normal individuals. $S_{JV}O_2 < 50\%$ is indicative of inadequate cerebral oxygenation. A normal or near-normal $S_{JV}O_2$ value may, however, mask regional cerebral ischemia. $S_{JV}O_2$ monitoring has high specificity but low sensitivity for the detection of cerebral ischemia. $S_{JV}O_2$ monitoring has been used to assess the adequacy of cerebral cooling prior to DHCA using a target $S_{JV}O_2$ of >95%.

Pharmacologic Options for Neuroprotection

Despite an improved understanding of the mechanisms underlying neuronal injury after cardiac surgery,

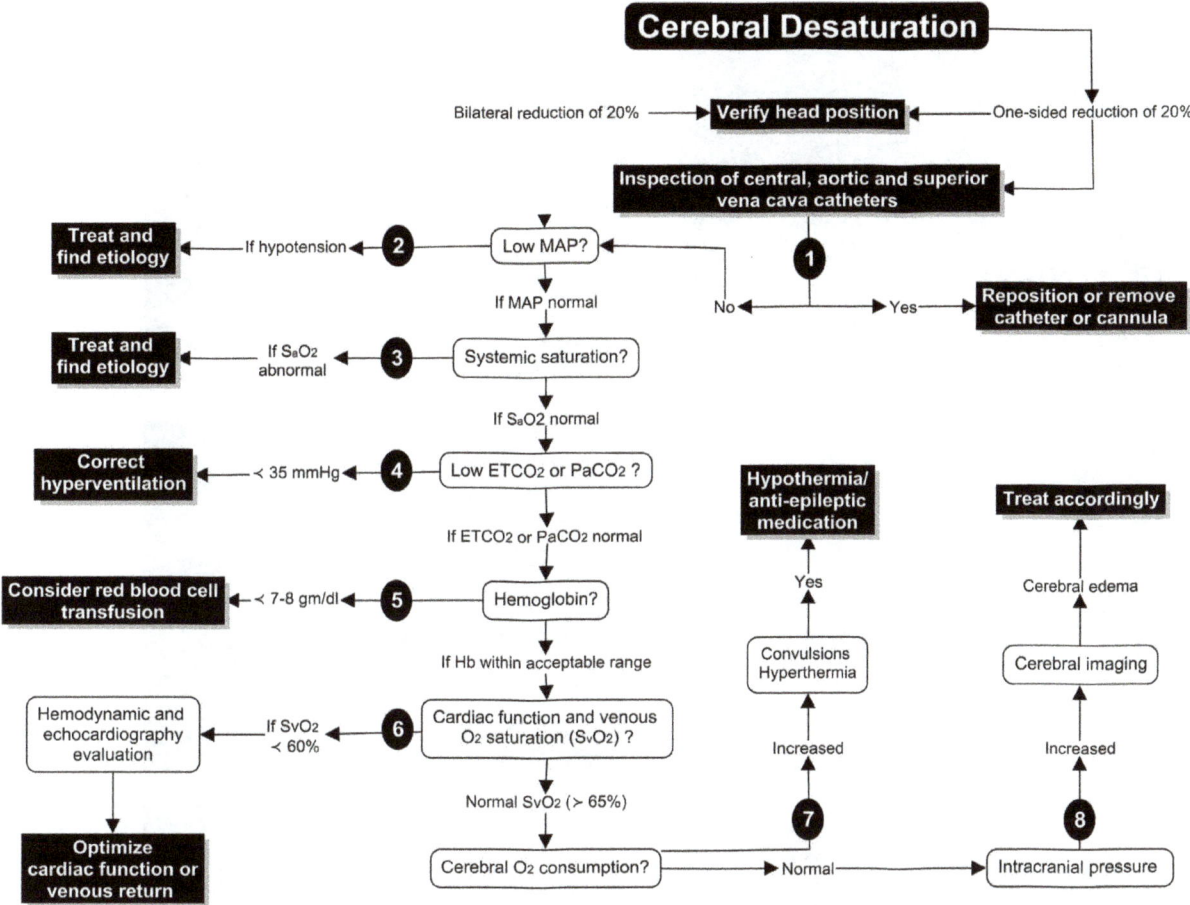

Figure 18.2 Intervention algorithm to manage decreases in cerebral oxygen saturation.
Step 1: Verify head position and position of vascular catheters. Step 2: Adjust blood pressure to within 20% of baseline values. Step 3: Increase inspired oxygen fraction to correct low oxygen saturation values. Step 4: Adjust ventilator parameters to increase arterial end tidal carbon dioxide levels within normal ranges (35–45 mmHg). Step 5: Consider giving blood transfusions to patients with low hemoglobin level when steps 1–4 have not increased cerebral oxygen saturation within 20% of baseline values. Step 6: Consider improving ventricular function in the presence of low output state. Step 7: Rule out hypothermia, seizures and light anesthesia. Step 8: Consider cerebral edema and increased intracranial pressure. Abbreviations: ETCO$_2$, end tidal carbon dioxide; Hb, hemoglobin; MAP, mean arterial pressure; O$_2$, oxygen; PaCO$_2$, arterial carbon dioxide tension; SaO$_2$, arterial oxygen saturation; SvO$_2$, mixed venous oxygen saturation. (Adapted from Deschamps et al.)

there are currently no recommendations regarding pharmacologic neuroprotection.

There is some evidence that the use of volatile anesthetics in cardiac anesthesia is associated with lower mortality compared to intravenous agents. A meta-analysis including 549 patients found that both calcium-binding protein S100β serum levels and cerebral oxygen metabolic rate were decreased after CPB in the group receiving inhaled anesthetic agents compared to those having total intravenous anesthesia. Patients in the inhalational anesthesia group had a higher intraoperative CBF and better postoperative Mini-Mental State Examination scores.

Inhalational anesthetic agents induce both pre- and post-conditioning neuroprotection via intracellular mechanisms. These include activation of adenosine receptors, K$_{ATP}$ channels and protein kinase C, inhibition of NF-kB activation and pro-inflammatory IL-1B cytokine production, as well as inhibition of N-Methyl D-aspartate (NMDA) receptors.

Ketamine is an NMDA receptor antagonist that decreases the intracellular calcium concentration, thereby reducing cerebral apoptosis. The exact mechanism remains unclear, but the neuroprotective effect of ketamine may be explained by the inhibition of inflammatory responses to surgery and CPB.

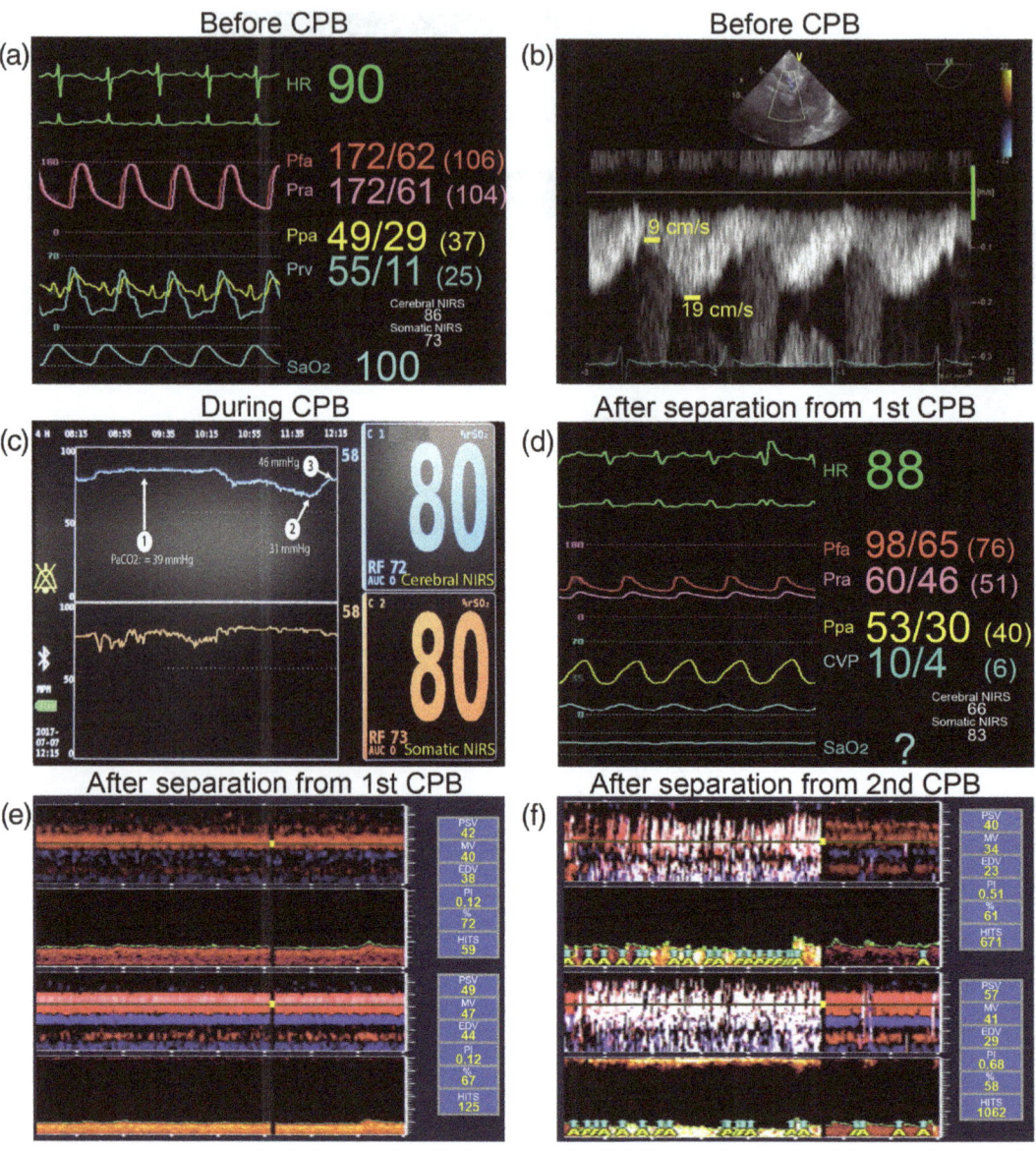

Figure 18.3 Hemodynamic monitoring including cerebral oximetry and transcranial Doppler. (a) Hemodynamic parameters prior to cardiopulmonary bypass (CPB). Pulmonary and systemic hypertension is present, with an abnormal systemic-to-pulmonary mean arterial pressure ratio (106/37 = 2.9; normal >4). The right ventricular (RV) pressure waveform (Prv, blue trace) shows an abnormal diastolic slope suggesting RV diastolic dysfunction. (b) Significant portal vein pulsatility ([19cm/s–9cm/s]/19cm/s = 52%; normal < 30%) was present in this patient initially. (c) Cerebral and somatic oxygen saturation monitoring using near-infrared spectroscopy (NIRS) during CPB. Baseline cerebral saturation was 72% on the right side and somatic saturation 73% on the right lower limb with an arterial carbon dioxide partial pressure ($PaCO_2$) of 39 mmHg (point 1). Cerebral desaturation to 66% upon initiation of CPB with unchanged somatic value (point 2) pointed to hypocapnia ($PaCO_2$ of 31 mmHg) as seen on subsequent arterial blood gas analysis; ventilation was corrected, and the cerebral saturation returned to baseline (point 3; $PaCO_2$ of 45 mmHg). (d) Hemodynamic parameters and transtemporal transcranial Doppler (TCD) ultrasound monitoring of both middle cerebral artery (MCA) blood velocities. (e) During the first CPB separation attempt. Note the significant gradient (mean of 25 mmHg) between the mean femoral arterial pressure (Pfa) and radial arterial pressure (Pra). The increase in the pulmonary artery pressure (Ppa) was secondary to aortic prosthetic valvular dysfunction. Transtemporal TCD velocities of both MCA after the first (e) and second (f) separation from CPB. Note the absence of high-intensity transient signals (HITS) upon the first separation attempt (59 and 125). (f) A significant increase in HITS was present upon the second CPB separation attempt (671 and 1062). This preceded the development of right ventricular dysfunction and implicated air embolization to the right coronary artery. Abbreviations: AUC, area under the curve; CVP, central venous pressure; EDV, end-diastolic velocity; HR, heart rate; MV, mean velocity; $PaCO_2$, arterial carbon dioxide partial pressure; PI, pulsatility index; PSV, peak systolic velocity; RF, baseline reference value; SaO_2, arterial oxygen saturation. (Adapted from Azzam et al.)

Ketamine also suppresses NF-kB expression and may therefore reduce the expression of genes encoding pro-inflammatory cytokines such as interleukin (IL)-6 and IL-8. A prospective randomized controlled study of 58 patients undergoing cardiac surgery with CPB proposed that the use of an intravenous bolus of ketamine (0.5 mg/kg) during anesthetic induction attenuates postoperative delirium. The authors hypothesize that ketamine may trigger a prolonged effect that renders NMDA receptors less susceptible to activation by ischemia and reperfusion injury during the postoperative period. These results were not supported in a larger multicenter, double-blind trial of 672 patients undergoing cardiac and non-cardiac surgery under general anesthesia. Ketamine was administered at low dose or high dose and compared to a placebo group. This second study did not demonstrate an effect on the incidence of postoperative delirium but showed an increase in the incidence of postoperative hallucinations and nightmares in both ketamine groups compared to the placebo group.

The neuroprotective effects of propofol remain unclear. Some of the evidence suggests that propofol protects neurons against mild ischemic injury by decreasing activity via gamma-aminobutyric acid (GABA) receptor activation, inhibition of NMDA receptors and reduction of calcium, sodium and potassium ion channel transport. In a prospective study of patients undergoing CABG on CPB, 40 patients were randomized to receive either propofol or desflurane during the anesthetic induction. The authors demonstrated that patients receiving propofol had lower S100β serum levels compared to desflurane anesthesia and suggest that propofol may thus reduce cerebral injury.

Calcium channel blockers such as nimodipine are thought to confer some neuroprotective effects by decreasing vasospasm after subarachnoid hemorrhage. Conversely, in one study including patients undergoing valve replacement surgery, nimodipine was believed to promote intracerebral hemorrhagic events through vasodilatation and antiplatelet effects.

Animal and in vitro studies suggest that lidocaine may protect against brain hypoxia and ischemia through multiple mechanisms. These include reduction of residual metabolism, decreased neuronal membrane depolarization, preservation of cerebral blood flow and modulation of excitotoxic cascades. In a randomized controlled trial of 277 patients undergoing cardiac surgery with CPB, low doses of intravenous lidocaine seem to have a protective effect in non-diabetic patients, while diabetic patients were more likely to develop postoperative neurocognitive dysfunction if they received lidocaine. The authors hypothesize that this detrimental effect in diabetic patients may be linked to lidocaine metabolism, more specifically its elimination through demethylation pathways, which are deficient in patients with diabetes. In a small randomized controlled study of 65 patients undergoing CABG, patients who had received a lidocaine infusion at the induction of anesthesia had less cognitive dysfunction after surgery. A follow-up study of 158 patients was not able to confirm any of the previous findings. Preliminary results of a larger trial currently underway suggest that an intraoperative lidocaine infusion does not confer any neuroprotective effects.

It is well known that surgery on CPB generates a cascade of inflammatory reactions due to activation of the complement system, leukocytes and pro-inflammatory cytokines. Corticosteroids given prior to commencing CPB or as part of the prime may help suppress systemic inflammation and have been shown to reduce postoperative neuron-specific enolase and S100β serum levels. As with other CPB related indications, the usefulness of glucocorticoids as a neuroprotective agent remains subject to debate.

Barbiturates are used as intravenous anesthetic induction agents. In some centers they are given as neuroprotective agents during DHCA. Barbiturates decrease the cerebral metabolic rate, lower cerebral oxygen consumption, and therefore provide protection during ischemia. The use of thiopental during DHCA seems to provide cerebral protection. When administered prior to DHCA, however, the available evidence suggests that thiopental may deplete the cerebral energy state before arrest, which may lead to ischemia and poorer neurological outcome.

Over the past decades, perioperative statin therapy before cardiac surgery has garnered interest. A retrospective study of 6,813 patients undergoing coronary artery bypass surgery concluded that patients who were given the combination of statin and beta-blockers before surgery had lower odds of postoperative stroke. Conversely, two retrospective studies including 9,430 patients did not find an association between statin use and reduced rates of neurologic complications following cardiac surgery.

Table 18.2. Summary of the recommendations for temperature management during cardiopulmonary bypass from the Society of Thoracic Surgeons, the Society of Cardiovascular Anesthesiologists and the American Society of ExtraCorporeal Technology

1. Optimal site for temperature monitoring

1.1. The oxygenator arterial outlet blood temperature is recommended to be used as a surrogate for cerebral temperature measurement during CPB. (Class 1, Level C)

1.2. To accurately monitor cerebral perfusate temperature during warming, it should be assumed that the oxygenator arterial outlet blood temperature underestimates cerebral perfusate temperature. (Class 1, Level C)

1.3. Pulmonary artery or nasopharyngeal temperature recording is reasonable for core temperature measurement. (Class IIa, Level C)

2. Avoidance of hyperthermia

2.1. Surgical teams should limit arterial outlet blood temperature to less than 37°C to avoid cerebral hyperthermia. (Class 1, Level C)

3. Peak cooling temperature gradient and cooling rate

3.1. Temperature gradients between the arterial outlet and venous inflow on the oxygenator during CPB cooling should not exceed 10°C to avoid generation of gaseous emboli. (Class 1, Level C)

4. Peak warming temperature gradient and rewarming rate

4.1. Temperature gradients between the arterial outlet and venous inflow on the oxygenator during CPB rewarming should not exceed 10°C to avoid outgassing when warm blood is returned to the patient. (Class 1, Level C)

4.2. Rewarming when arterial blood outlet temperature ≥ 30°C:

4.2.1. To achieve the desired temperature for separation from bypass, it is reasonable to maintain a temperature gradient between the arterial outlet and the venous inflow temperature of 4°C or less. (Class IIa, Level B)

4.2.2. To achieve the desired temperature for separation from bypass, it is reasonable to maintain a rewarming rate of 0.5°C/min or less. (Class IIa, Level B)

4.3. Rewarming when arterial blood outlet temperature < 30°C:

4.3.1. To achieve the desired temperature for separation from bypass, it is reasonable to maintain a maximal gradient of 10°C between the arterial outlet and venous inflow temperature. (Class IIa, Level C)

Magnesium is a non-competitive blocker of the NMDA glutamate receptor that modulates calcium, sodium and potassium ion influx. Magnesium sulfate decreases inflammatory cytokine levels and reduces the effect of hypoxia, therefore preventing cell death. A systematic review of seven studies with a total of 1,164 patients was conducted to present evidence of the neuroprotective effects of magnesium in adults with cardiac arrest or undergoing cardiac surgery. This review concludes that magnesium administration during cardiac surgery may improve functional neurological outcomes in patients who undergo cardiac surgery on CPB. The dosing regimen of magnesium varied between studies, with a maximum of 5 g in a 24-hour period.

Mannitol is a potent osmotic diuretic and reduces cerebral edema. It is also a free radical scavenger that may be beneficial after cerebral ischemia. Data

support mannitol administration, there is some evidence that it lowers 30-day mortality after acute type A aortic dissection. Many centers routinely use mannitol as part of their priming fluids for every cardiac case done on CPB.

Temperature Management and Cerebral Morbidity

Most elective cardiac surgery are done at mild hypothermia, between 34 and 36°C, or at normothermia; more complex cases are often done at moderate hypothermia, 28–32°C, to improve end-organ tolerance to ischemia.

Although there are various sites to measure core or cerebral temperature, it is now recommended to use the oxygenator arterial outlet blood temperature as a surrogate for cerebral temperature. During cooling, the difference between arterial outlet and venous inflow blood temperature should not exceed 10°C to discourage the formation of gaseous microemboli. During rewarming, the arterial outlet blood temperature should be limited to 37°C to avoid cerebral hyperthermia. Rapid rewarming and cerebral temperature in excess of 37°C are known to cause poor neurological outcomes. Table 18.2 summarizes the recommendations on temperature management from the Society of Thoracic Surgeons, the Society of Cardiovascular Anesthesiologists and the American Society of ExtraCorporeal Technology. Chapters 7 and 9 provide more in-depth discussion of this topic.

Epiaortic Ultrasound Scanning of the Ascending Aorta

The necessity of manipulating the ascending aorta for cannulation as well as complete cross-clamping, partial clamping or both has long been recognized as a significant source of cerebral emboli during cardiac surgery. In some cases atherosclerotic changes can be detected by carefully palpating the vessel, however this method is unreliable. For this reason an increasing number of surgeons advocate using epiaortic ultrasound (EAU) to identify areas of the ascending aorta that are free of disease and to allow safe cannulation and placement of clamps in adjacent disease free areas. A recent review including 11,496 patients showed the rate of stroke in CABG patients who underwent EAU to be significantly improved compared to those who did not (0.6% versus 1.9%).

Neurological complications after cardiac surgery are unfortunately common and generally the result of a combination of multiple factors. Both embolic and ischemic etiologies can adversely impact neurological outcome. Blood pressure control is essential to reduce the incidence of cerebral hypoperfusion and ischemic stroke, as is good temperature management during cooling and rewarming as well as careful manipulation of the ascending aorta for placement of cannulas and clamps. Despite some significant limitations, cerebral oxygen saturation can be utilized to assess cerebral perfusion and oxygenation. Multiple attempts to find a pharmacologic treatment to prevent neurologic injury have been unsuccessful.

Suggested Further Reading

1. Liu Y, Chen K, Mei W. Neurological complications after cardiac surgery: anesthetic considerations based on outcome evidence. *Curr Opin Anaesthesiol* 2019; 32: 563–567.

2. Joshi B, Ono M, Brown C et al. Predicting the limits of cerebral autoregulation during cardiopulmonary bypass. *Anesth Analg* 2012; 114: 503–510.

3. Sun X, Lindsay J, Monsein LH et al. Silent brain injury after cardiac surgery: a review: cognitive dysfunction and magnetic resonance imaging diffusion-weighted imaging findings. *J Am Coll Cardiol* 2012; 60: 791–797.

4. Vedel AG, Holmgaard F, Rasmussen LS et al. High-target versus low-target blood pressure management during cardiopulmonary bypass to prevent cerebral injury in cardiac surgery patients: a randomized controlled trial. *Circulation* 2018; 137: 1770–1780.

5. Hogue CW, Brown CH 4th, Hori D et al. Personalized blood pressure management during cardiac surgery with cerebral autoregulation monitoring: a randomized trial. *Semin Thorac Cardiovasc Surg* 2021; 33: 429–438.

6. Lewis C, Parulkar SD, Bebawy J et al. Cerebral neuromonitoring during cardiac surgery: a critical appraisal with an emphasis on near-infrared spectroscopy. *J Cardiothorac Vasc Anesth* 2018; 32: 2313–2322.

7. Biancari F, Santini F, Tauriainen T et al. Epiaortic ultrasound to prevent stroke in coronary artery bypass grafting. *Ann Thorac Surg.* 2020 January;109(1): 294–301.

8. Chen F, Duan G, Wu Z et al. Comparison of the cerebroprotective effect of inhalation anaesthesia and total intravenous anaesthesia in patients undergoing cardiac surgery with cardiopulmonary bypass: a systematic review and meta-analysis. *BMJ Open* 2017; 7: e014629.

9. Hudetz JA, Patterson KM, Iqbal Z et al. Ketamine attenuates delirium after cardiac surgery with cardiopulmonary bypass. *J Cardiothorac Vasc Anesth* 2009; 23: 651–657.

10. Engelman R, Baker RA, Likosky DS et al. The Society of Thoracic Surgeons, The Society of Cardiovascular Anesthesiologists, and The American Society of ExtraCorporeal Technology: Clinical practice guidelines for cardiopulmonary bypass – temperature management during cardiopulmonary bypass. *J Cardiothorac Vasc Anesth* 2015; 29: 1104–1113.

Renal Morbidity Associated with Cardiopulmonary Bypass

Juan Pablo Domecq and Robert C Albright

Acute kidney injury (AKI) is the most common major complication after cardiac surgery. The incidence of cardiac surgery-associated AKI (CSA-AKI) varies between 5 and 40% and leads to dramatically worse outcomes. The incidence of CSA-AKI requiring renal replacement therapy (RRT) after coronary artery bypass grafting (CABG) alone is roughly 1%. After valve surgery or combined CABG plus valve surgery, the risk of requiring RRT increases to 1.7 and 3.3% respectively. Regardless of its reversibility, CSA-AKI has been associated with increased mortality and risk of developing chronic or end-stage renal disease, and consequently generating substantial cost as well.

Definitions

AKI is the abrupt decline in the glomerular filtration rate (GFR), resulting in the accumulation of metabolic waste products and in the dysregulation of extracellular volume and electrolytes that normally would be excreted by the kidney.

For many years there was neither a standard definition nor staging system for AKI. In 2004, Bellomo et al proposed the RIFLE criteria (Risk, Injury, Failure, Loss and End-Stage Kidney Disease). They were revised in 2012, when the Acute Kidney Injury Network (AKIN) proposed a more sensitive definition for AKI, taking into account that even small elevations in serum creatinine are associated with increased mortality. In 2012 a multidisciplinary group proposed "The Kidney Disease: Improving Global Outcomes (KDIGO) definition and staging system," which is now widely used in research and clinical practice. Criteria for the diagnosis and staging of AKI are summarized in Table 19.1

These standard criteria are limited by their reliance on creatinine as the serum marker of decreased renal function (i.e. decreased GFR). Serum creatinine is a suboptimal biomarker for AKI recognition as it often lags 48–72 hours behind the onset of kidney injury. Abnormal serum creatinine is also confounded by its dependence on tubular secretion and its relationship to muscle mass, catabolism and fluid status. Fluid overload may negatively confound serum creatinine's ability to indicate AKI. CPB priming volume and/or heart failure often lead to fluid overload in the perioperative period, which might result in an underestimate of the incidence and severity of AKI by falsely lowering serum creatinine.

Several other biomarkers for the detection of AKI have been proposed:

- The increase of the serum and urine neutrophil gelatinase-associated lipocalin (NGAL) precedes an increase in creatinine by over two days. NGAL is an excellent predictor of AKI in the pediatric cardiac surgical population, and recent data has suggested that NGAL may also be of value in adult patients in the perioperative period.
- The combination of urine metalloproteinases-2/insulin-like growth factor-binding protein 7 (TIMP-2/IGFBP7) is FDA approved to assess the risk of moderate or severe AKI in critically ill adults post cardiac surgery.

Epidemiology and Outcomes Associated with AKI

Depending on the adopted definition, the incidence of CSA-AKI is up to 30% after cardiac surgery, while the requirement for RRT ranges between 1 and 6%. Any AKI occurring in the perioperative period carries an increased risk of short and long-term mortality (see Figure 19.1).

Even slight decreases in GFR imply an increased mortality risk: an increased mortality risk of four to five-fold with any increase in serum creatinine has been reported among patients followed for one year. A 30% decrease in GFR during the perioperative period is associated with a 6% overall mortality over

Table 19.1. Overview over the most commonly used renal failure scores

Classification	Definition of AKI	Stage	Serum Creatinine Criteria for AKI Staging
RIFLE	Increase in SCr ≥50% within 7 days	Risk	Increased creatinine x 1.5 or GFR decrease >25% or UO < 0.5 ml/kg/h for 6 h
		Injury	Increased creatinine x 2 or GFR decrease >50% or UO < 0.5 ml/kg/h for 12 h
		Failure	Increased creatinine x 3 or creatinine ≥ 4 mg/dL (Acute rise of ≥ 0.5 mg/dL) or GFR decrease >75% or anuria for 12 h
		Loss	Persistent ARF – complete loss of kidney function> 4 weeks
		End-Stage Kidney Disease	End-stage kidney disease > 3 months
AKIN score	Increase in SCr by ≥0.3 mg/dl or ≥50% within 48 h	1	Increase of ≥ 0.3 mg/dl or to 1.5–1.9 times baseline or UO < 0.5 ml/kg/h for 6 h
		2	To 2–2.9 times baseline or UO < 0.5 ml/kg/h for 12 h
		3	To ≥ 3 times baseline or ≥ 0.5 mg/dl increase to at least 4.0 mg/dl or the initiation of RRT or UO < 0.3 mL/kg/h for 24 h or anuria for 12 h
KDIGO score	Increase in SCr by ≥0.3 mg/dL within 48 hours, or increase in SCr to ≥1.5 times baseline, or UO <0.5 mL/kg/hour for 6 h	1	Increase in SCr ≥ 0.3 mg/dl within 48 h or to 1.5–1.9 times baseline or UO <0.5 ml/kg/h for 6–12 h
		2	Increase in SCr to 2.0–2.9 x baseline or UO < 0.5 ml/kg/h for ≥12 h
		3	Increase in SCr to 3.0 x baseline or at least 4.0 mg/dl or UOP <0.3 mL/kg/hour for ≥ 24 h, or anuria for ≥12 h, or initiation of RRT

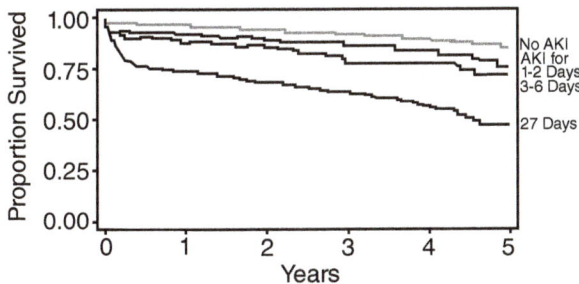

Figure 19.1 Survival by duration of acute kidney injury (AKI). The proportion of patients surviving from the time of cardiac surgery is plotted by the categories for the duration of AKI. From Giovanni Mariscalco, Roberto Lorusso, Carmelo Dominici et al. Acute Kidney Injury: a relevant complication after cardiac surgery; The Annals of Thoracic Surgery; Volume 92; Issue 4; pages 1539–1547 (October 2011)

the subsequent year, as compared with 0.4% mortality without an accompanying AKI. When RRT is required for AKI, recovery of renal function sufficient to discontinue chronic RRT occurs in less than half of these patients, leading to a dramatic decrease in quality of life and longevity (20% mortality rate per year).

Pathophysiology

The underlying mechanisms of CSA-AKI remain poorly understood and appear to be multifactorial. Cardiac surgery often leads to renal hypoperfusion due to CPB induced free radical production, increase in inflammatory

185

mediators, pigment nephropathy after hemolysis, activation of the complement cascade, low flow and hypoperfusion, or activation of the sympathetic and renin-angiotensin-aldosterone (RAA) system. Cardiac surgery is often complicated by bleeding and vasodilatory shock, both of which are associated with reduced renal perfusion.

If renal hypoperfusion persists long enough structural tubular injury will occur. Paradoxically, improving renal perfusion can perpetuate renal damage by inducing ischemia-reperfusion injury. Restoring renal perfusion in already injured renal cells induces opening of the mitochondrial permeability transition pore and increases the production of reactive oxygen species, the release of pro-inflammatory cytokines, neutrophils, macrophages and lymphocytes, causing renal parenchymal cellular infiltration.

Pulsatile blood flow is important to achieve adequate renal blood flow in the renal cortex and to preserve oxygen delivery to cortical and medullary areas of the kidney. Non-pulsatile perfusion increases renin secretion, leading to elevation of the systemic vascular resistance and redistribution of intra-renal blood flow. However evidence supporting a clinical benefit is limited.

Damage to red blood cells is common during pulsatile CPB, often seen as "pink urine." Hemolysis and increased levels of plasma-free hemoglobin encourage the production of reactive oxygen species and deposits of Tamm Horsfall protein in the renal collecting system. Patients developing CSA-AKI can have up to double the level the plasma-free hemoglobin at the end of CPB compared to those with no renal injury, suggesting that hemolysis significantly contributes to the incidence of renal failure.

Risk Factors

Generally, the risk factors for developing AKI can be separated into those that are patient-related versus those that are procedure and perfusion-related. Table 19.2 provides a summary of the main risks.

Patient-Related Factors

The single most important patient-related factor predicting AKI is preexisting chronic kidney disease (CKD). There is an overall 10–20% risk of AKI requiring RRT among cardiac surgical patients with a preoperative serum creatinine of 2–4 mg/dl. The

Table 19.2. Risk factors for postop AKI

Patient-related	CKD
	Diabetes mellitus
	Female sex
	Advanced age
	Obesity
	Preop heart failure
	Poor preop functional state
	Peripheral vascular disease
	Anemia
Procedure-related	CPB
	Urgent or emergency surgery
	Postop cardiogenic shock
	Bleeding (Hct < 24%)
	Transfusion
	Type of surgery:
	Valve < valve + CABG < redo surgery < aortic surgery other than ascending aorta
Perfusion-related	CPB duration
	Hemodilution
	Rewarming
	Oxygen delivery

risk of requiring RRT increases to nearly 28% with a preoperative serum creatinine greater than 4 mg/dl.

Even subclinical CKD is an independent risk factor for RRT in cardiac surgical patients. Patients with moderately reduced creatinine clearance (CrCl <60 ml/minute) have a similar risk as those undergoing redo sternotomy, considered by many a profound risk factor for perioperative RRT.

Other patient-related risk factors include preexisting diabetes mellitus, female gender, increased age, obesity, preoperative congestive heart failure and low ejection fraction, peripheral vascular disease, preoperative balloon pump requirements, hypoalbuminemia, chronic obstructive pulmonary disease, emergency surgery, anemia and, although somewhat controversial, decreased serum ferritin level (see Table 19.2)

Procedure-Related Factors

The type of cardiac surgical procedure plays a substantial role in renal outcomes and the need for RRT after surgery. Procedures such as valve replacement, valve repair, combined valve and coronary surgery, redo surgery and aortic arch surgery are associated with a substantially higher risk of CSA-AKI and a greater incidence of the need for RRT. As expected, patients undergoing urgent or emergency surgery have a higher incidence of AKI and need for RRT.

Low hematocrit values (<23%) during CPB are associated with an increased incidence of postoperative renal failure. Paradoxically, blood transfusion during bypass is also associated with developing renal failure. Both seem to be confounders to each other – the risk of renal failure doubles when hematocrit levels <23% occur in transfused patients.

Perfusion-Related Risk Factors

Despite preserving cardiac output, the use of CPB is associated with CSA-AKI.

The risks and benefits of several perfusion related interventions need to be considered:

- Temperature management – Hypothermia is often being used for organ protection during CPB through reduction of metabolic activity and amelioration of ischemic stress. However, there is evidence that hypothermia, particularly when the CPB inflow temperature is <27°C, may contribute to renal injury. It is also suggested that the temperature of the perfusate, rather than nasopharyngeal or bladder temperature, is the determining factor.
- Rewarming – Returning the patient to normothermia before weaning from CPB appears to equally influence the risk of renal injury. A large cohort study of nearly 8,500 patients demonstrated that an oxygenator arterial outlet temperature of >37°C was independently associated with developing AKI, while temperatures of 36 and 36.5°C were not.
- Hemodilution – As seen above, a low hematocrit during CPB is an independent risk factor for developing AKI postoperatively. The relative risk increases by 7% for each 1% decrease of nadir hematocrit on-pump. Strategies to minimize prime volume and other blood conservation techniques are discussed in Chapters 5, 8 and 16.
- Oxygen delivery – Low oxygen delivery while on bypass has been demonstrated to be an independent risk factor of the development of CSA-AKI. Ensuring that the NADIR oxygen delivery index (DO_{2i}) is kept above

$260–300$ ml/min/m^2 is reported to reduce the risk of developing kidney injury.

- Duration of CPB – Longer CPB times are associated with a higher incidence of developing CSA-AKI. A meta-analysis of nearly 12,500 patients showed that the mean difference of CPB duration between the AKI and non-AKI group was 25.65 minutes. A recent analysis of nearly 4000 patients confirmed these findings and demonstrated that the risk increased exponentially for patients with an estimated GFR of <30 ml/min/1.73m^2 (see Figure 19.2).
- Hemolysis – Blood cells' exposure to artificial surfaces and to shear forces during CPB can lead to varying degrees of cell lysis, potentially more so with pulsatile than with non-pulsatile flow. The mechanical destruction of erythrocytes and subsequent release of plasma-free hemoglobin can cause the occlusion of renal tubules and ultimately tubular cell necrosis.
- Pulsatile/non-pulsatile flow – Pulsatile flow during CPB has been advocated in some quarters as a means to reduce the incidence of CSA-AKI. There is an equipoise of low-grade evidence showing advantages and no change in renal outcomes when compared to laminar flow CPB. A 2019 retrospective review of 2,500 patients, however, found that there is either no association between pulsatile flow and reduced kidney injury or that the difference is extremely small.
- Pressure/flow – To this day the argument whether blood pressure or pump flow is more important to decrease the incidence of renal or other organ injury is not settled. There is an equipoise in the evidence and research is ongoing. An emerging, experimental concept is measuring bladder urine PO_2 and adjusting flow and/or pressure according to its value.

Blood Flow and Oxygen Delivery to the Kidneys

Autoregulation in the kidneys keeps blood flow constant despite variations in blood pressure in the range from 80 to 200 mmHg. The kidneys receive approximately 20% of the total cardiac output (about 1 L/minute). Oxygen delivery thus exceeds 80 ml/minute/100 g tissue. The distribution of blood flow within the kidney is not

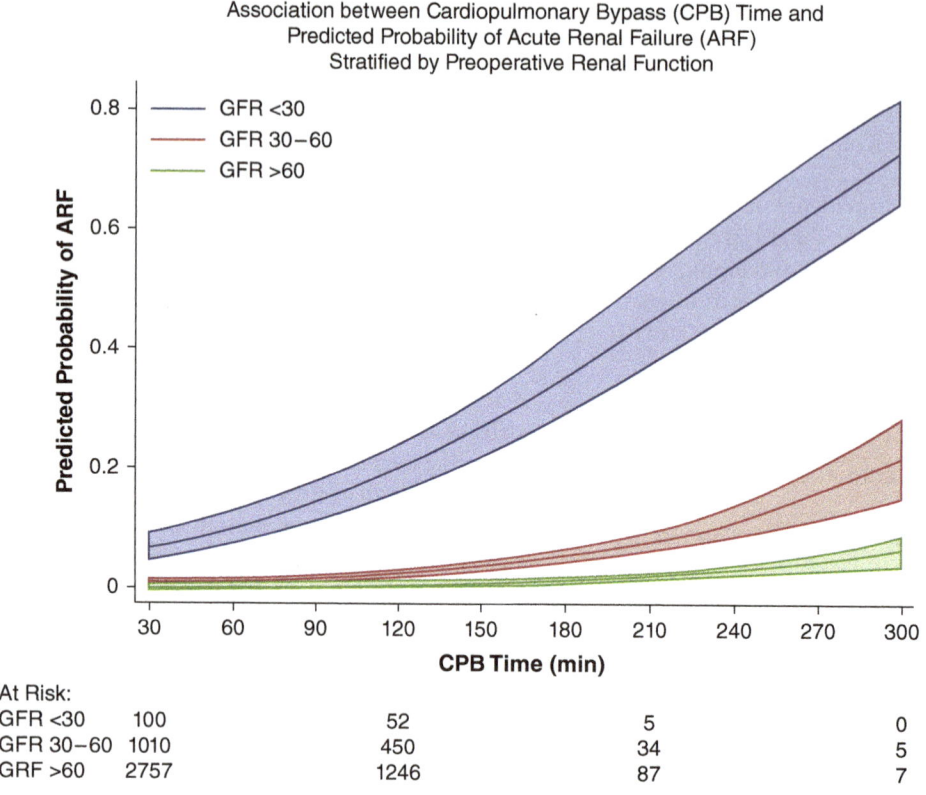

Association between Cardiopulmonary Bypass (CPB) Time and
Predicted Probability of Acute Renal Failure (ARF)
Stratified by Preoperative Renal Function

At Risk:

GFR <30	100	52	5	0
GFR 30–60	1010	450	34	5
GRF >60	2757	1246	87	7

Figure 19.2 From correlation of cardiopulmonary bypass duration with acute renal failure after cardiac surgery. (Axtell, Andrea L et al. *The Journal of Thoracic and Cardiovascular Surgery*, Volume 159, Issue 1, 170–178.e2.)

uniform, with the cortex receiving more than 90% (about 5 ml/minute/g) of total blood flow; therefore, there is lower blood flow (about 0.03 ml/minute/g) to the renal medulla. Although a high percentage of blood goes to the cortex, the cortex extracts only about 18% of total oxygen delivered to it. On the other hand, the medullary region has a far smaller blood flow, but has a far greater extraction (about 79% of the delivered oxygen), as a result of the high oxygen requirement for tubular reabsorption of sodium and chloride ions. Renal medullary hypoxia is an obligatory part of the process of urinary concentration as oxygen diffuses from arterial to venous vasa recta and the medullary thick ascending limb requires a large amount of oxygen to generate an osmotic gradient to maximize the concentration of the urine. These cells are therefore uniquely vulnerable to anoxic damage. Total renal oxygen consumption is less than 10% of total body utilization, and thus there is a low arteriovenous oxygen content difference (1.5 ml O_2 /100 ml blood). The low oxygen extraction by the kidney suggests that supply

exceeds demand and that there should be an adequate oxygen reserve. However, the kidney is highly sensitive to reduction in perfusion with AKI being a frequent complication of hypotension. The sensitivity of the kidney to damage as a result of hypoperfusion, despite its low overall oxygen consumption, is related to the physiological intra-renal oxygen gradient. Within the kidney, the cortex and medulla have widely disparate blood flows and patterns of oxygen extraction (see Figure 19.3).

Medullary oxygenation is normally strictly balanced by a series of control mechanisms which match regional oxygen supply and consumption. Failure of these controls renders the medullary region susceptible to acute or repeated episodes of hypoxic injury, which may lead to acute tubular necrosis (ATN). The differing requirements of cortex and medulla for blood flow and oxygen result in oxygen tension in the cortex of about 50 mmHg higher than that of the inner medulla. This explains why renal tubules are

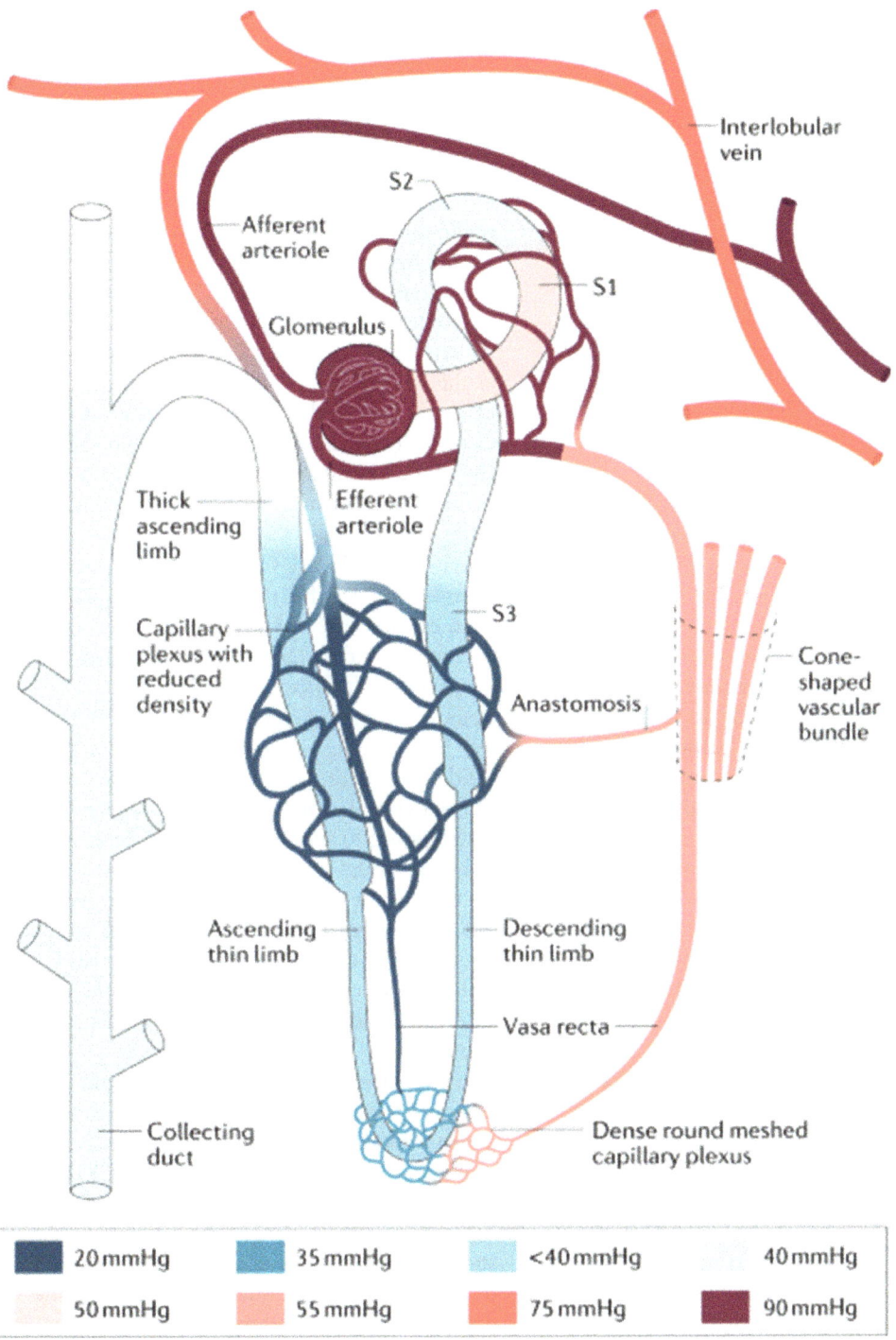

Figure 19.3 Distribution of renal blood flow and oxygen levels throughout the kidney. (From Scholz, H, Boivin, FJ, Schmidt-Ott, KM et al. Kidney physiology and susceptibility to acute kidney injury: implications for renoprotection. *Nat Rev Nephrol* 17, 335–349 (2021).)

extremely vulnerable to hypoxic injury and why ATN can be induced by as little as a 40–50% decrease in renal blood flow.

Prevention of AKI

Any strategies to minimize the risk of CSA-AKI need to focus on avoiding decreased oxygen delivery to the kidney, as it is the major mechanism of renal injury in patients undergoing cardiac surgery. The KDIGO guidelines recommend a bundle comprising of:

- discontinuation of nephrotoxic agents
- optimization of blood glycemic control
- close monitoring of serum creatinine level and urine output
- maintaining hemodynamic stability.

The PrevAKI trial published in 2017 showed that implementation of the KDIGO guidelines bundle compared against standard care resulted in a 23% relative reduction in CSA-AKI frequency. The implementation of the bundle led to significantly improved hemodynamic parameters, higher inotrope use, less hyperglycemia and reduced use of renin-angiotensin system (RAS) blockers compared to controls. However, there was no difference in secondary outcomes such as RRT requirements, ICU and hospital stay or all-cause mortality at 30, 60 and 90 days.

The discontinuation of nephrotoxic agents for AKI prevention has been previously investigated. A systematic review of six studies with 1,663 enrolled participants found low quality evidence that discontinuing ACE inhibitors or angiotensin receptor blockers prior to coronary angiography and cardiac surgery may reduce the incidence of AKI.

As the causes of AKI are multifactorial, a single intervention is unlikely to demonstrate significant benefits, but a combination of different non-pharmacological and pharmacological interventions is likely to offer better results in reducing the risk of CSA-AKI.

Non-pharmacological Interventions

As in any other type of AKI, ensuring adequate renal perfusion and adjusting potentially nephrotoxic medications are general measures to prevent CSA-AKI and need to be assessed for every patient individually.

- Avoidance of cardiopulmonary bypass: Off-pump cardiac surgery has been advocated to mitigate some issues related to CPB, such as the systemic inflammatory response, non-pulsatile flow and the impact of endothelial damage. A recent systematic review of 33 randomized controlled trials (17,322 patients) evaluated the use of off-pump coronary artery bypass (OPCABG) grafting surgery. OPCABG was associated with a 14% relative risk reduction of CSA-AKI compared to on-pump CABG surgery. However, no difference was noted in the risk of RRT or death. Long-term renal outcomes have also been studied showing no benefit from OPCABG. Current guidelines, such as the 2018 guidelines from the European Society of Cardiology and European Association for Cardio-Thoracic Surgery, suggest that OPCABG should be considered for subgroups of high-risk patients and performed by experienced off-pump teams.

- Pulsatile flow during CPB has been advocated as a means to reduce the incidence of CSA-AKI. There is an equipoise of low-grade evidence showing advantages and no change in renal outcomes when compared to laminar flow CPB.

- Remote ischemic preconditioning (RIPC): RIPC was initially considered a great promise, but later yielded conflicting results. RIPC is the induction of brief episodes of ischemia and reperfusion in distal tissues to induce the natural defenses to ischemia in the kidney and other organs to prevent further damage during the surgery. A Cochrane review including 28 RCTs with 6,851 patients showed that, disappointingly, RIPC leads to minimal or no difference in the incidence of CSA-AKI, need for RRT, length of hospital stay or mortality.

- Renal replacement therapy: Prophylactic RRT has been proposed for patients with preexisting advanced kidney disease. A small pilot RCT evaluated 88 non-dialysis dependent CKD patients and randomized them to either receiving hemodialysis three times before surgery or standard of care. The trial showed a 10-fold decrease in mortality but it did not affect the development of postoperative morbidities. Due to the small sample size and some methodological limitations further studies are required for a more accurate assessment of the effects of prophylactic dialysis in patients with underlying CKD undergoing cardiac surgery.

Pharmacological Interventions

Numerous pharmacological interventions to reduce the incidence and/or severity of CSA-AKI have been investigated over the years but for the most part showed no benefit. Levosimendan, statins, N-acetylcysteine, sodium bicarbonate, erythropoietin, theophylline, anti-oxidant supplements (selenium, zinc, vitamin C and vitamin B1), dexamethasone, pentoxyphyline, clonidine, diltiazem, dopamine, and melanocyte-stimulating hormone are among the interventions that have been studied but all have failed to demonstrate a reduction on CSA-AKI. It is important to highlight that hydroxyethyl starch has not only been associated with no benefits but an increase in mortality after CABG. A recent systematic review showed that the perioperative use of statins may be associated with an increased risk of CSA-AKI.

- Glycemic control: Intraoperative hyperglycemia is an independent risk factor for complications, including death, and increased ICU and hospital stay. Avoiding hyperglycemia with moderate, rather than tight, glycemic control, is recommended for patients undergoing cardiac surgery.

- Fluid management: The difficulty in achieving the right balance between fluid administration to optimize preload and preserve cardiac output on one side, and avoidance of fluid overload with pulmonary edema and excessive extracellular fluid accumulation on the other side, is key to avoiding CSA-AKI. Fluid overload worsens CSA-AKI and is associated with a higher risk for pulmonary edema and organ dysfunction.

- Liberal fluid administration pre-CPB has been shown to exacerbate bypass associated hemodilution to hematocrit <23% and leads to a higher rate of blood transfusion and postoperative renal failure.

- Diuretics and mannitol: Currently the recommendation is to avoid intraoperative loop diuretics as they increase oxygen consumption in the renal medulla.

  A recent systematic review found that the intraoperative use of mannitol, which is widely added to CPB priming fluids, cannot be considered an evidence-based intervention to prevent AKI.

- Inhaled anesthetics, propofol and dexmedetomidine: A systematic review of 58 trials including 6,105 patients undergoing cardiac surgery showed that inhaled anesthetics were associated with lower mortality, minimal reduction of the cardiac index and less vasoactive support compared to propofol. Another similar review in 2014 showed that inhaled anesthetics are potentially protective against CSA-AKI.

  Dexmedetomidine is a highly selective α2 adrenoceptor agonist, used for perioperative anxiolysis, sedation and analgesia. A number of small trials suggest that it reduces the incidence and severity of CSA-AKI after cardiac surgery. A recent randomized controlled trial evaluated the effects of dexmedetomidine on renal function in patients undergoing valve replacement against a placebo group. It found that the drug significantly increased intraoperative urine output and decreased postoperative incidence of AKI, however it did not report on the incidence of RRT.

- Fenoldopam: Fenoldopam is a selective agonist of dopamine D1 receptors and is responsible for relaxation of smooth muscle, vasodilatation and inhibition of tubular reabsorption of sodium in the kidney. The evidence supporting its use is equivocal. Some studies demonstrate that intraoperative fenoldopam may reduce CSA-AKI, others demonstrated no benefit but showed an increased number of hypotensive episodes.

- Avoiding potential nephrotoxins:

  o RAS blockers – The perioperative use of RAS blockers is controversial. Two systematic reviews found 29 and 13 observational studies demonstrating that patients who were continued on RAS blockers on the day of surgery had an increased risk of CSA-AKI, more episodes of intraoperative hypotension and higher mortality. Another review of three randomized controlled and three observational trials found low quality evidence that withdrawal of RAS at least 24 hours prior to cardiac surgery may reduce the incidence of CSA-AKI. These facts plus the unlikely risk of increasing cardiovascular events after a short, temporary suspension of RAS blockers led experts to recommend stopping these drugs 24 hours before cardiac surgery.

  o iv contrast – Early cardiac surgery after contrast administration is also controversial. Several observational studies found a higher incidence of CSA-AKI when surgery was commenced within 24 hours of coronary angiography. It seems widely accepted that surgery should be delayed for 24–72 hours after contrast administration, the clinical situation permitting. There is some observational data suggesting that cardiac surgery can be performed safely within a day of contrast administration in appropriately selected patients with a low risk of AKI.

- Nonsteroidal anti-inflammatory drugs (NSAIDs) – It is generally recommended that NSAIDs should be avoided perioperatively in patients undergoing cardiac surgery. There is, however, more recent data showing that their use in CABG patients might be safe.

Management of Patients with Chronic Kidney Disease

The number of patients with chronic kidney disease or on dialysis presenting for cardiac surgery has steadily increased in the last decade. Their perioperative management is challenging, both clinically and logistically.

RRT-dependent Patients

Cardiac surgical patients with CKD who are already RRT-dependent should be dialyzed close to the time of operation; generally, this is best done in the 1–2 days preceding surgery, to optimize their metabolic and volume status. Arrangements should also be made for RRT to recommence in the early postoperative period. Intraoperative ultrafiltration can be used in case of emergency surgery or if additional fluid removal is needed. Zero balance ultrafiltration can help with removing toxins, electrolytes (particularly potassium after cardioplegia administration) or drugs. In some cases, RRT may be required in the immediate postoperative period to manage fluid balance as well as biochemical parameters.

There is no need to use normal saline instead of balanced solutions such as Lactated Ringer's to prime the CPB pump for patients with end-stage renal disease. The small amount of extra potassium (4–5 mEq/L) is unlikely to generate significant hyperkalemia, particularly compared to the large potassium load administered through cardioplegia. Also, large volumes of normal saline are associated with causing a hyperchloremic acidosis that in turn will aggravate any hyperkalemia.

Patients with Non-RRT-dependent CKD

Patients with chronic renal impairment, but who do not have sufficiently advanced renal disease to warrant RRT, may benefit from intraoperative hemofiltration/ultrafiltration while on CPB to optimize acid-base and electrolyte status during surgery. Such patients, as discussed above, have a higher likelihood of developing AKI in the postoperative period and may require RRT postoperatively until their renal function returns to a viable level.

CSA-AKI portends a grave outcome both acutely and in the long-term. As non-remediable demography and preexisting illnesses play such a large role in the development of perioperative kidney injury, appropriate identification of high-risk patients and preoperative counseling are critically important. All efforts should be undertaken to prevent adverse outcomes by maximizing general supportive measures and specifically avoiding nephrotoxins. Application of panels of biomarkers of AKI may offer some hope of earlier recognition and intervention. Prompt, but not rushed, initiation of medical and extracorporeal therapy, coordination of care among the multiple care teams and avoidance of further iatrogenic complications will maximize positive outcomes in these high-risk patients.

Suggested Further Reading

1. Cheungpasitporn W, Thongprayoon C, Kittanamongkolchai W et al. Comparison of renal outcomes in off-pump versus on-pump coronary artery bypass grafting: a systematic review and meta-analysis of randomized controlled trials. *Nephrology*. October 2015;20(10):727–735.

2. Chew STH, Hwang NC. Acute kidney injury after cardiac surgery: a narrative review of the literature. *J Cardiothorac Vasc Anesth*. August 7, 2018.

3. Cole SP. Stratification and risk reduction of perioperative acute kidney injury: an update. *Anesthesiol Clin*. December 2018;36(4):539–551.

4. Hoste EAJ, Vandenberghe W. Epidemiology of cardiac surgery-associated acute kidney injury.

Best Pract Res Clin Anaesthesiol. September 2017;31(3):299–303.

5. Kim WH, Hur M, Park SK et al. Pharmacological interventions for protecting renal function after cardiac surgery: a Bayesian network meta-analysis of comparative effectiveness. *Anaesthesia.* August 2018;73 (8):1019–1031.

6. Nadim MK, Forni LG, Bihorac A et al. Cardiac and vascular surgery-associated acute kidney injury: The 20th International Consensus Conference of the ADQI (Acute Disease Quality Initiative) Group. *J Am Heart Assoc.* June 1, 2018;7(11).

7. Wang Y, Bellomo R. Cardiac surgery-associated acute kidney injury: risk factors, pathophysiology and treatment. *Nat Rev Nephrol.* November 2017;13(11):697–711.

8. Whiting P, Morden A, Tomlinson LA et al. What are the risks and benefits of temporarily discontinuing medications to prevent acute kidney injury? A systematic review and meta-analysis. *BMJ open.* April 7, 2017;7 (4):e012674.

9. Ranucci M, Biagioli B, Scolletta S et al. Lowest hematocrit on cardiopulmonary bypass impairs the outcome in coronary surgery: nn Italian multicenter study from the National Cardioanesthesia Database. *Tex Heart Inst J.* 2006;33(3):300–305.

10. Newland RF, Baker RA, Mazzone AL et al. Perfusion downunder collaboration. rewarming temperature during cardiopulmonary bypass and acute kidney injury: a multicenter analysis. *Ann Thorac Surg.* May 2016;101(5):1655–1662.

Common and Uncommon Disasters during Cardiopulmonary Bypass

Gregory M Janelle, Jane Ottens and Michael Franklin

Cardiopulmonary bypass (CPB) is highly technical and complex. No matter the degree of team preparedness, accident and error can occur due to malfunction of equipment and/or human factors. Since its first successful clinical use in 1953 by John Gibbon, incremental improvements in the heart lung machine (HLM) – such as the introduction of low-level and bubble alarms, one-way valves, servo regulation of pump controllers along with the acceptance of a culture centered around safety – have resulted in a decline of perfusion-related accidents. In contrast to aviation, however, where many secondary systems are available should one fail, the modern day HLM is not designed with sufficient internal redundancy to compensate for many potential primary device failures. It is therefore imperative that a support system is in place and that countermeasures are practiced and employed to minimize any potential negative impact on our patients.

These safety practices need to be constantly reviewed and their implementation should be regularly rehearsed by all members of the intraoperative team and not only by the perfusion team. Safety practices such as the use of protocols, bypass checklists, failure modes and effects analyses (FMEAs) have been demonstrated to reduce the incidence of error and equipment fault. Where an error or a fault is detected, the repetitive nature of perfusion practice and the high degree of competency of trained perfusionists often lead to a "good catch" before patients actually come to harm.

Still, unforeseen events occur, no matter how much preparation is undertaken. Institutional protocols, compliance with instructions for use (IFUs) of equipment and step-by-step processes to deal with error and unforeseen events will minimize their impact.

Incident Reporting and Safety Culture

In 2000, James Reason devised a Swiss cheese model of accidents which portrays that multiple contributors (the holes in cheese slices) need to be in alignment for adverse events to occur. He also advocated that *"Incident reporting allows us to be aware of mishaps, incidents, near misses and are in fact 'free lessons' on safety."* For over 20 years the Australian and New Zealand College of Perfusionists (ANZCP) has been running a voluntary, de-identified perfusion incident reporting system (PIRS) for perfusion accidents (Australian and New Zealand Perfusion Incident Reporting System Version 1). This was first developed after the publication in 1997 of a survey, which found that incidents in the field of perfusion occur at a rate of 1:2,500 and are 10-fold more prevalent than incidents in anesthesia. Similar perfusion incident surveys have followed and the frequency of common and uncommon incidents seems to be fairly similar across continents and cultures. Recently the ANZCP updated PIRS, to incorporate the Safety 2 concept with a focus on what went well, rather than what went wrong (PIRS-2, https://anzcp.org/pirs-ii). Figures 20.1–20.4 give an overview of the most recent PRIS findings. Similarly, the Society of Clinical Perfusion Scientists of Great Britain and Ireland maintain a web based incident reporting system with archived safety reports documented.

Incident reports, while providing valuable insight into adverse events, are based on random events and cannot be used to measure safety (error rates) due to inherent potential bias. Event reports are low in number, submitted from a limited number of reporters and represent a snapshot of activity. These reports, however, highlight the error type and incidents that do occur. While the variety of errors that can occur is vast, this chapter includes a discussion of the most commonly reported perfusion incidents along with potential prevention strategies and treatment options.

A culture of safety dictates that all common and uncommon disasters that occur during

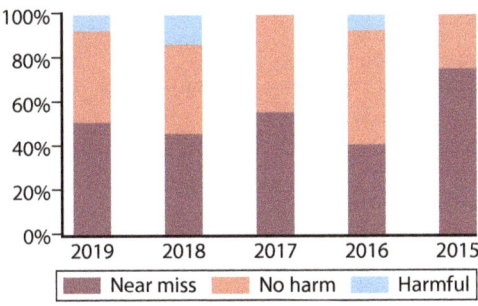

Figure 20.1 Incident type reported to ANZCP PIRS -2 for the period 2015–2019. Incidents are categorized into "a near miss event," a "no harm incident" and "harmful." ANZCP.org/PIRS-ii.

cardiopulmonary bypass should be treated with a team approach. Several broad general principles based on a team approach should be followed in any identified or evolving safety event during CPB:

- Notify everyone in the room that the potential safety issue exists
- Get help (from another perfusionist preferably: two sets of eyes are better than one)
- Consider coming off bypass if possible (if near the beginning or end of the CPB)
- If the cause is not immediately reversible, change out faulty equipment if possible (need appropriate backup and properly maintained devices)
- Minimize risk of harm to the patient

Pre-bypass checklists will help to reduce the incidence of error and equipment fault but must be undertaken diligently as a perform/verify process.

Simulation can be a valuable part of ongoing training for all perfusionists as it fosters critical thinking and provides the ability to practice the response to common and uncommon events in a non-clinical environment. Simulation and training for the whole intraoperative team has been validated as an effective tool for improving the response time to the resolution of many catastrophic emergencies.

Common and Uncommon Disasters

Any minor issue may lead to one of many common and uncommon disasters during CPB. Although there is significant overlap between sections they are grouped into:

i. oxygenator failures
ii. equipment failures
iii. clinical events.

Oxygenator Failures

The first sign of failure to oxygenate is usually the arterial blood appearing dark. The surgeon may comment on this as often they notice this first because the operating room lights shine on the lines. Blood gas analysis or online measurements will confirm a low pO_2; the SaO_2 measured by the pulse oximetry probe on the patient's finger or earlobe is generally unreliable on CPB.

Failure to oxygenate during CPB has numerous potential etiologies, some of which will be further explored in subsequent sections. The two main categories of oxygenation failure are gas supply issues and membrane oxygenator failures. While uncommon, as with anesthesia gas supply issues, errors in hospital and/or tank supplies have been reported. With the introduction of pipeline supply low-pressure alerts and pin-indexing of oxygen and other gas connectors, many such errors have been avoided over the past several decades. The inclusion of oxygen sensors can mitigate against delivering hypoxic or even normoxic mixtures when supplemental oxygen is intended. Issues related to gas supply will be discussed within Clinical Events later in this chapter.

Membrane oxygenator failure may similarly result from several causes. Diffusion membrane oxygenators utilize hollow-fiber technology or a folded silicone membrane. A countercurrent flow of oxygen-rich gas is typically passed across the oxygenator, allowing the perfusionist to control the patient's PaO_2 by setting the FiO_2 and the $PaCO_2$ by adjusting the rate fresh gas flow, or "sweep," to accomplish ventilation. The FiO_2 is set using a gas blender that mandates a supply of oxygen and air. Failure at the blender (connections, inlet or outlet patency, or calibration) may result in hypoxemia. Any leak along the pathway, from the wall source through the blender (including the in-line anesthetic gas vaporizer) to the oxygenator may result in insufficient gas exchange at the membrane oxygenator. Occlusion or impairment of efferent gas exhaust from the oxygenator can cause the same issues.

Oxygenators vary in size in accordance with the surface area of the gas/fluid interface, which allows matching supply and demand with patients' sizes and needs. The advantage of size-matched oxygenators is that the priming volume is directly proportional to the size of the oxygenators, allowing for judicious blood conservation in smaller patients. Conversely,

Table 20.1. Prevention and recognition of failure to oxygenate

Complete pre-bypass checklist	• Verify oxygen/air source • Review patient size and reference IFU to choose appropriately sized oxygenator • Ensure all gas supply pathways are connected, secured and patent. • Ensure gas analyzers are calibrated
Record pump settings/line pressures/flows to recognize serial changes for progressive oxygenator failures	
Monitor serial blood gases to determine adequacy of oxygenation/ventilation	
Countermeasures	
If immediate failure upon bypass initiation, determine if CPB can be safely discontinued while solving the problem	• Add a gas line from a spare oxygen cylinder or from the anesthetic machine • Hold volume in the right heart to allow RV ejection and pulmonary blood flow (partial bypass) and ventilate lungs to reduce shunt
Gas supply interruption	• Start from one end of the gas circuit, i.e. from the wall gas, work along toward the oxygenator, to methodically find where the issue is • Consider incorrectly seated anesthetic gas vaporizer
Blender failure	• Obtain a spare blender from another machine

Oxygenator failure	• Consider oxygenator changeout versus pump exchange
	  ○ Cognitive aids/checklists may prevent errors or omissions in steps
	  ○ Simulation and training will improve efficiency, sterility, success rates and decrease stress

choosing an oxygenator of insufficient surface area to support full CPB of a larger individual leads to tissue hypoxia.

Prolonged mechanical support can lead to progressive oxygenator failure, as can insufficient systemic anticoagulation. Fibrin clot deposition may develop insidiously and may be evidenced by a progressive decline in the ability to oxygenate/ventilate, requiring a steady increase of FiO_2 or sweep. Visible fibrin deposits may appear and the pressure on the pre-oxygenator line from the pump may increase for any set speed of the pump.

The appearance of water condensation in the oxygenator may indicate oxygenator failure and, while uncommon with newer oxygenators, plasma leak through the membrane can occur. Periodic monitoring of the adequacy of systemic anticoagulation,

typically at 20–30 minute intervals, is imperative as multiple factors (consumption, redistribution, hemodilution, heparin resistance, volume loss) can lead to the need to readminister anticoagulant medications (see Chapter 6).

Similarly, occlusion (cannula position, tubing kinked, air lock) or visible thrombus in the venous inflow and/or the reservoir can prevent blood flow to the oxygenator, while any outflow occlusion (occluded downstream filter, kinked line, malpositioned arterial cannula) can prevent oxygenated blood from reaching the patient.

Violation of the integrity of the gas/fluid membrane interface, either from a manufacturing defect or inappropriate handling, can predispose to catastrophic arterial gas embolism or diminish the membrane's ability to transfer oxygen and CO_2. Table 20.1

Table 20.2. Prevention and recognition of failure to achieve adequate flow

Complete pre-bypass checklist	• Ensure the cardiopulmonary bypass circuit is continuous, free of air and unobstructed prior to clamping and dividing lines • Review cannulation strategies during time-out process and prior to institution of CPB • Ensure appropriate tubing, connectors and splitters are present and available for planned cannulation strategies • Verify position of cannulas, test arterial cannula prior to initiating bypass for patency and pressure ("good swing")
Record pump settings/line pressures/flows to recognize serial changes	

Countermeasures

If immediate failure upon bypass initiation, determine if CPB can be safely discontinued while solving the problem	• Start from one end of the CPB circuit, visually inspect pathway for air, clamps, kinks, occlusions
	  ○ Remove obstructions and/or occlusions
	  ○ "Milk" air along venous line back to venous reservoir if an air lock has occurred; secure cannula snares to prevent further air entrapment
	  ○ Determine whether cannulas remain appropriately positioned (surgeon: visually and by palpation; anesthesiologist: imaging if present)

summarizes strategies for prevention and recognition of the problem and suggests appropriate countermeasures.

Blood Path Obstruction

Arterial blood path obstruction can lead to the inability to provide adequate flow of oxygenated blood to the patient during CPB. Venous blood path obstruction can lead to impaired venous drainage of the head, heart and visceral organs. Impaired drainage of the pulmonary venous system, either directly or through a vent in the pulmonary artery, the left atrium or the left ventricle, can result in pulmonary edema. Table 20.2 provides an overview of prevention, recognition and countermeasures.

Falling Cerebral Saturation

Institutions use cerebral oximetry (RSO_2) with varying frequency and for varying indications and apply different thresholds for intervention if cerebral saturation drops. Measuring RSO_2 during CPB is currently not considered universal standard of care. There is no convincing evidence that cerebral oximetry is sensitive or specific enough to determine the absolute value of cerebral oxygen saturation or if a certain percentage decline from baseline mandates the need for an intervention, although case reports of ipsilateral decreases in RSO_2 may indicate issues related to cannula misplacement or venous obstruction. Several randomized controlled studies investigating all-cause morbidity and mortality or the association of low intraoperative RSO_2 values with postoperative delirium have returned mixed results. See Table 20.3 for suggested troubleshooting when cerebral saturation drops.

Equipment Failure

Errors with and failure of equipment are either of a technical nature (related to equipment and/or software) or are due to human factors (error or violations in practice). Equipment failure can occasionally be attributed to conditions prevalent within the system they need to function in. These are usually organizational and result from inadequate policies, procedures

Table 20.3. Potential causes of falling cerebral oximetry saturation

Exclude monitoring failure	• Devices functioning properly? • Sensors properly affixed (symmetrically and not overlying superior sagittal sinus)?
Patient issues	• Extracranial tissue edema? • Shift in patient position?
O_2 supply impaired	• Arterial cannula position? • Aortic dissection? • Venous/SVC cannula obstructed or poor venous drainage (increasing CVP will decrease cerebral blood flow at any given MAP)? • CPB flow adequate?
Physiological issues	• Hypocapnia (may lead to cerebral vasoconstriction)? • Low hemoglobin? • Methemoglobinemia? • Light anesthesia? • Temperature effect? o Rewarming (increased O_2 demand)?

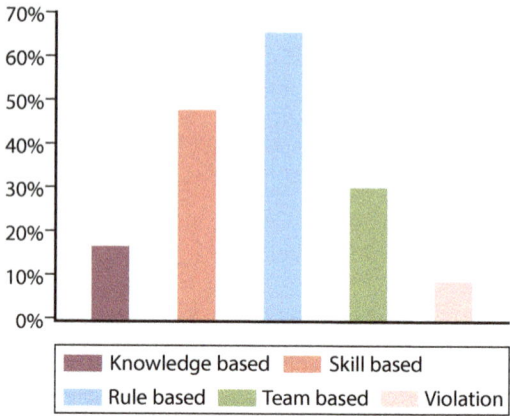

Figure 20.3 Human factor reports may be divided into different human factor types. The breakdown of report types, associated with the incidents for the period 2010–2020 are shown. ANZCP.org/PIRS-ii.

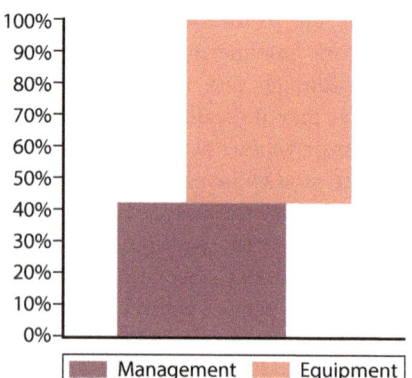

Figure 20.2 The reports of incidents may be grouped into either management or equipment failure. Management can be due to protocol, managerial or organizational failures. ANZCP.org/PIRS-ii.

and/or protocols or pressure on clinicians (see Figures 20.2 and 20.3).

Ideally, "backup" equipment should be available for all devices used in the operating room. While this is not always possible, there should be a documented contingency plan when there is no backup. An extra perfusion staff member (or other adequately trained staff) is also advisable to improve safety and to help out in a crisis. All equipment, including backup devices, have to be properly maintained and serviced, uninterrupted power supply systems need to be checked and charged routinely.

The following should be accessible and readily available as backup:

- Spare HLM with all monitoring devices (n + 1 for the number of cardiac operating rooms in use)
- Spare heater/cooler
- Spare gas cylinders/regulators and gas lines
- Hand-cranks for centrifugal and roller pumps – easily accessible and operable
- Spare oxygenators/tubing/change out kit with sterile scissors
- Portable lighting and flashlights (inexpensive "head lights" allow for freeing up hands when needed)
- Spare disposable tubing and connectors for circuit disruptions.

An ECMO circuit may also be used if no backup HLM is available. Although there is no reservoir, a patient on CPB can be transferred onto ECMO until the failed CPB system is fixed or an alternative has been found.

Circuit Disruption

Circuit disruption is the most commonly reported incident in surveys (see recent PIRS-2 reporting in

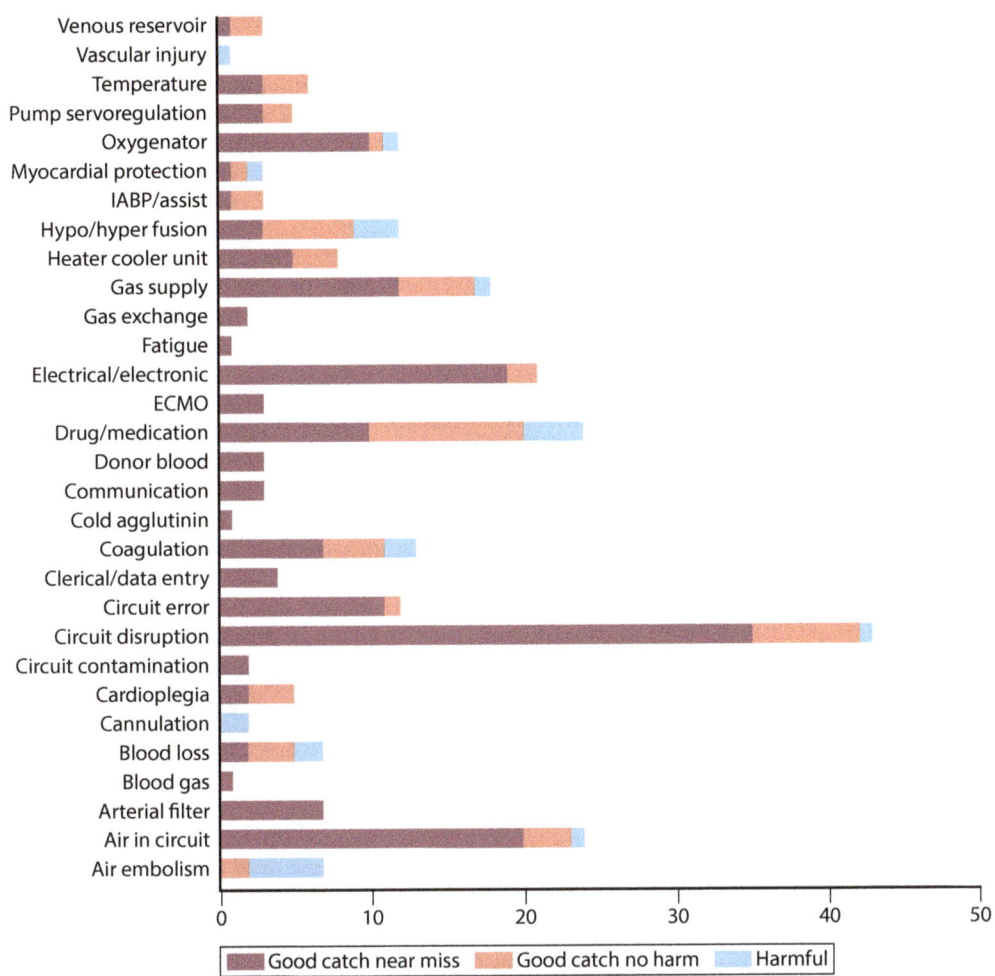

Figure 20.4 Incident category and severity of PIRS 2 reports for the 10-year period 2010 to 2020 are shown. Each subgroup is divided into good catch near miss, good catch no harm, harmful events. The large number of good catch events highlights that most incidents are "caught" before they can cause harm. ANZCP.org/PIRS-ii.

Figure 20.4). The CPB circuit is complex and has many components that can disconnect or leak. The use of checklists during setup and priming can help identify errors during setup. Securing connections with cable ties and having spare connectors in the room in case of failure helps mitigate against avoidable accidents. Finally, having a second perfusionist verify the use of a checklist and the circuit setup helps against making easily rectifiable mistakes.

The most common sources of leaks are:

- Faulty components (filters, vent valves, gas/hemoglobin saturation cells)
- Connections not secure (cable ties and cross threading, non-heat sealed)
- Lines not connected in setup
- Split tubing from roller pump raceways, in particular pump boots
- Reservoir ports snapped off
- Temperature thermistors leaking
- Taps snapping off, destroying the threaded Luer-lock connection
- Lines blown apart due to over-pressurization
- Excessive use of suckers or vents connected to an unvented reservoir can cause pressure to build up and will eventually blow the lid off the reservoir.

Air in Circuit

The third most common, and potentially disastrous, event that occurs during CPB is air entrainment into the circuit. Macrobubbles, or visible gross collections

199

of air in the arterial circuit, can result in occlusion of major arteries and arterioles, resulting in end-organ ischemia. Air in the coronary arteries presents as acute ST-elevation ischemia and may result in profound myocardial dysfunction and inability to separate from CPB, while cerebral arterial gas embolism may result in stroke, seizure, or impaired neurocognitive function postoperatively. Any microbubbles can transfer directly into the patient's microcirculation with the potential to cause harm through diffuse impairment of gas exchange in the capillary bed. Air in the venous lines can cause an air lock, preventing venous drainage and necessitating a rapid reduction of forward flow in order to prevent emptying of the venous reservoir.

Air embolism during cardiac surgery is a complication with potentially severe or fatal consequences. Even if recognized and treated immediately, it can cause significant and irreversible neurological injury. A sudden and rapid drop in the cerebral oximetry readings without an obvious alternative explanation should give rise to a high index of suspicion for cerebral arterial gas embolism. Transesophageal echocardiography can potentially help in identifying air in the aorta.

The primary goal for managing this complication is protecting the brain. Measures include:

- Identifying the location of air entry and preventing further air from entering the circulation.
- Supine positioning. Steep Trendelenburg positioning had previously been thought to help expel air bubbles from the cerebral circulation, however, this is now not recommended, as placing the patient head-down can exacerbate cerebral edema.
- Decreasing cerebral oxygen demand, which can be achieved pharmacologically with medications such as propofol, as well as by actively cooling the patient. Cerebral oxygen demand decreases by approximately 7% for each degree Celsius that the patient is cooled (see also Chapter 18). Active cooling is easily achieved on CPB once the source of air has been identified and eliminated and flow has been reestablished. Emergent initiation of deep hypothermia has also been successfully supplemented with retrograde cerebral perfusion in several cases, whereby oxygenated blood is run retrograde via superior vena cava cannulation

with resultant purge of arterial gas into the arch effluent.

- Treatment with IV methylprednisolone has been considered with the goal of minimizing the inflammatory damage secondary to ischemia and subsequent reperfusion, although the efficacy is not clear.
- Intravenous lidocaine may be beneficial.
- Definitive treatment for cerebral arterial gas embolism includes hyperbaric oxygen therapy.

In addition to decreasing oxygen demand, the other goal in this situation is to maintain adequate oxygen delivery to tissues, which can be achieved with normovolemia and adequate perfusion pressure. Hemodilution to a hematocrit of ~30% may be beneficial. The most common causes leading to air in the CPB circuit are summarized in Table 20.4.

Electrical Failure

All hospitals should have multiple levels of power supplies, with backup generators that switch in without delay when mains power fails. While the incidence of multi-level power failures is rare, they do occur, and strategic planning needs to be included in local protocols.

Most contemporary HLMs have a battery backup built into the system. These need to be maintained to assure best battery performance. Keeping a hand crank on each HLM is mandatory in case of total electrical failure. Although practices such as making sure the HLM's battery is fully charged, that the machine is plugged into a wall socket that is fed by the hospital backup system and that the hand crank is present seem totally intuitive, it is advised to include them in the pre-CPB checklist to assure high reliability.

On occasions where a single pump dies, a spare pump module should be available for immediate use. Clinicians need to make sure during setup that the tubing is long enough to be moved to a different module. Failure of the electronic control panel or the recording system are mostly software issues and can often be dealt with by rebooting the system. Modern HLMs should be able to be run with just manual control, independent of the electronic system.

Heater Cooler Failure

The heating/cooling device is a major component of cardiopulmonary bypass. A backup device or an

Table 20.4. Causes of air entrainment into CPB circuit

Vent tubing backwards

Purge lines open

Failure/inactivation of low-level alarm or bubble detectors; venous line occlusion with subsequent draining of reservoir

Membrane fiber leak

Vacuum drainage with excessive negative pressure

Inattention/distraction of perfusionist

Countermeasures

Vent tubing	• Pre-bypass checklist • Check suckers with blood/saline before commencing CPB • One-way valve in all vents
Level alarm, bubble detectors	Tested, connected and servo regulated
Positive and negative pressure valves intact	
Positive and negative pressure is measured and alarmed when vacuum is used	
Decrease venous embolic load	• Snare venous cannula to prevent (further) air from entering • Partially clamp venous line

Table 20.5. Common drug errors

Incorrect drug labeling

Out of date drugs used

Heparin not given or given in wrong dose or at inappropriate time

Protamine given while pump suckers activated

Cardioplegia solution with too much/too little potassium

Cardioplegia delivered systemically before cross-clamping of aorta

Incompatible blood group transfusion

Anesthetic gas vaporizer on HLM left open after CPB

Countermeasures

Double-check drugs including reading label and dates on vials and syringes, use of appropriate labeling system

Commence CPB only after all team members have confirmed safe ACT

Suckers are turned off and removed from chest when anesthesiologist announces that protamine is about to start

Confirm blood/cardioplegia ratio before operation; check potassium concentration with blood gas analysis

Use end-of-CPB checklist to ensure HLM is stripped down correctly

Clinical Events

Numerous clinical events may result in CPB disasters. The following are summaries of some of the more prevalent clinical events that have been previously reported in the Australian and the UK perfusion incident reporting systems.

Drug and Medication Error

This topic represents the second highest number of incidents reported to PIRS-2 (Figure 20.4). Teamwork and excellent communication, preferably in the form of closed loop communication, are important so each member of the team is aware of allergies, religious beliefs (e.g. Jehovah's Witness) and when drugs are given (especially heparin and protamine). Table 20.5 compiles a select few of the more common drug errors and ways to prevent them.

alternative method to rewarm a patient should be available. These devices must be maintained in accordance with their IFU to minimize mycobacterial growth. Meticulous maintenance is particularly important, highlighted by the impact of mycobacterium chimaera, as continual disinfection may cause faults due to the corrosive nature of chemicals used.

A backup heater/cooler or similar device from an ECMO circuit should be available at all times. If this is not the case a roller pump with a loop of tubing attached to 2 Hansen connectors, sitting in a bucket of warm water can allow some temperature control until a more permanent solution has been found.

Heparin Resistance

Heparin is the most common anticoagulant used for cardiopulmonary bypass. The standard heparin dose is 300–500 IU/kg, the target ACT varies between institutions but generally is somewhere between 400 and 550 seconds. Failure to achieve the ACT goal despite repeated heparin doses up to 600 IU/kg is defined as heparin resistance. In the event of an inadequate response to heparin, it is a Class 1A recommendation of the Society of Thoracic Surgeons and Society of Cardiovascular Anesthesiologists that recombinant antithrombin III be used to improve heparin sensitivity. If not treated adequately, heparin resistance could result in subtherapeutic anticoagulation, potentially leading to oxygenator failure, thromboembolic phenomena and patient death. Alternative anticoagulants such as bivalirudin or argatroban should be considered in cases where heparin resistance is not due to inadequate antithrombin III levels (see also Chapter 6 for more detail).

Cold Agglutination

Cold agglutinins are IgM antibodies directed against red blood cells. They are inert at physiological body temperatures and have a variable temperature threshold below which they become active (thermal amplitude). Depending on this threshold they might become activated during hypothermic bypass. Once activated they agglutinate erythrocytes, which in turn fix to activated complement, leading to irreversible cell damage. Severe hemolysis occurs when the blood temperature is (i) cold enough for the antibody to be active and (ii) warm enough for complement to be active. Surgeons wearing magnifying loops or perfusionists observing their cold cardioplegia circuit are often the first ones to spot any agglutination. Normothermia, avoiding cold cardioplegia and flushing the coronaries with warm cardioplegia before removing the aortic cross clamp are the mainstays of managing patients with known cold agglutinins or sudden onset of hemolysis (see Chapter 16 for more detail).

Malignant Hyperthermia

Malignant hyperthermia (MH) is the result of a reaction to specific triggering agents in patients with myopathies typically affecting the type 1 ryanodine receptor. This condition is hereditary and transmitted in an autosomal dominant pattern. There often is a family history of malignant hyperthermia that will be reported in preoperative assessment. When a malignant hyperthermia crisis is triggered, a hypermetabolic state is induced in which there is a massive and unchecked release of calcium from the sarcoplasmic reticulum of skeletal muscle. This triggers a cascade of derangements, including hyperthermia, tachycardia, hyperkalemia, hypercapnia, muscular breakdown and metabolic acidosis. It is often noticed first by the surgeon, noticing unusual chest wall rigidity or that the patient feels warm. Blood gases confirm that CO_2 rises fast despite increasing sweep gas flow. Metabolic acidosis, excessive temperature despite cooling and hematuria are also typical warning signs.

In cases of preoperatively known or suspected malignant hyperthermia the anesthesiologist and perfusionist should discuss the anesthetic plan, including avoidance of all triggering agents such as succinylcholine and volatile anesthetic agents, as well as flushing the anesthesia machine with O_2 and removing the vaporizer from HLM.

In the event of a MH crisis all potential triggering agents have to be stopped immediately and removed from continuity with the patient. The ventilator circuit and CO_2 absorber canister should be replaced with new components, the patient has to be treated with dantrolene and the surgical procedure should be terminated as soon as reasonably possible. The Malignant Hyperthermia Association of the United States maintains a 24-hour hotline and additional resources to help prepare for and provide real time assistance to acutely manage a malignant hyperthermia crisis. Similar helplines are available in most countries around the world.

Vasoplegic Shock

Systemic vasodilation, often refractory to standard therapies, is a dangerous complication of cardiopulmonary bypass. It is thought to be associated with a systemic inflammatory response that can be precipitated by the patient's circulation interacting with the foreign materials of the bypass circuit. It may also result from a reaction of common anesthetics with certain drug classes, including but not limited to angiotensin converting enzyme inhibitors and angiotensin II receptor blockers. The vasoplegic patient is unable to achieve adequate end-organ perfusion due to hypotension in spite of adequate or supra-normal cardiac output. In some cases, this can make it impossible to safely separate from CPB if not adequately treated. Treatment options include vasopressors, such as norepinephrine, vasopressin, intravenous methylene blue and vitamin B12 (hydroxycobalamin), as well as newer agents such as angiotensin II.

Aortic Dissection

Manipulation or instrumentation of the aorta can cause disruption of the intima and acute dissection of the vessel. This occasionally occurs during aortic cannulation or at proximal coronary graft anastomosis sites. It is critical to identify this complication early. As a consequence of cannulating a dissected aorta, there may be loss of radial arterial line waveform or elevated line pressure when attempting to go on bypass and the aorta may begin to appear dilated and discolored. Intraoperative transesophageal echocardiography, as well as epiaortic ultrasound, can be used to identify or confirm this diagnosis.

This complication needs to be treated immediately. Depending on the extent of the damage done this can require surgery ranging from an ascending aortic interposition graft to a complete aortic arch replacement.

Over-pressurization during Cardioplegia

Over-pressurization during anterograde or retrograde cardioplegia can occur. Monitoring the pressure in the delivery system and taking the pressure drop in the aortic root or the coronary sinus into account can avoid cardiac injury. Consequences of over-pressurization of the retrograde system include coronary sinus rupture, and more commonly, epicardial petechiae and myocardial edema from extravasation of high pressure cardioplegia. Over-pressurization of the aortic root during antegrade cardioplegia can result in direct injury to the aortic root or valve. The root is typically monitored visually by the surgeon and a Y-connector can be used to vent the root when needed. Anterograde cardioplegia catheters with integrated overpressure relief valves are commercially available.

Inadvertent Cannulation of Hepatic Vein during Bi-caval Venous Cannulation

Advancing the inferior vena cava cannula too far during bi-caval cannulation is not uncommon. Inadvertent placement into the hepatic vein can lead to poor venous drainage, hepatic venous congestion with potential hepatic dysfunction and efferent venous obstruction of visceral organs and the kidneys. Transesophageal echocardiography can be used to confirm proper cannula placement and assist with repositioning.

This chapter highlights commonly reported incidents in current perfusion practice. New forms of complications arise as our HLMs become more complex and feature integration with monitoring and electronic medical records. In order to run a highly reliable perfusion service it is essential that protocols and procedures for dealing with accidents and unforeseen events are regularly updated to include new equipment or technology as it is added to our arsenal of tools.

Suggested Further Reading

1. Reason J. Human error: models and management. BMJ. 2000; 320 (7237):768–770.

2. Wilcox TW, Baker RA. Incident reporting in perfusion: current perceptions on PIRS-2. J Extracorp Tech 2020; 52:7–12.

3. Darling E, Searles B. Oxygenator change-out times: the value of a written protocol and practice simulation exercises. Perfusion 2010 May; 25(3):141–143; discussion 144–145.

4. Uysal S, Lin HM, Trinh M et al. Optimizing cerebral oxygenation in cardiac surgery: a randomized controlled trial examining neurocognitive and perioperative outcomes. J Thorac Cardiovasc Surg 2020; 159(3):943–953.e3

5. Ferraris VA, Brown JR, Despotis GJ et al. Special report: STS workforce on evidence based surgery. 2011 update to the Society of Thoracic Surgeons and the Society of Cardiovascular Anesthesiologists blood conservation clinical practice guidelines * The Society of Thoracic Surgeons Blood Conservat. ATS. 2011;91 (3):944–982.

6. Shore-lesserson L, Baker RA et al. The Society of Thoracic Surgeons, The Society of Cardiovascular Anesthesiologists and The American Society of ExtraCorporeal Technology: Clinical practice guidelines – anticoagulation during cardiopulmonary bypass. Ann Thorac Surg. 2018;105 (2):650–662.

7. Gulabani M, Gurha P, Ahmad S et al. Intra-operative post-induction hyperthermia, possibly malignant hyperthermia: anesthetic implications, challenges and management. J Anaesthesiol Clin Pharmacol. 2014;30 (4):555–557.

8. Still RJ, Hilgenberg AD, Akins CW et al. Intraoperative aortic dissection. Ann Thorac Surg. 1992;53(3):374–379.

9. Assaad S, Geirsson A, Rousou L et al. The dual modality use of epiaortic ultrasound and transesophageal echocardiography in the diagnosis of intraoperative iatrogenic type-a aortic dissection. J Cardiothorac Vasc Anesth. 2013 Apr;27(2):326–328.

Index

205

For EU product safety concerns, contact us at Calle de José Abascal, 56–1°,
28003 Madrid, Spain or eugpsr@cambridge.org.

www.ingramcontent.com/pod-product-compliance
Ingram Content Group UK Ltd.
Pitfield, Milton Keynes, MK11 3LW, UK
UKHW060333090126
466816UK00014B/264